Comprehensive Evidence Analysis for Interventional Procedures Used to Treat Chronic Pain

Editor

AMEET NAGPAL

PHYSICAL MEDICINE AND REHABILITATION CLINICS OF NORTH AMERICA

www.pmr.theclinics.com

Consulting Editor
SANTOS F. MARTINEZ

May 2022 • Volume 33 • Number 2

ELSEVIER

1600 John F. Kennedy Boulevard ● Suite 1800 ● Philadelphia, Pennsylvania, 19103-2899

http://www.theclinics.com

PHYSICAL MEDICINE AND REHABILITATION CLINICS OF NORTH AMERICA Volume 33, Number 2
May 2022 ISSN 1047-9651, 978-0-323-84965-4

Editor: Lauren Boyle
Developmental Editor: Diana Grace Ang

Reprints. For copies of 100 or more of articles in this publication, please contact the Commercial Reprints Department, Elsevier Inc., 360 Park Avenue South, New York, NY 10010-1710. Tel.: 212-633-3874; Fax: 212-633-3820; E-mail: reprints@elsevier.com.

Physical Medicine and Rehabilitation Clinics of North America (ISSN 1047-9651) is published quarterly by Elsevier Inc., 360 Park Avenue South, New York, NY 10010-1710. Months of issue are February, May, August, and November. Business and Editorial Offices: 1600 John F. Kennedy Blvd., Suite 1800, Philadelphia, PA 19103-2899. Customer Service Office: 3251 Riverport Lane, Maryland Heights, MO 63043. Periodicals postage paid at New York, NY and additional mailing offices. Subscription price per year is $332.00 (US individuals), $905.00 (US institutions), $100.00 (US students), $377.00 (Canadian individuals), $932.00 (Canadian institutions), $100.00 (Canadian students), $477.00 (foreign individuals), $932.00 (foreign institutions), and $210.00 (foreign students). Foreign air speed delivery is included in all *Clinics* subscription prices. All prices are subject to change without notice. **POSTMASTER:** Send address changes to *Physical Medicine and Rehabilitation Clinics of North America*, Customer Service Office: Elsevier Health Sciences Division, Subscription Customer Service, 3251 Riverport Lane, Maryland Heights, MO 63043. **Customer Service: 1-800-654-2452 (US). From outside of the United States, call 314-447-8871. Fax: 314-447-8029. E-mail: JournalsCustomer Service-usa@elsevier.com (for print support); JournalsOnlineSupport-usa@elsevier.com (for online support).**

Physical Medicine and Rehabilitation Clinics of North America is indexed in *Excerpta Medica, MEDLINE/ PubMed (Index Medicus), Cinahl,* and *Cumulative Index to Nursing and Allied Health Literature.*

Contributors

CONSULTING EDITOR

SANTOS F. MARTINEZ, MD, MS
Physical Medicine and Rehabilitation, Assistant Professor, Department of Orthopaedic Surgery and Biomedical Engineering, University of Tennessee College of Medicine, Campbell Clinic Orthopaedics, Memphis, Tennessee

EDITOR

AMEET NAGPAL, MD, MS, MEd
Division Chief, Pain Medicine, Department of Anesthesiology, UT Health San Antonio, San Antonio, Texas, USA; Incoming Division Chief, Physical Medicine & Rehabilitation, Department of Orthopaedics & Physical Medicine, Medical University of South Carolina, Charleston, South Carolina

AUTHORS

MICKEY E. ABRAHAM, MD
Koman Family Outpatient Pavilion, Center for Pain Medicine, La Jolla; Resident Physician, Department of Neurosurgery, University of California, San Diego, California

JOHN ALM, DO
Assistant Professor, Department of Physical Medicine & Rehabilitation, University of Kansas School of Medicine, Kansas City, Kansas

MAGDALENA ANITESCU, MD, PhD, FASA
Professor of Anesthesia and Pain Medicine, Section Chief, Division of Pain Management, Director, Pain Medicine Fellowship Program, Department of Anesthesia and Critical Care, University of Chicago Medical Center, Chicago, Illinois

MALATHY APPASAMY, MBBS
Department of Physical Medicine & Rehabilitation, Main Line Health System, Glen Mills, Pennsylvania

RYAN ASCHENBRENER, MD
PM&R board-eligible, current Interventional Spine & Musculoskeletal Medicine Fellow, International Spine, Pain & Performance Center, Washington, DC

BRIAN T. BOIES, MD
Associate Professor of Anesthesiology and Pain Medicine, University of Texas Health Science Center at San Antonio, San Antonio, Texas

SHERIEF BOSS, MD
Neurology Resident, Previous Neurocritical Fellow, University of Chicago, Chicago, Illinois

EDUARDO J. CARRERA, MD
PM&R Resident, University of Colorado, School of Medicine, Department of Physical Medicine and Rehabilitation, Aurora, Colorado

DAVID J. CARROLL, MD
Resident, Department of Anesthesiology, University of Texas Health Science Center at San Antonio, San Antonio, Texas

JOEL P. CASTELLANOS, MD
Koman Family Outpatient Pavilion, Center for Pain Medicine, La Jolla; Associate Clinical Professor, Department of Anesthesiology, Center for Pain Medicine, University of California, San Diego, San Diego, California

ANDREA L. CHADWICK, MD, MSc, FASA
Associate Professor, Department of Anesthesiology, University of Kansas School of Medicine, Kansas City, Kansas

GEORGE CHANG CHIEN, DO
Attending Physician, Director of Pain Medicine, Department of Physical Medicine and Rehabilitation, Ventura County Medical Center, Ventura, California

COLE CHENEY, MD
Division of Physical Medicine and Rehabilitation, University of Utah, Salt Lake City, Utah

NATE CLEMENTS, MD
Department of Anesthesiology, University of Texas Health Science Center, San Antonio, Texas

AARON CONGER, DO
Division of Physical Medicine and Rehabilitation, University of Utah, Salt Lake City, Utah

QUINN WONDERS CONVERY, BCPS, PharmD
Physical Medicine and Rehabilitation Department,; Clinical Pharmacy Specialist, Department of Pharmacy, Veterans Administration Greater Los Angeles Health Care System, Los Angeles, California

MEHUL J. DESAI, MD, MPH
Medical Director, International Spine, Pain & Performance Center, Clinical Associate Professor, School of Medicine and Health Sciences, The George Washington University, Washington, DC

MAXIM S. ECKMANN, MD
Professor of Anesthesiology and Pain Medicine, University of Texas Health Science Center at San Antonio, San Antonio, Texas

TYLER ERICSON, MD
Anesthesiology Resident, Department of Anesthesiology, University of Virginia, Charlottesville, Virginia

SAMANTHA C. EROSA, MD
Chronic Pain Fellow, Department of Anesthesiology, Center for Pain Medicine, University of California, San Diego, San Diego; Koman Family Outpatient Pavilion, Center for Pain Medicine, La Jolla, California

YASHAR ESHRAGHI, MD
Department of Interventional Pain Management, Ochsner Health System, New Orleans, Louisiana

BENJAMIN GILL, DO, MBA
Department of Physical Medicine and Rehabilitation, University of Missouri, Columbia, Missouri

MAGED GUIRGUIS, MD
Department of Interventional Pain Management, Ochsner Health System, New Orleans, Louisiana

APARNA JINDAL, MBBS
Resident, Department of Anesthesia, University of Iowa Hospitals and Clinics, Iowa City, Iowa

ADAM KEMP, MD
Anesthesiology and Critical Care, Duke University, Durham, North Carolina

DAVID J. KENNEDY, MD
Department and Physical Medicine and Rehabilitation, Vanderbilt University Medical Center, Vanderbilt Stallworth Rehabilitation Hospital, Nashville, Tennessee

LYNN KOHAN, MD
Associate Professor of Anesthesiology, Program Director, Pain Medicine Fellowship, Pain Management Center, Fontaine Research Park, Charlottesville, Virginia

CHRISTOPHER LAM, MD
Assistant Professor, Department of Anesthesiology, University of Kansas School of Medicine, Kansas City, Kansas

LEILANI MANSY, BS
University of Missouri-Kansas City School of Medicine, Kansas City, Missouri

AUSTIN MARCOLINA, DO
Resident Physician, Department of Physical Medicine and Rehabilitation, University of Texas Southwestern Medical Center, Dallas, Texas

ZACHARY L. McCORMICK, MD
Division of Physical Medicine and Rehabilitation, University of Utah, Salt Lake City, Utah

SCOTT MILLER, MD
Resident Physician, Physical Medicine and Rehabilitation, Vanderbilt University Medical Center, Vanderbilt Stallworth Rehabilitation Hospital, Nashville, Tennessee

ROYA S. MOHEIMANI, MD
Chronic Pain Fellow, Department of Anesthesiology, Center for Pain Medicine, University of California, San Diego, San Diego; Koman Family Outpatient Pavilion, Center for Pain Medicine, La Jolla, California

LORNE D. MUIR II, DO
Resident, Department of Anesthesiology, University of Texas Health Science Center at San Antonio, San Antonio, Texas

AMEET NAGPAL, MD, MS, MEd
PM&R Board Certified and Pain Medicine, Department of Anesthesiology, UT Health San Antonio, San Antonio, Texas

UDAI NANDA, DO
Director, Headache Center of Excellence, Department of Physical Medicine and
Rehabilitation, Interventional Pain Service, Veterans Administration Greater Los Angeles
Health Care System; Associate Program Director, Pain Medicine Fellowship Program,
Division of Physical Medicine and Rehabilitation, Department of Medicine, University of
California, Los Angeles, Los Angeles, California

NENNA NWAZOTA, MD
University of Texas at Southwestern, Dallas, Texas

JESSICA C. OSWALD, MD, MPH
Koman Family Outpatient Pavilion, Center for Pain Medicine, La Jolla; Department of
Anesthesiology, Center for Pain Medicine; Department of Emergency Medicine,
University of California, San Diego, San Diego, California

ARTI ORI, MD
Department of Anesthesiology and Perioperative Medicine, Pain Medicine Division,
Brigham and Women's Hospital, Boston, Massachusetts

SANJOG PANGARKAR, MD
Director, Inpatient and Interventional Pain Service, Department of Physical Medicine and
Rehabilitation, Veterans Administration Greater Los Angeles Health Care System;
Professor of Medicine, Division of Physical Medicine and Rehabilitation, Department of
Medicine, University of California, Los Angeles, Los Angeles, California

AMY C. S. PEARSON, MD
Assistant Professor, Department of Anesthesia, Pain Division, University of Iowa
Hospitals and Clinics, Iowa City, Iowa

MELISSA E. PHUPHANICH, MD, MS
Department of Physical Medicine and Rehabilitation, UCLA/Veterans Administration
Greater Los Angeles Healthcare System, Los Angeles, California

STEVEN T. POTTER, DO, MS
Physical Medicine & Rehabilitation (PM&R) Resident, Department of Rehabilitation
Medicine, UT Health San Antonio, San Antonio, Texas

SETH PROBERT, DO
PM&R Resident, Department of Rehabilitation Medicine, UT Health San Antonio,
San Antonio, Texas

ALLISON GLINKA PRZYBSYZ, MD
Department of Orthopedics and Rehabilitation, University of Wisconsin-Madison,
Madison, Wisconsin

CHRISTIAN ROEHMER, MD
Department and Physical Medicine and Rehabilitation, Vanderbilt University Medical
Center, Vanderbilt Stallworth Rehabilitation Hospital, Nashville, Tennessee

BYRON J. SCHNEIDER, MD
Vanderbilt Stallworth Rehabilitation Hospital, Associate Professor, Vanderbilt University
Medical Center, Nashville, Tennessee

NATHANIEL M. SCHUSTER, MD
Koman Family Outpatient Pavilion, Center for Pain Medicine, La Jolla; Associate Clinical
Professor, Department of Anesthesiology, Division of Pain Medicine, University of
California, San Diego, San Diego, California

JAY D. SHAH, MD
Department of Interventional Pain Management, Ochsner Health System, New Orleans, Louisiana

PRIYANKA SINGLA, MD
Chronic Pain Fellow, Department of Anesthesiology, University of Virginia, Charlottesville, Virginia

VIDHAN SRIVASTAVA, MD
Anesthesia Resident, University of Chicago, Chicago, Illinois

FAYE TATA, DO
PM&R Resident, Department of Rehabilitation Medicine, UT Health San Antonio, San Antonio, Texas

NIRGUNA THALLA, MD
PM&R Resident, Department of Rehabilitation Medicine, MedStar Georgetown University, MedStar National Rehabilitation Hospital, Physical Medicine and Rehabilitation, Washington, DC

KEVIN VORENKAMP, MD, FASA
Chief, Division of Pain Medicine, Associate Professor, Duke University, Durham, North Carolina

KEVIN VU, MD
Resident Physician, Department of Physical Medicine and Rehabilitation, Spaulding Rehabilitation Hospital, Boston, Massachusetts

SEAN WELCH, MD
PM&R Resident, Department of Rehabilitation Medicine, UT Health San Antonio, San Antonio, Texas

JOSEPH WILLIAM, DO, MPH
Department and Physical Medicine and Rehabilitation, Vanderbilt University Medical Center, Vanderbilt Stallworth Rehabilitation Hospital, Nashville, Tennessee

BHAVANA YALAMURU, MBBS, MD
Assistant Professor, Pain Division, Department of Anesthesiology, University of Virginia Health System, Charlottesville, Virginia

AARON J. YANG, MD
Associate Professor, Physical Medicine and Rehabilitation, Vanderbilt University Medical Center, Vanderbilt Stallworth Rehabilitation Hospital, Nashville, Tennessee

PETER YI, MD, MSEd
Assistant Professor, Anesthesiology and Critical Care, Duke University, Durham, North Carolina

Contents

Foreword: A Maturing Field xv

Santos F. Martinez

Preface: (Needle) Jockeying for the Evidence xvii

Ameet Nagpal

Epidural Steroid Injections 215

Joseph William, Christian Roehmer, LeiLani Mansy, and David J. Kennedy

Epidural steroid injections (ESI) can be an effective treatment of radicular pain, while also providing potential for functional improvement. There are 3 main interventional approaches including: interlaminar (IL), transforaminal (TF), and caudal. The risks and efficacy data vary between these routes of injection and the underlying pathology with the TF route having the most robust efficacy data. However, selecting an injection approach should be based on a patient's clinical presentation, pathology, anatomy, consideration of the natural course of pain, and the unique risks and benefits of the particular technique.

Radiofrequency Ablation for Zygapophyseal Joint Pain 233

Benjamin Gill, Cole Cheney, Nate Clements, Allison Glinka Przybsyz, Zachary L. McCormick, and Aaron Conger

Radiofrequency ablation for spinal zygapophyseal joint pain is a safe and effective procedure in carefully selected patients when an appropriate technique is used. The equipment and techniques for performing this procedure have evolved over the past several decades. Likewise, the selection criteria have been refined to optimize results. This article provides an overview of the epidemiology of zygapophyseal joint pain, patient selection and outcomes data associated with RFA, and risks and contraindications of the procedure.

Sacroiliac Joint Interventions 251

Aaron J. Yang, Byron J. Schneider, and Scott Miller

The sacroiliac joint complex (SIJC) is composed of complex anatomy of numerous potential pain generators that demonstrate varying pathophysiology and differing innervations. This heterogeneity has been a challenge to advancing research and clinical care. Moving forward, individualized approaches taking these factors into account may be a path forward to improved outcomes. Thus, as we move toward precision medicine in interventional spine care, it is imperative to investigate more targeted diagnostic and therapeutic approaches to the SIJC.

Peripheral Joint Injections   267

Austin Marcolina, Kevin Vu, and George Chang Chien

> Peripheral joint injections are a common interventional treatment of peripheral joint–mediated pain, including arthritis, tendinopathy, and bursitis that are not responsive to conservative management. Degenerative changes of articular joints are often related to these symptoms through chronic inflammatory changes, which typically arise due to repetitive trauma, autoimmune disease, or metabolic abnormalities. The primary diagnosis for degenerative disease in the peripheral joints is osteoarthritis but can also include rheumatoid arthritis, gout, and other less common etiologies. Chronic inflammatory damage to the articular surfaces and joint capsules can lead to pain and functional decline. As such, the use of peripheral joint injections after the failure of typical conservative treatment, including physical therapy and oral medications, is common. Although these injections are typically not curative in nature, their primary objective is to decrease pain to allow functional improvement concurrently with physical and pharmaceutical modalities. Common injectates used for peripheral joint injections include local anesthetic, corticosteroid, hyaluronic acid, platelet-rich plasma, and mesenchymal stromal cells.

Trigger Point Injections   307

Malathy Appasamy, Christopher Lam, John Alm, and Andrea L. Chadwick

> Myofascial pain and myofascial pain syndromes are among some of the most common acute and chronic pain conditions. Many interventional procedures can be performed in both an acute and chronic pain setting to address myofascial pain syndromes. Trigger point injections can be performed with or without imaging guidance such as fluoroscopy and ultrasound; however, the use of imaging in years past has been recommended to improve patient outcome and safety. Injections can be performed using no injectate (dry needling), or can involve the administration of local anesthetics, botulinum toxin, or corticosteroids.

Spinal Cord Stimulation: A Psychiatric Perspective   335

Mehul J. Desai, Ryan Aschenbrener, Eduardo J. Carrera, and Nirguna Thalla

> The rapid development of neuromodulation specifically as it pertains to spinal cord stimulation (SCS) has ushered in an era of new and novel waveforms and programming methodologies. Accompanying this evolution has been a significant investment in clinical trials and outcomes-based research solidifying the foundation of SCS while investing in future indications and therapy expansion. Critically evaluating the existing literature to apply these therapies diligently remains vital to the future of neuromodulation.

Dorsal Root Ganglion Stimulation   359

Steven T. Potter, Sean Welch, Faye Tata, Seth Probert, and Ameet Nagpal

> The recent development and Food and Drug Administration approval in 2016 of dorsal root ganglion stimulation is a relatively new and novel form of target neuromodulation that promises improved outcomes compared with the current standard of care. Current literature is limited

and dependent on industry evaluation. Future independent investigation will help clarify existing data and refine techniques to improve safety, effectiveness, and expand application.

Peripheral Nerve Stimulation for Chronic Pain and Migraine: A Review 379

Samantha C. Erosa, Roya S. Moheimani, Jessica C. Oswald, Joel P. Castellanos, Mickey E. Abraham, and Nathaniel M. Schuster

Interventional pain procedures offer treatments for chronic pain conditions refractory to conservative measures. Neuromodulation, including peripheral nerve stimulation (PNS), applies electrical stimuli to neural structures to treat pain. Here we review the literature on PNS for various chronic pain conditions including neuropathic pain, postamputation pain, musculoskeletal pain, migraine, and pelvic pain.

Intrathecal Pumps 409

Tyler Ericson, Priyanka Singla, and Lynn Kohan

Intrathecal drug delivery systems are a well-established intervention for chronic pain. The localized delivery of analgesics allows for reduced side effect profiles and pain scores in patients with chronic pain. Given their proven benefits and the development of novel intrathecal medications, intrathecal drug delivery systems are being used earlier in chronic pain management treatment pathways. Success is reliant on proper patient selection and mitigating the risks of various adverse events stemming from the implantation procedure, medications, and the device itself. This article discusses patient selection criteria, medication selection, risks, complications, supporting data, and future directions of intrathecal drug delivery systems.

Vertebroplasty and Kyphoplasty 425

Sherief Boss, Vidhan Srivastava, and Magdalena Anitescu

Vertebral fractures are a common problem in the United States, which is why copious research has been performed to determine the best approaches to repair such fractures—including determining the least invasive procedures with the greatest benefits and fewest complications. In the past 3 decades, vertebral augmentation procedures (VAP) have been very effective, with new techniques appearing in the field that has very reasonable outcomes and marked improvement in patients' quality of life. This article highlights the different VAP approaches—comparing the advantages, disadvantages, and potential side effects of each approach.

Sympathetic Blocks for Sympathetic Pain 455

Melissa E. Phuphanich, Quinn Wonders Convery, Udai Nanda, and Sanjog Pangarkar

The sympathetic nervous system (SNS) is an integral component of the body's response to stress. Once activated, the SNS has broad-reaching effects on multiple organ systems that modulate pain, behavior, and mood. Blockade of the system can improve pain associated with multiple etiologies, including vascular, visceral, and neuropathic pain. Multiple techniques are available to block the SNS and provide options that improve analgesia and can be individualized to a particular patient's needs and disease state.

Sympathetic Blocks for Visceral Pain

475

Kevin Vorenkamp, Peter Yi, and Adam Kemp

For patients with chronic pain or cancer-related pain, the most common indication for sympathetic block is to control visceral pain arising from malignancies or other alterations of the abdominal and pelvic viscera. When it is recalcitrant to conservative care, or if the patient is intolerant to pharmacotherapy, consideration of sympathetic blocks or neurolytic procedures is considered. Potential advantages of a neurolytic procedure, compared with spinal and epidural anesthetic infusions, include cost savings and avoidance of hardware. Interventional therapies that target afferent visceral innervation via the sympathetic ganglia offer effective and durable analgesia and improve multiple metrics of quality of life.

Peripheral Nerve Injections

489

Arti Ori, Aparna Jindal, Nenna Nwazota, Amy C.S. Pearson, and Bhavana Yalamuru

Ultrasound techniques and peripheral nerve stimulation have increased the interest in peripheral nerve injections for chronic pain. The knowledge of anatomy and nerve distribution patterns is paramount for optimal use of peripheral nerve blocks in the management of chronic pain conditions. They are an important tool in an interventional pain physician's armamentarium and can be integrated into pain practices effectively to offer patients pain relief.

Peripheral Joint Radiofrequency Ablation

519

Maxim S. Eckmann, Brian T. Boies, David J. Carroll, and Lorne D. Muir II

This article provides a detailed description of peripheral joint radiofrequency ablation and its contemporary use in the treatment of chronic knee, hip, and shoulder pain. Special attention is given to anatomy and innervation of the joints discussed, technical approach, selection criteria, contraindications, and patient outcomes.

Novel Technologies in Interventional Pain Management

533

Yashar Eshraghi, Jay D. Shah, and Maged Guirguis

This article comprehensively covers 3 major novel technologies and techniques in the management of chronic lower back pain. The first 2 procedures, percutaneous interspinous spacer implantation, and minimally invasive lumbar decompression have shown significant impact in the management of lumbar spinal stenosis (LSS), especially in patients who are not great surgical candidates or are otherwise not amenable to open spinal surgery. The wealth of data for these procedures continues to increase, with up to 4 to 6-year follow-up data recently being made available. A novel solution for vertebrogenic back pain is also discussed as follow-up data emphasizes the safety and sustainability of the procedure. This article also establishes a framework for evaluating novel technologies in interventional pain management.

PHYSICAL MEDICINE AND REHABILITATION CLINICS OF NORTH AMERICA

FORTHCOMING ISSUES

August 2022
Wound and Skin Care
Xiaohua Zhou and Cassandra Renfro,
Editors

November 2022
Functional Medicine
Elizabeth Bradley, *Editor*

February 2023
Orthobiologics
Michael Khadavi and Luga Podesta,
Editors

RECENT ISSUES

February 2022
Cycling
Angela N. Cortez and Dana H. Kotler,
Editors

November 2021
Non-Spine Ablation Procedures
Santos F. Martinez, *Editor*

August 2021
Post-Polio Syndrome: Background,
Management and Treatment
Darren C. Rosenberg and Craig Rovito,
Editors

SERIES OF RELATED INTEREST

Orthopedic Clinics
https://www.orthopedic.theclinics.com/
Neurologic Clinics
https://www.neurologic.theclinics.com/
Clinics in Sports Medicine
https://www.sportsmed.theclinics.com/

Foreword
A Maturing Field

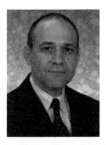

Santos F. Martinez, MD, MS
Consulting Editor

I thank Dr Nagpal for this update on treatment parameters, which should help guide our options in treating a difficult patient population. Interventional approaches for pain management is truly an art, continues to expand, and certainly complements other rehabilitation services. This presentation hits on many of the most common bread-and-butter procedures with objective data so that an informed approach can best benefit the patients. This informational approach confirms further basis and reasoning when offering such strategies and also raises attention to additional needed research to further our efforts. Interventional pain management procedures have earned a solid place among our *Physical Medicine and Rehabilitation Clinics of North America* series and are an integral part of Physical Medicine and Rehabilitation.

Santos F. Martinez, MD, MS
Physical Medicine and Rehabilitation
Department of Orthopaedic Surgery and
Biomedical Engineering
University of Tennessee College of Medicine
Campbell Clinic Orthopaedics
Memphis, TN 38104, USA

E-mail address:
smartinez@campbellclinic.com

Phys Med Rehabil Clin N Am 33 (2022) xv
https://doi.org/10.1016/j.pmr.2022.02.006
1047-9651/22/© 2022 Published by Elsevier Inc.

pmr.theclinics.com

Preface

(Needle) Jockeying for the Evidence

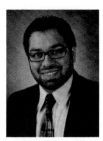

Ameet Nagpal, MD, MS, MEd
Editor

It is not unusual for physicians, including physiatrists, to question the role and utility of interventional procedures in the treatment of chronic pain. Much of this skepticism is driven by overutilization of these procedures, which has been well documented by analyses of Center for Medicare and Medicaid Services claims data.[1-3] Those of us who perform these procedures are well aware of the improvement in pain and function that they have the potential to provide, but most of us are also aware that the data informing our use of these procedures are often inadequate.

This issue of *Physical Medicine and Rehabilitation Clinics of North America* is designed to critically evaluate the evidence for each of the major procedural categories that physiatrists may utilize in their treatment of a patient with chronic pain. I strategically chose this incredibly strong group of authors because of their comprehensive knowledge of the literature surrounding their respective topics. I believe that this issue will be a great resource for any physiatrist who is interested in referring a patient for these procedures, as each article has a "Patient Selection" section that describes appropriate referral criteria. Each article also contains an "Outcome Data" section that has attempted to describe the extant research on each of these topics so as to guide interventionalists on when it is (or is not) appropriate to perform these procedures.

While our field is young, the growth potential is enormous. It is of utmost importance that we, the gatekeepers to these procedures, are judicious in their use. This issue is *not* designed to be a technical manual; rather, it is designed to inform the reader of the fact that these procedures can be effectively used in the treatment paradigm of those patients with chronic pain. It is my hope that by putting all of these data in one location,

Phys Med Rehabil Clin N Am 33 (2022) xvii–xviii
https://doi.org/10.1016/j.pmr.2022.02.001
1047-9651/22/© 2022 Published by Elsevier Inc.

my colleagues and I will no longer have to (needle) jockey to find the evidence to inform our decision making.

Ameet Nagpal, MD, MS, MEd
Department of Anesthesiology
UT Health San Antonio
San Antonio, TX 78229, USA

Department of Orthopaedics & Physical Medicine
Medical University of South Carolina
Charleston, SC 29425, USA

E-mail address:
nagpal@musc.edu

REFERENCES

1. Manchikanti L, Sanapati MR, Soin A, et al. An updated analysis of utilization of epidural procedures in managing chronic pain in the Medicare population from 2000 to 2018. Pain Physician 2020;23(2):111–26.
2. Manchikanti L, Sanapati MR, Pampati V, et al. Update of utilization patterns of facet joint interventions in managing spinal pain from 2000 to 2018 in the US fee-for-service Medicare population. Pain Physician 2020;23(2):E133–49.
3. Manchikanti L, Pampati V, Vangala BP, et al. Spinal cord stimulation trends of utilization and expenditures in fee-for-service (FFS) Medicare population from 2009 to 2018. Pain Physician 2021;24(5):293–308.

Epidural Steroid Injections

Joseph William, DO, MPH[a],*, Christian Roehmer, MD[a],
LeiLani Mansy, BS[b], David J. Kennedy, MD[a]

KEYWORDS

- Epidural steroid injections • Intervertebral disc displacement • Spinal stenosis
- Radicular pain • Radiculopathy

KEY POINTS

- Epidural steroid injections (ESIs) are a commonly used treatment modality for radicular pain.
- The quality of the efficacy data varies between different underlying anatomic pathologies for radicular pain.
- When performed according to guidelines, ESIs are relatively safe procedures. Nonetheless, clinicians should be familiar with the anatomy, risks, and benefits of the various routes of administration.

INTRODUCTION

Lumbar radiculopathy is one of the most common spine conditions seen by the spine specialist, with its prevalence being 3-5% of the population.[1] First-line treatment of radicular pain generally consists of conservative measures including motion-based therapy progressing to formal exercise and oral medications for symptom relief.[2] If conservative treatments do not lead to clinical improvement, or if they are not tolerated by the patient, this may be an indication for an interventional treatment such as an ESI.

During an epidural steroid injection (ESI), a solution of anti-inflammatory corticosteroid, typically paired with a local anesthetic or preservative-free normal saline, is injected into the epidural space to aid in pain relief. ESIs were first used for radicular pain due to a herniated nucleus pulposus from the intervertebral disc, but their indications now include radicular pain from a variety of causes (see section later in discussion on patient selection criteria). The 3 most commonly used approaches to access

[a] Department and Physical Medicine and Rehabilitation, Vanderbilt University Medical Center, Vanderbilt Stallworth Rehabilitation Hospital, 1221 Children's Way, Suite 1318, Nashville, Tennessee, USA; [b] University of Missouri-Kansas City School of Medicine, 2411 Holmes Street, Kansas City, Missouri, USA
* Corresponding author: Vanderbilt Stallworth Rehabilitation Hospital, 2201 Children's Way, Suite1318, Nashville, TN 37212, USA
E-mail address: joseph.william@vumc.org

Phys Med Rehabil Clin N Am 33 (2022) 215–231
https://doi.org/10.1016/j.pmr.2022.01.009
1047-9651/22/© 2022 Elsevier Inc. All rights reserved.

pmr.theclinics.com

the epidural space include interlaminar (IL), transforaminal (TF), and caudal; each of which will be discussed in detail throughout this article.

Mechanism of Action for Pain Relief in Epidural Steroid Injections

Corticosteroids are felt to diminish pain by blocking prostaglandin synthesis and the conduction of pain signals through nociceptive c fibers (nerve fibers that mediate dull, aching pain).[3] Phospholipase A2, an enzyme involved in the arachidonic acid pathway that produces the precursors to inflammatory molecules such as prostaglandins and leukotrienes, is also inhibited, decreasing cell-mediated inflammation and edema along the nerve roots.[4] Local anesthetic, often injected in combination with the corticosteroid, also aids in reducing transmission along unmyelinated c fibers due to sodium channel blockade. In turn, this diminishes ectopic nerve discharges, collagen scar formation, and excess neurotransmitter and pro-inflammatory cytokine release.[5]

Patient Selection Criteria

The main indication for an ESI involves etiologies that cause radicular pain. Radicular pain can be caused by the compression, inflammation, or irritation of a nerve root, leading to the radiation of pain and numbness along the distribution of the affected spinal nerve root. While radicular pain is the most common appropriate reason for an ESI, it is different than a documented radiculopathy. Radiculopathy is defined by any of the following: focal concordant decrement in reflexes, concordant weakness, sensation loss in the affected distribution, or at times a positive dural tension sign.[6] While it is a clinical diagnosis, radiculopathy can be confirmed by electrodiagnostic testing.[7]

Radiculopathy is most commonly caused by the pathology of the intervertebral discs. With a disc herniation, the gelatinous inner portion of the disc (nucleus pulposus) herniates through the fibrous outer layer (annulus fibrosus). The herniated disc can cause irritation of the associated spinal nerve and can cause radicular pain and/or neural deficits if significant nerve root compression is present. Stenosis of either the spinal canal itself or of the canals of exiting nerve roots (neural foramen) are other common causes of radiculopathy and radicular pain.[8]

Unresolving or severe radiculopathy is a strong indication for an ESI. However, it is important to realize that radicular pain alone, without the neural damage associated with radiculopathy, is an equally strong indication for an ESI. This is especially true as most studies show positive outcomes from an ESI enrolled subjects with radicular pain alone, not just the subset with radiculopathy.[9] Limiting the indications to radiculopathy only would be a gross mischaracterization of the literature and evidence-based medicine. Radicular pain is multifactorial and chronic mechanical compression of a nerve may subsequently lead to microvascular changes, including ischemia of the nerve, venous congestion, as well as to inflammatory changes such as intraneural edema and demyelination, further contributing to pain.[5] Additional conditions that can be considered for treatment with ESIs include radicular pain from the following:

- Postlaminectomy syndrome/postsurgery syndrome/failed back surgery syndrome
- Spondylolisthesis
- Scoliosis
- Postherpetic or posttraumatic neuralgia
- Facet synovial cysts that result in nerve root compression
- Epidural lipomatosis

Determining appropriate candidates for an ESI is critical, as the procedure is not without risks. Although the relative strength of the efficacy data does vary between the various etiologies for radicular pain, the indication for an ESI is patients with radicular pain who have not had adequate relief or are unable to tolerate conservative management.

Further diagnostics studies may also be warranted to properly localize the pathology including but not limited to x-ray (XR), computed tomography (CT), myelography, electromyography (EMG), nerve conduction studies (NCS), and magnetic resonance imaging (MRI). Generally, three-dimensional imaging from an MRI or CT scan is considered standard of care before receiving an ESI, with the MRI being preferred due to better visualization of soft tissues and lack of radiation.[10] Subsequent injections should be predicated on the response to the first injection. If there is no immediate or durable clinical improvement in symptoms from the first injection, repeating the same injection without modification is not likely indicated.[11] Additionally, a series of injections, historically known as a series of 3 injections, has no place in modern medicine.[12,13]

Procedural Subtypes

There are various techniques and approaches when performing an ESI and many factors should be considered when determining which approach would be the most effective for each patient. These factors include but are not limited to the patient's unique anatomy, nature, and location of the patient's pathology, the provider's comfort in performing the technique, the patient's medical comorbidities, all combined with the known outcome literature for effectiveness and the potential of a specific technique to deliver the medication to the target tissue. The standard of care for ESIs is the use of fluoroscopic or CT guidance, unless there is an absolute contraindication to fluoroscopy such as pregnancy. Additionally, the standard of care requires verifying that the injectant is being delivered to the correct site with the visualization of the needle tip and through the use of live, real-time fluoroscopy contrast medium.[9,10] This technique also allows for increased accuracy of drug delivery while also decreasing the risks associated with inappropriately placed medications.[14] Some ESIs (namely IL and caudal approaches) can also be delivered using anatomic landmarks alone or with ultrasound guidance. However, these techniques do not allow for the confirmation of the injectate properly being delivered to the correct location (ie, epidural space) and, most importantly, not an unintended location (ie, intrathecal, subdural, or vascular). Thus, they should not be routinely used and reserved for the rare cases in which fluoroscopy or CT guidance is contraindicated.[15]

Regarding the injectant itself, there are multiple options at various concentrations including particulate corticosteroids (ie, betamethasone, methylprednisolone, triamcinolone), and nonparticulate corticosteroids (ie, dexamethasone). Particulate corticosteroids have been linked to cases of spinal cord infarctions in the event of inadvertent intra-arterial injection.[16] Studies have shown short- and long-term equivalence between the particulate and nonparticulate formulations.[16,17] Thus, dexamethasone, a nonparticulate corticosteroid, is typically indicated as the first-line therapy for TF ESIs throughout the spine.[18] Refer to **Table 1** for the equipment setup for ESIs in general, as well as specific equipment differences related to each interventional approach.

Interlaminar Epidural Steroid Injection

Interlaminar injections (ie, injections through the posterior space between adjacent lamina) are performed to deliver the medication to the posterior epidural space. Ventral spread to the disc and dorsal root ganglion is unpredictable. There are a

Table 1
Typical epidural steroid injection equipment setup[16,18]

Fluoroscope Compatible Procedure Table
C-Arm Fluoroscope
Sterile Gloves
Surgical Mask
Prep Tray
Absorbent Towels or Fenestrated Drape
Chlorhexidine Gluconate (ChloraPrep), Iodine, Isopropyl Alcohol, or Betadine for Skin prep
4-inch x 4-Inch Gauze Dressings
Medication Labels
Band-Aids
One 18-Gauge x 1.5 inch Needle (Medication Aspiration)
One 25-Gauge x 1.5-inch Needle (Transdermal/intramuscular Infiltration if Desired)
Extension Tubing
One 3–5 cc Luer lock Syringe (Contrast Media)
One 5 cc Luer lock Syringe (Treatment Medication)
One 10 cc Luer lock Syringe (Local Anesthetic Transdermal/intramuscular Infiltration)
Preservative-Free Normal Saline
Contrast Medium (eg, Isovue 200, OmniPaque 240/300)
Local Anesthetic (eg, 1%–2% Lidocaine) *Note long-acting agents* such as *bupivacaine are generally*
  avoided in the epidural space due to the possibility of a prolonged motor block, and ropivacaine
  has been shown to cause spiculation when mixed with dexamethasone raising potential safety concerns
Steroid (eg, Dexamethasone, Methylprednisolone)

Caudal	**Interlaminar**	Transforaminal
One 22-gauge or 25-gauge 3.5–8 inch spinal needle	One 18-, 20, or 22-gauge x 3.5–8 inch Tuohy Epidural Needle	One 22-gauge or 25-gauge 3.5–8 i nch spinal needle
Optional: 18-gauge or 16-gauge epidural introducer needle with a 19-gauge or 21-gauge catheter, respectively	Loss of Resistance (LOR) Syringe with air or preservative-free normal saline	Steroid: Nonparticulate
Steroid: Particulate or Nonparticulate	Steroid: Particulate or Nonparticulate	

couple of studies showing a far lateral or parasagittal IL injections have better efficacy than midline IL injections and are comparable to the TF approach.[19,20] It is possible that with a parasagittal approach the medication is more likely to reach the ventral epidural space, which is closer to the dorsal root ganglion and may be the nidus of pain. The IL approach is also typically conducted with a larger volume of injectate than the TF approach, which may make them advantageous for multi-level and/or bilateral pathology although the literature for this group is limited.[14] It is a general contraindication to do an IL-ESI at the level of a previous laminectomy due to the lack of a ligament flavum and clear landmarks for safety. Some also argue that it is not ideal to do an IL-ESI at a level affected by severe central stenosis due to the lack of space for appropriate needle placement. Additionally, IL-ESIs are associated with a higher risk of dural puncture and epidural hematoma compared with TF ESIs.[21]

IL-ESIs are generally performed with the patient in the prone position. The IL window (ie, the space between the lamina of adjacent vertebrae) is then located on fluoroscopy using an anterior–posterior radiograph with or without a small degree of cranial or caudal tilt based on the patient's unique anatomy. Safety is paramount and clear images of the corresponding laminae are necessary to ensure safe epidural access. A small amount of local anesthetic is injected at the needle insertion site and along the planned needle trajectory is then taken with the Tuohy needle. The interventionalist must understand what tissue layers they will encounter between the skin and the target. While these will vary between the approach taken, the IL injection goes through the ligamentum flavum immediately before reaching the epidural space. To maximize safety, it is imperative that the interventionalist knows whereby their needle tip is at all times.[10] The depth of the needle is best assessed via lateral or contralateral oblique fluoroscopic imaging, also known as the depth or safety view. With the depth view on imaging, the needle is advanced. It is generally assisted with an air or saline loss of resistance (LOR) technique, which helps indicate passage through the ligamentum flavum and entrance into the epidural space. LOR alone is insufficient as it has both a false negative and false positive rate, thus it should be combined with live imaging. Once appropriate placement is suspected by the interventionalist, contrast medium is injected through extension tubing under live fluoroscopic visualization to confirm placement in the epidural space and absence of vascular, subdural, or intrathecal spread (**Fig. 1**). Once appropriate flow is confirmed, the treatment medication is delivered via the extension tubing to avoid advancing the needle. Subsequently, the needle is removed, and a sterile dressing is placed.[10,22]

Transforaminal Epidural Steroid Injection

Transforaminal injections enter the epidural space through the intervertebral foramen. This approach is typically chosen for patients with neural foraminal stenosis, disc herniation, or lateral recess stenosis. The TF approach also allows for selective nerve root injections, with the potential for the injectant to reach the anterior/ventral epidural space. This is a procedural advantage with the TF approach compared with the IL approach as the target for the injectant becomes the ventral epidural space which is felt to be the main source of pain in most of the patients.[23] This combined with a more robust body of literature showing efficacy, leads many to suggest these are generally the preferred route for most of the patients.[13] The TF approach may also be the preferred approach for patients that have undergone surgical laminectomies or those who have anatomic limitations in accessing the posterior epidural space. Additionally, because the medication is injected closer to the affected nerve root, less volume of medication is needed with this method, decreasing the possible

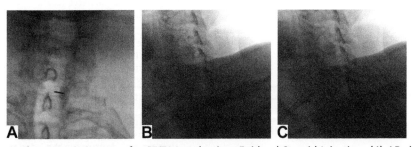

Fig. 1. Fluoroscopic Images of a C7/T1 Interlaminar Epidural Steroid Injection; (*A*) AP view showing a needle in the interlaminar space, (*B*) Contralateral oblique view showing needle placement after the loss of resistance obtained, (*C*) Contralateral oblique view showing appropriate contrast spread in the epidural space. Note in addition to contra-lateral oblique the contrast should be injected under live fluoroscopy using an AP view.

adverse events related to the procedure.[23] Despite these advantages, TF ESIs are associated with a risk of intra-arterial uptake, which can lead to rare but significant complications such as spinal cord infarction and paralysis if not recognized and subsequently injected with a particular corticosteroid.[24] In animal data, this specific risk is completely mitigated by the use of a nonparticulate corticosteroid.[25,26]

There are 4 unique approaches that can be used when performing a TF-ESI (ie, subpedicular, supraneural, retroneural, and infraneural). The specific targets and approximate fluoroscopic angles for these 4 approaches can be found in **Table 2**. The supraneural lumbar TF approach will be described in detail but note there are other approaches that can be used based on the patient's unique anatomy and pathology. The patient is generally placed in the prone position and the target vertebral foramen is identified. The ipsilateral foraminal space is then located between 2 vertebrae using an oblique XR. The trajectory of the needle should be toward the neural foramen, which is located just inferior to the pedicle. A small amount of local anesthetic may be injected at the needle insertion site and along the planned needle trajectory, although this is not necessarily shown to decrease procedural-related pain.[27]

Next, a spinal needle is aimed inferior to the pedicle of the more superior vertebrae, near the top of the intervertebral foramen. The needle position is determined using both lateral and antero-posterior (AP) views on fluoroscopy. In contrast to the IL approach whereby the depth view is considered the safety view, for the L1–L5 levels, the AP view is the safety view to assure the needle does not go too medial. On the AP view, to decrease the chances of an intradural injection, the needle should not go medial to the 6 O'clock position under the pedicle. For the S1–S2 approach, the lateral view is again the safety view to assure the needle does not go ventral to the spinal canal.[10,22]

Once the needle is in appropriate position confirmed by both AP and lateral views, contrast dye is injected through extension tubing under live fluoroscopy under the AP view to confirm placement in the epidural space and the absence of vascular,

Table 2
Transforaminal epidural steroid injection approaches[16,18]

Technique	Target
Subpedicular (Classic "safe triangle" approach)	Six o'clock position of the pedicle on the AP view, above the target nerve
Retroneural	Dorsal to the spinal nerve (useful in cases of upward displacement of the target nerve).
Supraneural	Just above the target nerve, below the pedicle (to avoid the floor of the intervertebral foramen in the "safe triangle").
Infraneural (Otherwise known as the "Kambrins Triangle")	Center of the lower half of the intervertebral foramen, between the intervertebral disc anteriorly and facet joint posteriorly. Studies have shown less arterial structures in the inferior portion of the foramen, thus decreasing the likelihood of intraarterial injection, but at the risk of increased intradiscal injection.

subdural, or intrathecal spread (**Fig. 2**). Digital subtraction imaging (DSI) may be used to further confirm appropriate spread if needed. Another safety option is an anesthetic test dose, in which local anesthetic is injected before the instillation of a more dangerous particulate corticosteroid.[28] Once appropriately confirmed, the treatment medication is delivered. Procedural images should be saved per routine care.[10] Subsequently, the needle is removed, and a sterile dressing is placed.[10,22] Again, while the lumbar TF-ESI is described in detail here, please note that similar procedures can be performed in the thoracic and cervical spine. However, the techniques in these locations are different due to the unique anatomy in these regions.

Caudal Epidural Steroid Injection

Caudal ESIs are placed into the most inferior portion of the epidural space through the sacral hiatus and caudal canal. Due to the nature of the sacral anatomy, caudal ESIs are the least specific of the three epidural techniques described requiring a larger amount of injectant with a smaller proportion of medication reaching the target level.[29] They also cannot be advanced proximal to the S2 level due to a risk of intrathecal injection. This pitfall can be somewhat overcome using an epidural introducer needle with a catheter directed to the target level, although in the theory this would increase the risks of an epidural hematoma.[30] This combined with a lack of strong efficacy data suggests that they have a limited utility for routine first-line use in a modern medical practice.

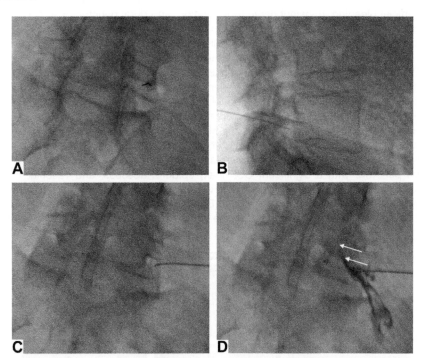

Fig. 2. Fluoroscopic Images of an L5/S1 Transforaminal Epidural Steroid Injection; (*A*) Oblique view showing needle placement for supraneural approach, (*B*) Lateral view showing proper needle placement within the neural foramen, (*C*) AP view showing proper needle placement approaching the 6 o'clock position beneath the pedicle, (*D*) AP view showing appropriate contrast spread in the epidural space medial to the pedicle as demonstrated by the arrows.

To perform a caudal ESI, the patient generally assumes the prone position. The sacral hiatus is located on fluoroscopy using an AP view, and local anesthetic is applied to the skin at the injection site. The spinal needle is inserted into the sacral hiatus via a midline approach using a lateral view is used to assure the needle is both in the hiatus and remains caudal to the S2–S3 level to decrease the risk of a dural puncture.[10] Subsequently, contrast is injected through an extension tube under live fluoroscopy to confirm accurate needle placement into the sacral epidural space (**Figure 3**). This is followed by the injection of a corticosteroid solution. Subsequently, the needle is removed, and a sterile dressing is placed.

Risks and Contraindications

Contraindications to ESIs can be categorized into absolute and relative contraindications. Absolute and relative contraindications can be found in **Table 3**.[10,31–33] Interestingly, factors that can negatively affect outcomes of an ESI include opioid dependence, smoking, chronic pain syndromes, and patients who have pending legal or disability claims.[5] These factors should be considered when determining if a patient would be an appropriate candidate for an ESI. As with any procedure, the risks and benefits should be clearly discussed with the patient and informed consent obtained. Expertise and a thorough understanding of the precise techniques involved, and relevant anatomy are necessary to perform an ESI safely. Adverse events documented from an ESI can range from mild to severe (**Table 3**). Minor adverse events such as superficial bleeding, transient nerve root irritation, and dural puncture with minor cerebral spinal fluid (CSF) leak occur in less than 1% of ESIs. Major events such as an epidural hematoma or infection that result in neurologic impairment and sequelae occur in significantly less than 0.01% of these procedures.[32,33]

The most common adverse events from ESIs include nausea/vomiting after the procedure and pain at the injection site.[33] Allergic reactions to the components of the injection may also occur. Patients should be screened for previous reactions to anesthetic, contrast solutions, or preservatives associated with steroids before the procedure.[10] Due to the proximity of the needle to the nerve roots, there is a risk of nerve injury, and transient lower or upper extremity numbness, weakness, or pain may occur.[10] More severe adverse events include traumatic nerve injury, paralysis, dural puncture with a significant CSF leak, epidural abscess, and vascular injury resulting in an epidural hematoma.[18,26,32] Retroperitoneal abscesses and hematomas have also been documented following an ESI though these are rare.[30] Regarding injections to the cervical spinal region, the risks are somewhat increased given the

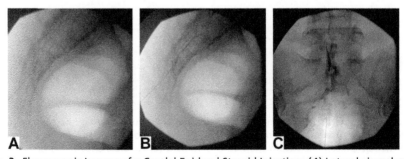

Fig. 3. Fluoroscopic Images of a Caudal Epidural Steroid Injection; (A) Lateral view showing a needle in the caudal canal, (B) Lateral view showing appropriate contrast spread in the epidural space, (C) AP view showing appropriate contrast spread in the epidural space.

Table 3
Epidural steroid injection contraindications and adverse events[4,24,25]

Relative:	Most Common:
Uncontrolled diabetes mellitus	Nausea and vomiting
Congestive heart failure	Pain at the injection site
Hepatitis C and other liver diseases	Dural puncture headache (with the
Chronic immunosuppression	IL approach)
Cushing syndrome	Less Common:
Improvement with conservative	Allergy/anaphylaxis to contrast
therapy	solution
Local injection site malignancy	Damage to surrounding structures
Myelopathy or cauda equina	Transient upper or lower extremity
syndrome (note ESI do not treat these	numbness/weakness
conditions)	Severe:
Known allergy or hypersensitivity to	Dural puncture requiring blood
contrast, anesthetic, or corticosteroid	patch
Acute spinal cord compression	Epidural abscess
Absolute:	Epidural hematoma
Systemic or local (injection site)	Traumatic nerve injury
infection	Paralysis
Infectious spondylosis	
Uncorrectable bleeding or clotting	
disorders	
Patient refusal	

unique anatomic considerations including less space if an epidural hematoma were to occur and the presence of the vertebral artery at most levels in the intervertebral foramen.[10,22]

Relevant Outcome Data for Epidural Steroid Injections

The data on efficacy can be challenging due to the wide variety of study designs, the variable inclusion criteria, and the outcomes reported.[34] The results can be complicated by differences in efficacy between approaches (ie, IL, TF, and caudal), pathology enrolled (ie, stenosis vs disc herniation) and other anatomic considerations (ie, cervical, thoracic, or lumbar), as well as the overall quality of the studies. Additionally, the natural history of radicular pain, differences in inclusion and exclusion criteria, type, and volume of steroid and/or anesthetic used, and debate regarding what a true placebo may be, often confound the assessment of clinical outcomes after intervention. Sometimes due to these variables, a placebo-controlled explanatory study may be of less value than a well-done pragmatic study or even a cohort study.[35] This section will highlight a selection of blinded, well-controlled, and randomized studies, on which much of the current practice models are based. See **Table 4** for a detailed summary of the relevant outcome data.

Interlaminar Epidural Steroid Injection Outcomes

Three important randomized controlled studies demonstrate the benefits and limitations of IL ESIs. Wilson-MacDonald et al. conducted a prospective randomized trial on IL-ESI for 92 patients with "lumbar nerve root compression." Patients included in the study had MRI evidence of disc prolapse or spinal stenosis and were randomized to undergo either IL epidural injection or intramuscular injection, both with 80 mg of methylprednisolone and 0.5% bupivacaine. Significant differences in pain, as rated by the Oxford pain chart, were seen in the IL group after 35 days, but no differences

Table 4
Selected comparison studies of epidural steroid injection techniques[1]

Author	Study Design	Participants	Indication	Treatment	Primary Outcomes	Summary of Findings
Ackerman and Ahmad	RCT	ILESI - 30 TFESI - 30 CESI - 30	Lumbar disc herniation and radicular pain	40 mg triamcinolone	Pain relief	Significant improvement in pain relief with TFESI at 24 wk
Pandey	RCT	ILESI - 18 TFESI - 40 CESI - 82	Lumbar disc herniation and back pain (with or without radiation)	ILESI & CESI - 80 mg methylprednisolone TFESI - 40mg methylprednisolone	JOA Score	Improvement in JOA in all 3 approaches, significant improvement with TFESI over others
Gharibo et al.	RCT	ILESI - 21 TFESI - 21	Lumbar back pain with unilateral radicular symptoms	80mg triamcinolone and 2mL of 0.25% bupivacaine	NRS, ODI	Significant improvement in pain after 2 wk with TFESI, no difference in ODI or other measures
Rados et al.	RCT	ILESI – 32 TFESI - 32	Lumbar disc herniation, unilateral lumbar radicular pain	ILESI - 80mg methylprednisolone and 8mL of 0.5% lidocaine TFESI - 40mg methylprednisolone and 3mL of 0.5% lidocaine	VAS, ODI	Improvement in VAS and ODI with both injection methods, no significant differences between groups
Friedly et al.	RCT	ILESI (T) - 143 ILESI (C) - 139 TFESI (T) - 56 TFESI (C) - 61	Lumbar central spinal stenosis and leg pain	Four different steroids used, variable amounts given per injection	RMDQ, Leg pain	No significant differences between groups at 6 wks

Legend: ILESI = Interlaminar Epidural Steroid Injection, TFESI = Transforaminal Epidural Steroid Injection, CESI = Caudal Epidural Steroid Injection, RCT = Randomized Controlled Trial, T = Treatment, C= Control, JOA = Japanese Orthopedic Association, NRS = Numeric Pain Rating Scale, ODI = Oswestry Disability Index, VAS = Visual Analog Scale, RMDQ = Roland–Morris Disability Questionnaire

were noted thereafter, including the rate of subsequent operations.[36] Arden and colleagues randomized 228 patients with "unilateral sciatica" to undergo either lumbar IL ESIs with 80 mg of triamcinolone acetonide and 10 mL of 0.2% bupivacaine or interligamentous injections with 2 mL of normal saline.[37] The primary outcome measure was the Oswestry low back pain disability questionnaire (ODQ), which at 3 weeks, reflected significant benefits for the treatment group. Beyond 3 weeks, there were no other sustained improvements.[37] Carette and colleagues performed a randomized controlled trial (RCT) of 156 patients with "sciatica due to herniated nucleus pulposus."[38] Participants were randomized to receive a lumbar IL epidural injection with either 80 mg of methylprednisolone acetate or 1 mL of isotonic saline. After 6 weeks, this study found a significant improvement in leg pain in the treatment group, but no statistically significant improvement in ODI score. Carette concluded that IL-ESI offers benefits for radicular pain due to herniated disc pathology, but no significant functional benefits.[38] There is a paucity of literature for the efficacy of IL ESIs in both the cervical and thoracic regions.[39]

Transforaminal Epidural Steroid Injection Outcomes

There is a growing trend among practitioners toward favoring the use of TF ESIs so as a result, this injection technique has been the most widely studied.[13] Karppinen and colleagues studied TF-ESIs in 160 patients with "sciatica," as defined by unilateral pain radiating from the back to below the knee.[40] Patients were randomized to a treatment group receiving 2 to 3 mL of methylprednisolone 40 mg/mL and bupivacaine 5 mg/mL, or a control group receiving 2 to 3 mL of normal saline. The treatment group showed significant improvement in leg pain based on the visual analog scale (VAS) at 2 weeks but experienced no significant improvements in pain at 4 weeks, or thereafter.[40] Ghahreman and colleagues performed a RCT on 150 patients with "lumbar radicular pain."[41] This study compared outcomes with the TF injection of steroid and anesthetic, anesthetic alone, or normal saline, versus intramuscular injection with steroid or normal saline. Patients in the transformational epidural steroid group were injected with 70 mg of triamcinolone and/or 2 mL of 0.5% bupivacaine. Patients randomized to the normal saline group were injected with a total of 2 mL. After 1 month, results were notable for significant improvement in the primary outcome measure of relieving at least 50% of pain for the treatment group (TF injection with steroid), as compared with all other groups. Improvements were also correlated with functional gain, as measured by the 36-Item Short Form Survey (SF-36), Roland Morris Disability Questionnaire (RMDQ), and decreased use of health care resources. Beyond the 1-month time frame, statistically significant improvements between groups regarding pain relief and secondary outcome measures were diminished.[41]

In contrast to these studies on TF-ESI, Riew and colleagues and Ng and colleagues both conducted RCTs of TF-ESI using anesthetic as a control group.[42,43] Riew and colleagues conducted a well-known study investigating the efficacy of TF injections in the treatment of 55 patients with "lumbar radicular pain."[42] The treatment group was injected with 6 mg of betamethasone and 1mL of 0.25% bupivacaine, and the control group was injected with 1 mL of 0.25% bupivacaine alone. Primary outcome measures of 13-month and 28-month postinjection operation rates were significantly lower in the treatment group, averting the need for decompression surgery.[42] Later, Ng and colleagues completed a similar RCT for TF injection in 86 patients with "chronic radicular pain."[43] Half of the participants were randomized to receive 40 mg of methylprednisolone and 2 mL of 0.25% bupivacaine, while the others were given 2 mL of 0.25% bupivacaine alone. After 3 months, the authors found subjective improvements in the major outcomes of Oswestry Disability Index (ODI), VAS, and walking distance; however, there were no statistically significant differences noted between the groups.[43] Given the relative risk differences between particulate and nonparticulate corticosteroids, Kennedy and colleagues studied the comparative efficacy of triamcinolone versus dexamethasone for lumbar radicular pain due to a single level herniated nucleus pulposus.[17] In this study they showed a high proportion of patients reporting successful outcomes at all-time points (2 weeks, 3 months, and 6 months), with no significant differences between groups aside from a slight increase in the number of injections received by those who received dexamethasone.[17] A similar finding of equivalence was found in the cervical spine,[44] but there is a dearth of quality data for outcomes from these procedures in the thoracic spine.

Overall, there is a strong consensus regarding the efficacy of TF-ESI in the treatment of radicular pain due to a herniated nucleus pulposus.[13] Moderate evidence exists showing that TF injections may offer improvements in function and decreased need for health care interventions.[13] It is imperative to understand the natural history of radicular pain to determine the goals of treatment, as recurrence rates in this population can be high regardless of the treatment given thus confounding the true efficacy of the intervention.[45]

Caudal Epidural Steroid Injection Outcomes

Randomized control studies for a Caudal ESI are limited. Bush and Hillier randomized a small cohort of 23 patients with "lumbar nerve root compromise" to a treatment and a placebo group.[46] The treatment group underwent caudal epidural injections with 80 mg of triamcinolone acetonide, plus 0.5% procaine hydrochloride, while the placebo group received caudal injections of 25 mL of normal saline. At the 4-week follow-up, the treatment group had statistically significant improvement in both pain relief, as scored by the VAS, and lifestyle, as measured by the Grogono and Woodgate Symptomatology Questionnaire.[46] Recently, Nandi and Chowdhery published a RCT on the efficacy of caudal injections for 93 patients with "lumbosacral sciatica."[47] Patients were randomized to a caudal epidural group injected with 80 mg of methylprednisolone or to a caudal epidural group injected with 20 mL of isotonic saline. The primary outcome measure was the patient's self-evaluation of improvement. The treatment group had a statistically significant success rate as compared with the placebo group after 4 weeks, but no statistical difference was seen at 12 weeks.[47] While these studies show some evidence regarding the effectiveness of caudal injections when used for lumbosacral radicular pain, there is a significant lack of evidence compared with the other approaches.

DISCUSSION

All 3 injection techniques have some data demonstrating benefits for the management of radicular pain, and several trials have been conducted to determine which method is the most effective (**Table 2**). TF-ESIs are often regarded as providing the strongest evidence of improvement in the treatment of lumbar radicular pain. Two well-controlled randomized studies demonstrate this.[48,49] Both studies compared all 3 injection methods (ie, TF, IL, and caudal) for the treatment of radicular pain due to disc pathology. Ackerman and Ahmad found that TF injections offered a statistically significant improvement in pain relief and required the fewest number of injections, as compared with the other injection techniques at 24 weeks.[48] Furthermore, Pandey concluded that all 3 injections were effective, but that the TF technique caused a statistically significant improvement in patients' symptom severity based on the Japanese Orthopedic Association (JOA) score at the 1-year follow-up.[49] These studies attributed the success with the TF technique to be due to a higher amount of steroid placement into the ventral epidural space.[48,49]

In contrast to the aforementioned studies, which showed significant benefits using the TF technique, several RCTs have shown little to no statistical difference between TF and IL techniques. Gharibo and colleagues randomized 42 patients with "lumbar radicular pain" to receive either TF or IL injections, with 80 mg of triamcinolone and 2 mL of 0.25% bupivacaine.[50] The study found statistically significant improvement in the numerical rating score (NRS) for pain with the TF method at the 2-week follow-up; however, all other measures, including ODI, NRS for depression, and opioid consumption, reflected no demonstrable difference.[50] Similarly, Rados and colleagues published a randomized, prospective study on 64 patients with "chronic unilateral radicular pain," comparing TF-ESIs and IL-ESIs.[51] As per common practice protocols, patients in the TF group were injected with 40 mg of methylprednisolone, while patients in the IL group were injected with 80 mg of methylprednisolone. Improvements were seen in primary outcome measures of VAS and ODI throughout 2 to 24 weeks; however, neither injection technique was statistically superior.[51] The studies that found no differences between the TF and IL approach generally had looser inclusion criteria. This manifested as the inclusion of "lumbar radicular pain" due to any etiology, which was in contrast to the studies that demonstrated the TF approach to be superior which focused on those with disc herniations.

Lastly, the randomized controlled study by Friedly and colleagues deserves discussion.[52] The 16-site study randomized 400 patients with radiographic spinal stenosis and associated neurogenic claudication, to receive an injection into the epidural space with either a corticosteroid and lidocaine or a lidocaine. These were conducted via either the TF or IL approach using 4 different steroid types, as well as variable amounts of injectant were used as treatments throughout the study. The only statistically different findings in the groups were increased patient satisfaction favoring those that received steroids, and more people who received only lidocaine crossed over to receive the steroids in a blinded fashion due to the lack of effectiveness of the injection. The authors noted no statistical differences at 6 weeks regarding the primary outcome measures of pain-related functional disability (as rated by the Rolland Morris Disability Questionnaire) and leg pain intensity.[52] Long term analysis did show a group of patients that had long-term resolution of their pain after a single injection, but the results were similar between the lidocaine and corticosteroid groups.[53]

SUMMARY

There is an overall consensus that ESIs provide a transient benefit for the relief of radicular pain in the setting of lumbar disc pathology and to a lesser degree spinal stenosis.[12,13,54] Lumbar ESIs may also be a surgery-sparing technique when used in conjunction with conservative care.[55] There is insufficient evidence for ESIs in the setting of axial back pain, and there are limited controlled studies available for cervical ESIs.[56] As indicated above, TF-ESIs have more robust outcomes data favoring efficacy. However, selecting the right approach should be based on the individual the patient's needs, with the consideration of adverse effects and contraindications.

CLINICS CARE POINTS

- ESIs are commonly used treatment approach for radicular pain and multiple RCTs have demonstrated their efficacy.

- Evidence indicates that ESIs are a relatively safe procedure when performed by trained physicians following appropriate guidelines.[10] Nonetheless, clinicians should be familiar with the anatomy, risks, and benefits associated with each interventional approach (ie, IL, TF, and caudal).
- Patient selection is key and further advancing imaging (ie, MRI) is generally standard of care to properly localize the pathology and for procedural planning.
- Nonparticulate steroids are first line for TF-ESIs in the lumbar spine, and the only safe option for thoracic and cervical TF-ESI. Particulates can be a second-line option for a lumbar TF-ESI. Particulates may also be used for the IL and caudal approaches.

DISCLOSURE

The authors have no competing conflicts of interest to disclose.

REFERENCES

1. Berry JA, Elia C, Saini HS, et al. A review of lumbar radiculopathy, diagnosis, and treatment. Cureus 2019;11:e5934.
2. Kennedy DJ, Noh MY. The role of core stabilization in lumbosacral radiculopathy. Phys Med Rehabil Clin N Am 2011;22:91–103.
3. Oliveira CB, Maher CG, Ferreira ML, et al. Epidural corticosteroid injections for sciatica: an abridged cochrane systematic review and meta-analysis. Spine 2020;45:E1405–15.
4. Murakami M, Kudo I. Phospholipase A2. J Biochem (Tokyo) 2002;131:285–92.
5. Palmer WE. Spinal injections for pain management. Radiology 2016;281:669–88.
6. Dillingham TR. Evaluating the patient with suspected radiculopathy. PM&R 2013; 5:S41–9.
7. Dillingham TR, Lauder TD, Andary M, et al. Identifying lumbosacral radiculopathies: an optimal electromyographic screen. Am J Phys Med Rehabil 2000; 79:496.
8. Patel EA, Perloff MD. Radicular pain syndromes: cervical, lumbar, and spinal stenosis. Semin Neurol 2018;38:634–9.
9. Kennedy DJ, Levin J, Rosenquist R, et al. Epidural steroid injections are safe and effective: multisociety letter in support of the safety and effectiveness of epidural steroid injections. Pain Med 2015;16:833–8.
10. Bogduk N. International spine intervention society, & standards committee. *Practice guidelines for spinal diagnostic and treatment procedures.* San Francisco, CA: International Spine Intervention Society; 2004.
11. Murthy NS, Geske JR, Shelerud RA, et al. The effectiveness of repeat lumbar transforaminal epidural steroid injections. Pain Med 2014;15:1686–94.
12. MacVicar J, King W, Landers MH, et al. The effectiveness of lumbar transforaminal injection of steroids: a comprehensive review with systematic analysis of the published data. Pain Med 2013;14:14–28.
13. Smith CC, McCormick ZL, Mattie R, et al. The effectiveness of lumbar transforaminal injection of steroid for the treatment of radicular pain: a comprehensive review of the published data. Pain Med 2020;21:472–87.
14. Sharma AK, Vorobeychick Y, Wasserman R, et al. The effectiveness and risks of fluoroscopically guided lumbar interlaminar epidural steroid injections: a systematic review with comprehensive analysis of the published data. Pain Med 2017; 18:239–51.

15. Ehsanian R, Schneider BJ, Kennedy DJ, et al. Ultrasound-guided cervical selective nerve root injections: a narrative review of literature. Reg Anesth Pain Med 2021;46:416–21.

16. McCormick ZL, Cushman D, Marshall B, et al. Pain reduction and repeat injections after transforaminal epidural injection with particulate versus nonparticulate steroid for the treatment of chronic painful lumbosacral radiculopathy. PM R 2016; 8:1039–45.

17. Kennedy DJ, Plastaras C, Casey E, et al. Comparative effectiveness of lumbar transforaminal epidural steroid injections with particulate versus nonparticulate corticosteroids for lumbar radicular pain due to intervertebral disc herniation: a prospective, randomized, double-blind trial. Pain Med 2014;15:548–55.

18. Rathmell JP, Benzon H, Dreyfuss P, et al. Safeguards to prevent neurologic complications after epidural steroid injections: consensus opinions from a multidisciplinary working group and national organizations. Anesthesiology 2015;122: 974–84.

19. Makkar JK, Gourav KK, Jain K, et al. Transforaminal versus lateral parasagittal versus midline interlaminar lumbar epidural steroid injection for management of unilateral radicular lumbar pain: a randomized double-blind trial. Pain Physician 2019;22:561–73.

20. Ghai B, Vadaje KS, Wig J, et al. Lateral parasagittal versus midline interlaminar lumbar epidural steroid injection for management of low back pain with lumbosacral radicular pain: a double-blind, randomized study. Anesth Analg 2013;117: 219–27.

21. Choi E-J, Park SJ, Yoo Y-M, et al. Comparison of the oblique interlaminar and transforaminal lumbar epidural steroid injections for treatment of low back and lumbosacral radicular pain. J Pain Res 2021;14:407–14.

22. Furman M. Atlas of image-guided spinal procedures. Philadelphia, PA: Elsevier Saunders; 2013.

23. Lee JH, Shin K-H, Bahk SJ, et al. Comparison of clinical efficacy of transforaminal and caudal epidural steroid injection in lumbar and lumbosacral disc herniation: a systematic review and meta-analysis. Pain Physician 2018;18:2343–53.

24. Chang-Chien GC, Knezevic NN, McCormick Z, et al. Transforaminal versus interlaminar approaches to epidural steroid injections: a systematic review of comparative studies for lumbosacral radicular pain. Pain Physician 2014;17:E509–24.

25. Okubadejo GO, Talcott MR, Schmidt RE, et al. Perils of intravascular methylprednisolone injection into the vertebral artery. an animal study. J Bone Joint Surg Am 2008;90:1932–8.

26. Kennedy DJ, Dreyfuss P, Aprill CN, et al. Paraplegia following image-guided transforaminal lumbar spine epidural steroid injection: two case reports. Pain Med 2009;10:1389–94.

27. Bakshi R, Berri H, Kalpakjian C, et al. The Effects of local anesthesia administration on pain experience during interventional spine procedures: a prospective controlled trial. Pain Med 2016;17:488–93.

28. Smuck M, Maxwell MD, Kennedy DJ, et al. Utility of the anesthetic test dose to avoid catastrophic injury during cervical transforaminal epidural injections. Spine J 2010;10:857–64.

29. Kao S-C, Lin C-S. Caudal epidural block: an updated review of anatomy and techniques. Biomed Res Int 2017;2017:9217145.

30. Palmer E. Management of cervical epidural hematoma after cervical epidural steroid injection using a catheter technique. Pain Med 2020;21:1301–2.

31. Ehsanian R, Rosati RM, Kennedy DJ, et al. Antiplatelet and anticoagulant risk for select spine interventions: a retrospective cohort. Pain Med 2020;21:910–7.
32. El-Yahchouchi CA, Plastaras CT, Maus TP, et al. Adverse event rates associated with transforaminal and interlaminar epidural steroid injections: a multi-institutional study. Pain Med 2016;17:239–49.
33. Carr CM, Plastaras CT, Pingree MJ, et al. Immediate adverse events in interventional pain procedures: a multi-institutional study. Pain Med 2016;17:2155–61.
34. Kennedy DJ, Schneider BJ. The challenges of research on interventions for low back pain. Ann Intern Med 2017;166:601–2. https://doi.org/10.7326/M17-0556.
35. Bogduk N, Kennedy DJ, Vorobeychik Y, et al. Guidelines for composing and assessing a paper on treatment of pain, Pain Med, 18(11), 2017, 2104–2096, https://doi.org/10.1093/pm/pnx121.
36. Wilson-MacDonald J, Burt G, Griffin D, et al. Epidural steroid injection for nerve root compression. a randomised, controlled trial. J Bone Joint Surg Br 2005;87:352–5.
37. Arden NK, Price C, Reading I, et al. A multicentre randomized controlled trial of epidural corticosteroid injections for sciatica: the WEST study. Rheumatology (Oxford) 2005;44:1399–406.
38. Carette S, Marcoux S, Truchon R, et al. A controlled trial of corticosteroid injections into facet joints for chronic low back pain. N Engl J Med 1991;325:1002–7.
39. Cohen SP, Bicket MC, Jamison D, et al. Epidural steroids: a comprehensive, evidence-based review. Reg Anesth Pain Med 2013;38:175–200.
40. Karppinen J, Malmivaara A, Kurunlahti M, et al. Periradicular infiltration for sciatica: a randomized controlled trial. Spine 2001;26:1059–67.
41. Ghahreman A, Ferch R, Bogduk N. The efficacy of transforaminal injection of steroids for the treatment of lumbar radicular pain. Pain Med 2010;11:1149–68.
42. Riew KD, Yin Y, Gilula L, et al. The effect of nerve-root injections on the need for operative treatment of lumbar radicular pain. a prospective, randomized, controlled, double-blind study. J Bone Joint Surg Am 2000;82-A:1589–93.
43. Ng L, Chaudhary N, Sell P. The efficacy of corticosteroids in periradicular infiltration for chronic radicular pain: a randomized, double-blind, controlled trial. Spine 2005;30:857–62.
44. Dreyfuss P, Baker R, Bogduk N. Comparative effectiveness of cervical transforaminal injections with particulate and nonparticulate corticosteroid preparations for cervical radicular pain. Pain Med 2006;7:237–42.
45. Kennedy DJ, Zheng PZ, Smuck M, et al. A minimum of 5-year follow-up after lumbar transforaminal epidural steroid injections in patients with lumbar radicular pain due to intervertebral disc herniation. Spine J 2018;18:29–35.
46. Bush K, Hillier S. A controlled study of caudal epidural injections of triamcinolone plus procaine for the management of intractable sciatica. Spine 1991;16:572–5.
47. Nandi J, Chowdhery A. A Randomized controlled clinical trial to determine the effectiveness of caudal epidural steroid injection in lumbosacral sciatica. J Clin Diagn Res 2017;11:RC04–8.
48. Ackerman WE, Ahmad M. The efficacy of lumbar epidural steroid injections in patients with lumbar disc herniations. Anesth Analg 2007;104:1217–22.
49. Pandey RA. Efficacy of epidural steroid injection in management of lumbar prolapsed intervertebral disc: a comparison of caudal, transforaminal and interlaminar routes. J Clin Diagn Res JCDR 2016;10:RC05–11.
50. Gharibo CG, Varlotta GP, Rhame EE, et al. Interlaminar versus transforaminal epidural steroids for the treatment of subacute lumbar radicular pain: a randomized, blinded, prospective outcome study. Pain Physician 2011;14:499–511.

51. Rados I, Sakic K, Fingler M, et al. Efficacy of interlaminar vs transforaminal epidural steroid injection for the treatment of chronic unilateral radicular pain: prospective, randomized study. Pain Med 2011;12:1316–21.
52. Friedly JL, Comstock BA, Turner JA, et al. A randomized trial of epidural glucocorticoid injections for spinal stenosis. N Engl J Med 2014;371:11–21.
53. Friedly JL, Comstock BA, Turner JA, et al. Long-term effects of repeated injections of local anesthetic with or without corticosteroid for lumbar spinal stenosis: a randomized trial. Arch Phys Med Rehabil 2017;98(8):1499–507. https://doi.org/10.1016/j.apmr.2017.02.029.
54. Ghahreman A, Bogduk N. Predictors of a favorable response to transforaminal injection of steroids in patients with lumbar radicular pain due to disc herniation. Pain Med 2011;12:871–9.
55. Riew KD, Park J-B, Cho Y-S, et al. Nerve root blocks in the treatment of lumbar radicular pain. A minimum five-year follow-up. J Bone Joint Surg Am 2006;88:1722–5.
56. DePalma MJ, Slipman CW. Evidence-informed management of chronic low back pain with epidural steroid injections. Spine J 2008;8:45–55.

Radiofrequency Ablation for Zygapophyseal Joint Pain

Benjamin Gill, DO, MBA[a], Cole Cheney, MD[b], Nate Clements, MD[c],
Allison Glinka Przybsyz, MD[d], Zachary L. McCormick, MD[b], Aaron Conger, DO[b],*

KEYWORDS

- Facet joint • Neurotomy • Medial branch • Low back pain • Neck pain

KEY POINTS

- Zygapophyseal joints may be the source of cervical and lumbar spine pain in 25% to 45% and 5% to 50% of individuals, respectively.
- Medial branches of the primary dorsal ramus provide sensory innervation to the typical zygapophyseal joints and may be denervated through radiofrequency ablation (RFA) in carefully selected patients.
- Selection for medial branch RFA is based on a thorough history and physical examination and is confirmed with fluoroscopically guided medial branch blocks (MBBs).
- Strict dual-block paradigms have been shown to predict higher rates of treatment success but also exclude a proportion of patients who may benefit from the procedure.
- Serious complications are rare when the procedure is performed in accordance with established standards.

INTRODUCTION
Epidemiology

Zygapophyseal (facet) joints have been implicated as the primary origin of symptoms in 25% to 45% of patients with cervical pain,[1–3] and between 5% and 50% of those presenting with low back pain.[4–6] Although the prevalence of thoracic facet pain has been estimated between 34% and 48%,[7,8] anatomic studies have called into question the location and course of the thoracic medial branches and therefore these estimates may not be accurate.[9] Further, because of the differing definitions of facet-mediated pain and methods used for diagnosis, the definitive incidence is controversial.

[a] Department of Physical Medicine and Rehabilitation, University of Missouri, Columbia, MO, USA; [b] Division of Physical Medicine and Rehabilitation, University of Utah, Salt Lake City, UT, USA; [c] Department of Anesthesiology, University of Texas Health Science Center, San Antonio, TX, USA; [d] Department of Orthopedics and Rehabilitation, University of Wisconsin-Madison, Madison, WI, USA
* Corresponding author. University of Utah, Department of Physical Medicine and Rehabilitation, 590 Wakara Way, Salt Lake City, UT 84108.
E-mail address: aaron.conger@hsc.utah.edu

Phys Med Rehabil Clin N Am 33 (2022) 233–249
https://doi.org/10.1016/j.pmr.2022.01.001

Anatomy

Facet joints are synovial structures that allow dynamic movement and load transmission throughout the spine. They are composed of the inferior articular process of a cephalad vertebra and a superior articular process (SAP) of the immediately caudal vertebra. Facet joints receive dual sensory innervation from the articular branches originating at the medial branch of the primary dorsal ramus of spinal nerve roots from C3/C4 to L4/L5. There are important exceptions to these patterns. The C2/C3 facet joint is innervated solely by the third occipital nerve (TON, the superficial C3 medial branch) and the L5/S1 facet joint is innervated by the L4 medial branch and L5 dorsal ramus. C1/C2 facets are innervated by the anterior rami of the first and second spinal nerves. The C0/C1 joints (craniocervical articulations) are innervated by branches of the C1 ventral ramus. Throughout the thoracic region, cadaveric studies suggest the articular branches may originate from the primary dorsal ramus itself.[9] Due to anatomic convention, at typical cervical levels the sensory innervation comes from corresponding facet levels, while in the thoracic and lumbar spine the innervation is from the same level and one level above. This is due to the presence of a C8 spinal nerve root (and medial branch nerve) in the absence of a C8 vertebra. Spinal medial branches also provide innervation to the multifidus muscles, interspinous muscles and ligament, and the periosteum of the neural arch.[10] In the lumbar spine, the medial branch traverses over the sequentially inferior vertebra at the confluence of the transverse process and SAP. The medial branch bifurcates through its course across the lamina with both ascending and descending articular projections before the medial branch's muscular innervation (**Fig. 1** and **2**)

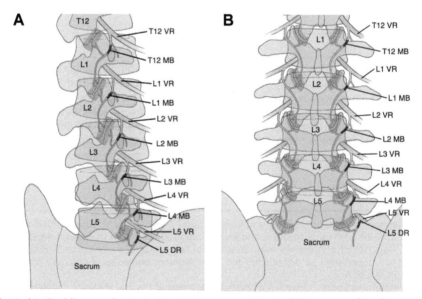

Fig. 1. (*A, B*), oblique and anterior/posterior representations of the course of lumbar medial branches (MB) and the L5 dorsal ramus (DR) after arising from their respective spinal nerve roots (VR). Red lines indicate the location used for targeting during MBBs and RFA. (*From Furman, Michael B. Atlas of Image-guided Spinal Procedures. Second ed. 2018. Chapter 15 E, 285 to 290.*)

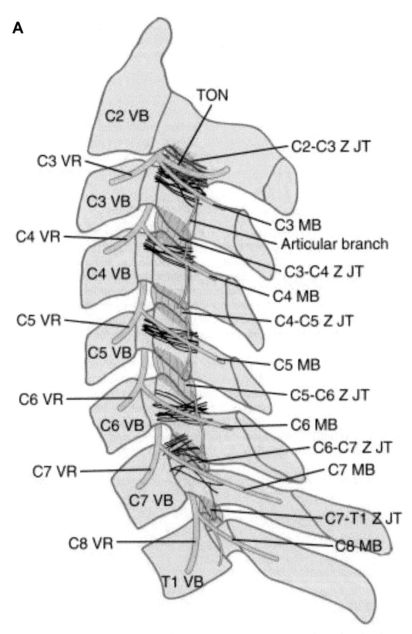

Fig. 2. A, lateral representation of the course of cervical medial branches (MB) at corresponding vertebral body (VB) levels including the third occipital nerve (TON). Black and blue lines represent the variable courses of these nerves seen in cadaveric studies.[11]. (*From* Furman, Michael B. Atlas of Image-guided Spinal Procedures. Second ed. 2018. Chapter 30H, 505-514.)

In the cervical spine, the medial branches run near the C2/C3 facet joint line (the TON), across the centroid of the articular pillars at C3–C6, and over the superior aspect of the SAP of C7.

History and Advancements

The conceptual basis for medial branch RFA to address pain originating at these joints was introduced in the 1970s. The initial technique for neurotomy involved surgically severing the lumbar medial branches.[12] Shortly thereafter, Shealy proposed a less invasive, percutaneous approach with electrode insertion to the intertransverse ligament.[13] Subsequent advancements have included variations in electrode placement, introduction of nontraditional RFA technology, enhanced safety precautions for the patient and physician, and refinement of selection paradigms. Utilization of RFA is increasing, especially in the lumbar spine. Overall, lumbar facet interventions are one of the most prevalent procedures among pain practices in the United States, second to epidural steroid injections, with some data showing a 130.6% increase in lumbar RFA claims between 2007 and 2016.[14]

Technical Considerations

Lesion size and geometry are dependent on the electrode/active tip gauge and length, ablation time and temperature, and the specific RFA technology used.[15] Conventional monopolar electrodes are known to create an ovoid lesion along the length of the active tip of the cannula, which does not substantially project beyond the distalmost aspect of the active tip.[15] As such, conventional monopolar electrodes must be placed in parallel to the targeted nerve(s) to produce an effective neurotomy (**Fig. 3**).[16] There are well-known violations of this principle that have resulted in substandard outcomes after conventional monopolar RFA performed in the lumbar spine.[17,18]

Cooled and deployable multi-tined electrodes are also commercially available. Cooled RFA involves pumping sterile saline to the lesion location thereby reducing tissue impedance and facilitating the projection of the ablation zone. Cooled lesions are spherical and project beyond the tip of the electrode, thereby allowing for alternative approaches to neural targets, such as the perpendicular approach (**Fig. 4**).[15]

Modern equipment for RFA procedures includes insulated cannulas, electrodes, and a radiofrequency generator (**Fig. 5**).

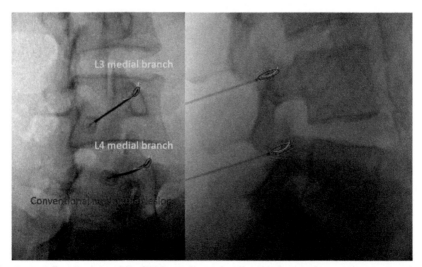

Fig. 3. A right L3 and L4 medial branch monopolar RFA procedure using conventional electrodes.

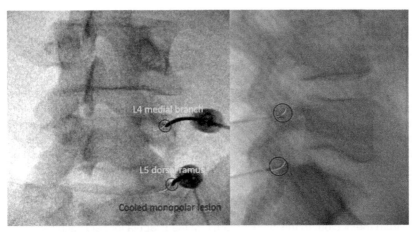

Fig. 4. A right L4 medial branch and L5 dorsal ramus monopolar RFA procedure using cooled electrodes.

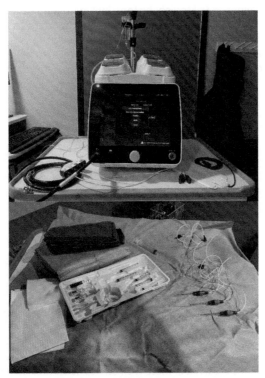

Fig. 5. Radiofrequency generator, grounding pad, and typical procedure tray with electrodes.

PATIENT SELECTION CRITERIA

Appropriate patient selection increases the probability of significant pain relief and functional improvement after RFA. Elements of history, physical examination, and imaging have demonstrated limited value for diagnosing facet-mediated pain and for predicting response to RFA.[19–21] According to the Spine Intervention Society, medial branch RFA may be considered for patients with complete pain relief on the anesthetization of the targeted nerves using a controlled diagnostic block, though in clinical practice less stringent criteria are often used.[16] However, before diagnostic blockade, an appropriate history and physical examination should be performed to appropriately evaluate the area for other mechanical and nonmechanical sources of spine pain.

History and Physical Examination

Elements of the patient history suggestive of facet joint pain include nonradicular symptoms, though not exclusive midline neck or back pain, with possible referral patterns from the occiput to the inferior margin of the scapula for cervical facet joint pain (**Fig. 6**) and gluteal to posterior thigh with infrequent radiation below the knee for lumbar facet pain (**Fig. 7**).

Symptoms typically should be present for more than 3 months, and recalcitrant to conservative management and substantially disrupt daily function and quality of life. Additional key elements of the history include a medical and surgical history with attention to anticoagulant use and previously placed implanted neuromodulation devices (eg, implantable cardioverter defibrillators, permanent pacemaker devices); although not absolute contraindications to RFA, they require special consideration to prevent complications.[22,23] Medical history, including depression, anxiety, chronic opioid utilization, and previous spine surgery are also important as they may influence outcomes of RFA.[24]

Physical examination findings suggestive of facet-mediated pain include paraspinal tenderness or tenderness to palpation along the tissue overlying the facet joints.[25,26]

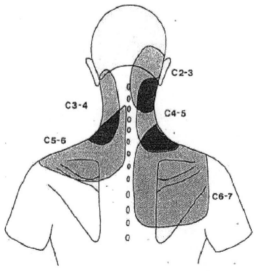

Fig. 6. Symptom patterns observed in those with cervical facet-mediated pain. (*From* Dwyer A, Aprill C, Bogduk N. Cervical zygapophyseal joint pain patterns. I: a study in normal volunteers. *Spine (Phila Pa 1976).* 1990;15(6):453-457.)

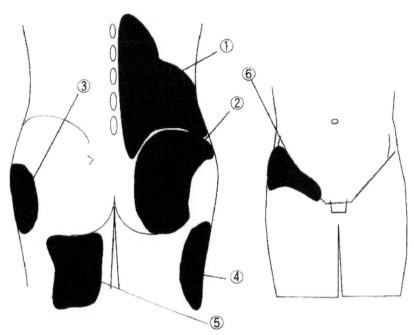

Fig. 7. Symptom patterns observed in those with lumbar facet-mediated pain. 1, lumbar spinal region; 2, gluteal region; 3, trochanter region; 4, lateral thigh region; 5, posterior thigh region; 6, groin region. (*From* Fukui S, Ohseto K, Shiotani M, Ohno K, Karasawa H, Naganuma Y. Distribution of Referred Pain from the Lumbar Zygapophyseal Joints and Dorsal Rami. The Clinical Journal of Pain. 1997;13(4).)

Facet-mediated pain is not typically reproduced with Valsalva maneuvers or spinal flexion.[27–29] Some evidence supports rotation-extension movements as predictive of RFA success,[27,30] while other studies have found negative associations with these maneuvers.[28,31] Physical examination findings associated with a negative result after MBB include evidence of adverse neural tension and increasing numbers of Waddell's signs.[32,33]

Radiographic Evaluation

Radiographs, combined with physical examination to identify points of maximal tenderness, are modestly helpful in detecting facet-mediated pain.[26] Despite their utility in visualizing posterior element structures, studies have failed to fully establish the relationship between radiographs, CT, and MRI and the confirmation of cervical or lumbar facet joint syndromes.[6,34] Some studies have used single-photon emission computed tomography (SPECT/CT) or planar bone scintigraphy to select patients for RFA;[35,36] however, a systematic review published in 2019 found only a single appropriately designed study showing poor diagnostic accuracy relative to the reference standard (medial branch blocks (MBBs)).[37] Although rarely used in clinical practice, some evidence supports the use of SPECT/CT to identify painful symptomatic cervical and facet joints.[35,36] While there is little evidence to support the use of imaging for determining the degree of facet joint pain, the importance of imaging lies in its ability to exclude other red flags, as well as to screen for sources of axial pain that may not be evidence without imaging such as the use of flexion-extension radiography to rule out significant dynamic spondylolisthesis.[34]

Medial Branch Nerve Blocks

Given that there are no pathognomonic, clinical, or radiographic findings associated with facet joint pain, MBBs remain the reference standard for establishing the diagnosis and serve to predict symptom improvement after RFA. Fluoroscopically guided MBBs have largely replaced intra-articular anesthetic injections due to their more favorable technical feasibility and diagnostic accuracy.[16] Factors that impact the predictive power of MBBs include the use of short and long-acting anesthetics, magnitude and timeframe of patient's subjective improvement following injection, and the number of blocks performed before RFA.[31]

It is generally accepted that higher thresholds of pain relief after MBBs predict greater success with RFA. This follows the reasoning that a higher level of pain relief suggests pain arising predominately from the targeted facet joint, and not other non-anesthetized structures. Patient age also impacts the likelihood of treatment success. For example, patients less than 40 years old may have a lower pretest probability of facet-mediated pain (compared with older patients) due to a lower prevalence of the condition in this age group.[38] Therefore, the posttest probability of facet-mediate pain will be lower with a higher risk of false-positive blocks in this population.[19] Confirmation of pain relief with MBB may be tested with different thresholds including a single injection or repeat injections. However, the false-positive rate of single MBB with diagnostic criteria of less than 70% pain relief may be as high as 45%.[39]

Despite the lower rate of successful outcomes after RFA when selected with single blocks, some physicians support the use of this paradigm as a compromise to increase access to patients with facet-mediated spinal pain.[31] However, guidelines from authoritative organizations often recommend dual comparative blocks with diagnostic criteria of 80% or higher pain relief before RFA to enhance diagnostic accuracy.[31,40,41]

RISKS AND CONTRAINDICATIONS

Serious adverse events associated with MBBs and RFA are rare. Procedure-related pain and dysesthesias occur with tissue disruption and subsequent release of proinflammatory cytokines, although these are often minor in severity and transient in duration.[42] Cases of injury to the spinal nerve roots have not been reported when the procedure is performed in accordance with established guidelines.[16] Interference with electrical devices (eg, pacemakers, cardioverter defibrillators, deep brain stimulators, spinal cord stimulators) has rarely been reported, manifest in only a single case report.[43]

Disruption in the electrical activity of implantable devices from magnetic fields created by RFA electrodes is another risk of this procedure, though bipolar RFA theoretically minimizes this risk as current is passed from one electrode to the second that is placed in close proximity, rather than from a single electrode to a grounding pad.[44,45] No study has compared the risk of disruption of the electrical activity of implantable devices when using monopolar versus bipolar RFA. Throughout the literature, device disruption risk has been described once, and this occurrence has not been reported in cohort studies.[43,44,46] Guidelines concerning cardiac implantable from a physician survey recommended screening all patients for cardiac devices, recent interrogation, magnet availability, active electrode to the ground be at least 15 cm away from the device, and cardiac monitoring during RFA.[47,48] Skin injury as a result of equipment misuse or defect can occur; the literature documents a second-degree skin burn from a radiofrequency adhesive electrical dispersive pad.[49] Infections are rare after MBBs and RFA but a case report of a lumbar epidural abscess in an immunosuppressed patient has been reported after MBBs.[50] Although it is not entirely clear how the abscess accumulated in the epidural space (MBBs are an extra-axial procedure), providers should be aware this hypothetical complication.

Studies that quantify adverse events have consistently demonstrated MBBs and RFA to be low-risk procedures. A large multicenter study that involved 181 MBBs and 86 RFA procedures did not document a single major adverse event, such as permanent neurologic deficit or clinically significant bleeding, and noted few minor events, including vasovagal reactions, allergic reactions, or pain aborting procedure; minor events occurred in 7% of MBBs and 3% of radiofrequency ablations (RFA).[51] Another large study found no bleeding complications in patients who continued antiplatelet and anticoagulants medications during these procedures.[52]

The American Society of Regional Anesthesia and Pain Medicine guidelines classify lumbar and thoracic RFA as "low-risk" and cervical RFA as "intermediate risk," consistent with guidelines published by the Spine Intervention Society (SIS).[16,53,54] Guidelines from these organizations allow for the continuation of platelet aggregation inhibitors. These guidelines also allow for anticoagulant use before these procedures in patients that are not at increased risk of bleeding (eg, old age, history of bleeding tendency, concurrent use of other anticoagulant or antiplatelet medications, liver cirrhosis, advanced liver disease, and advanced renal disease).[53,55] This reflects the findings of a large prospective cohort evaluating anticoagulation during interventional pain procedures that demonstrated no bleeding incidents in the cohort that continued anticoagulation and a larger number of adverse clotting events in the cohort that discontinued anticoagulation.[56] In the case of these increased bleeding risks, guidelines recommend shared patient–physician decision making on holding and restarting anticoagulation and antiplatelet medications (noting that the duration of discontinuation and medication restart varies depending on specific drug pharmacokinetics).[53]

Along with the typical considerations for percutaneous fluoroscopically guided procedures, the performance of spinal RFA may be contraindicated in the presence of the following conditions:

- Pregnancy
- Active infection
- Ongoing coagulopathies
- Acquired or congenital myopathy
- Neuromuscular disease (ALS, severe myasthenia gravis, and so forth).

OUTCOME DATA
Cervical

Outcomes from cervical medial branch RFA improve when strict patient selection with complete pain relief is reported from comparative diagnostic blocks (**Table 1**). In their 2016 systematic review with meta-analysis, Engel and colleagues reviewed 7 studies with pooled results, indicating that 63% of patients were pain free at 6-month follow-up and 38% were pain free at 1 year. It was concluded that there is moderate-quality evidence that patients selected using comparative blocks with 100% pain relief may expect a 61% chance of achieving complete pain relief.[65] However, a study by Burnham and colleagues compared patients with complete relief versus those with 80% to 99% relief and found no significant difference in response to cervical medial branch RFA.[64]

Thoracic

Systematic reviews have reported moderate-quality evidence for the use of diagnostic and therapeutic thoracic MBBs.[66,67] However, there are very limited data available in

Table 1
Summary of studies evaluating efficacy cervical medial branch RFA

Study	Design	Patients	% Relief from MBB*	Outcome (Pain Relief Threshold and Time points)	% Achieving outcome
Lord,[57] 1996	RCT	12	Placebo controlled 100%	100% at 6 mo	58%
McDonald,[58] 1999	Retrospective	Grp 1: 17 Grp 2: 11	Placebo controlled 100% Comparative 100%	100% at 6 mo	59% 55%
Sapir,[59] 2001	Prospective cohort	50	≥80%	≥50% at 12 mo	56%
Barnsley,[60] 2005	Prospective cohort	35	Placebo controlled 100%	100% for median duration 9 mo	74%
Shin,[61] 2006	Prospective cohort	28	≥50%	≥75% at ≥ 6 mo 100% at ≥ 6 mo	68% 29%
Speldewinde,[62] 2011	Prospective cohort	109	≥80%	≥50% at ≥ 6 mo 100% at ≥ 6 mo	78% 54%
MacVicar,[63] 2012	Prospective cohort	40 and 64 (2 practices)	100%	100% at median 17 and 20 mo (2 practices)	61% and 74% (2 practices)
Burnham,[64] 2020	Cross-sectional	50	≥80%	≥50% at ≥ 6 mo	54%

Abbreviations: *Medial, branch blocks were comparative if not otherwise specified; MBB, Medial branch block; RCT, randomized controlled trial.

the medical literature regarding outcomes for thoracic medial branch RFA.[68] A 2020 retrospective review of 23 patients who achieved more than 80% relief with dual diagnostic thoracic medial branch and subsequently underwent cooled RFA of the thoracic spine. Procedure was performed with targets as described per SIS guidelines with cooled ablation at 60° Celsius for 150 seconds.[16] This resulted in a 20.72% improvement in pain at 4 to 8 weeks, 53% improvement at 2 to 6 months, and 37% improvement at 6 to 12 months. Only 10% of the patients required repeat procedure within 6 to 12 months, 25% at 12 to 24 months, and 65% required repeat RFA at 24 to 36 months.[69]

Speldewinde and colleagues found that 46% of patients achieved greater than 6 months of 50% pain relief with benefits seen at all levels of the thoracic spine when treated with conventional monopolar RFA at 80° for 60 seconds.[70] In a study of 71 patients by Chen and colleagues 82% of patients reported greater than 50% pain relief at 12 months after bipolar RF neurotomy.[71] Joo and colleagues examined thermal ablation versus alcohol in a cohort of 40 patients with recurrent thoracolumbar pain after prior successful thermal RFA and found that the median effective period for alcohol ablation was significantly longer than that provided by thermal RFA.[72]

In summary, there are limited data regarding the effectiveness of thoracic RFA though small trials have demonstrated improvement in patient pain scores after treatment.

Lumbar

Many RCTs and cohort studies have demonstrated the effectiveness of lumbar RFA (**Table 2** below for notable examples). When using the preferred, parallel technique for conventional monopolar RFA, systematic reviews have demonstrated that 50% to 60% of patients achieve at least 50% relief after RFA when selected using the criterion of greater than 50% improvement with diagnostic blocks.[79] In the same analysis, 50% to 60% of patients were shown to achieve at least 50% relief when a stricter cut-off of 70% to 80% pain relief was applied. Further, patients in the more stringent groups were found to have an increased likelihood of achieving more than 80% pain relief. Alternatively, they found the use of single diagnostic blocks and the less preferred perpendicular approach resulted in lower success rates with no significant difference between sham treatment.[79]

Other systematic reviews have also noted the effectiveness of lumbar medial branch RFA. In a meta-analysis by Lee and colleagues, statistically significant improvements in the best responder (80% or greater) group when compared with controls at all time points (1–3 months, 6 months, 12 months) with reductions of 3.98, 4.55, and 5.65 in

Table 2
Summary of studies evaluating effectiveness lumbar medial branch RFA

Study	Design	Patients	Percentage of Relief from MBB*	Outcome (Pain Relief Threshold and Time points)	% Achieving outcome
Dreyfuss,[74] 2000	Prospective Cohort	15	≥80%	≥90% at 12 mo	60%
Cohen,[40] 2008	Retrospective	262	Single block Grp 1: 50%–79% Grp 2: ≥80%	≥50% at 6 mo	Grp 1: 52% Grp 2: 56%
Cohen,[24] 2007	Retrospective	92	Single block Grp 1: 50%–79% Grp 2: ≥80%	≥50% at ≥ 6 mo	Grp 1: 56% Grp 2: 58%
Stojanovic,[41] 2010	Retrospective	77	1 or 2 blocks 80%	≥50% at ≥ 3 mo	47%
Cohen,[75] 2013	Prospective Cohort	61	Single block ≥50%	≥50% at 12 mo	54%
MacVicar,[73] 2013	Prospective	106	100%	≥80% relief at 8 mo	55%
Mccormick,[76] 2015	Prospective	55	≥75%	≥50% relief at 6–12 mo	53%
Juch,[17] 2017	RCT	114	Single block ≥50%	≥ 2 point reduction in pain	57%
Conger,[77] 2020	Cross Sectional	85	≥80%	≥50% relief ≥ 6 mo	57%
McCormick,[78] 2019	RCT	43	Single block ≥75%	≥50% relief x 6 mo	49% (combined TRFA and CRFA groups)

Abbreviations: *Medial, branch blocks were comparative if not otherwise specified; CRFA, Cooled radiofrequency ablation; MBB, Medial branch blocks; RCT, randomized controlled trial; TRFA, Thermal radiofrequency ablation.

VAS pain scores at their respective time points.[80] At 12 months, 95% of patients in the RFA group exhibited improvements in back pain that exceeded the minimal clinically important difference (MCID).

DISCUSSION

Zygapophyseal joint pain is a relatively common source of spine pain encountered by musculoskeletal providers. RFA is safe and effective when performed in accordance with accepted technical standards in strictly selected patients. The published effectiveness of medial branch RFA varies widely with important differences noted in studies depending on patient selection and procedural characteristics. Benchmark studies using strict selection criteria based on response to diagnostic blocks have established the effectiveness of conventional RFA. For example, MacVicar et al. used SIS guidelines for dual comparative diagnostic MBBs with 100% relied on 2 occasions before RFA.[73] Success for RFA treatment was defined as at least 80% relief of pain for at least 6 months, restoration of all activities of daily living, require no other health care for back pain and return to work. In their study, 58% and 53% of patients (from 2 practices) met the requirements for treatment success.

Similarly, for the cervical spine, Lord and colleagues used stringent selection criteria and 3 MBBs requiring 100% relief of pain with anesthetic and no relief when saline was used and found a significant reduction in pain when cervical medial branch RFA was performed.[57,73] Alternatively, other studies using less stringent selection criteria for RFA have failed to show statistical or clinically significant differences.[17,81] Multiple studies have demonstrated that patients selected based on clinical features alone are less likely to achieve higher rates of relief from cervical medial branch RFA and that dual concordant medial branch with higher percentages of relief (80%–100%) have been shown to result in the best outcomes.[65]

SUMMARY

Zygapophyseal joints are frequently implicated in pain arising from the spine. RFA targeting the medial branch nerves (as a treatment of facet-mediated pain) was developed more than 50 years ago and continues to be an increasingly used procedure today. The sensory nerves that innervate these joints are the primary targets for treating facet-mediated spine pain using RFA. Fluoroscopically guided MBBs are necessary to diagnose facet mediated pain; dual-comparative MBBs with greater than 80% relief are more predictive of RFA success than less stringent block thresholds. RFA is both safe and effective when performed according to established technical standards in appropriately selected patients.

CLINICS CARE POINTS

- Radiofrequency ablation targeting medial branch nerves (as a treatment of facet-mediated pain) was developed more than 50 years ago and continues to be an increasingly used procedure today.
- The diagnosis of zygapophyseal pain is based on clinical evaluation and imaging and confirmed with fluoroscopically guided MBBs.
- It is generally accepted that greater magnitudes of pain relief with MBBs correlate with improved responses after RFA.
- Performance of spinal RFA in accordance with clinical practice guidelines improves the safety and effectiveness of the procedure.

DISCLOSURE

Dr Z.L. McCormick serves on the Board of Directors of the Spine Intervention Society and has received investigator-initiated research funding from Avanos Medical (paid directly to the University of Utah). None of the other authors have any financial conflicts of interest to disclose.

REFERENCES

1. Lord SM, Barmsley L, Wallis BJ, et al. Third occipital nerve headache: A prevalence study. J Neurol Neurosurg Psychiatr 1994;57:1187–90.
2. Barnsley L, Lord SM, Wallis BJ, et al. The prevalence of chronic cervical zygapophysial joint pain after whiplash. Spine (Phila Pa 1976) 1995;20(1):20–5.
3. Speldewinde GC, Bashford GM, Davidson IR. Diagnostic cervical zygapophysial joint blocks for chronic cervical pain. J Whiplash Relat Disord 2002;1:105–12.
4. Falco FJE, Manchikanti L, Datta S. An update of the systematic assessment of the diagnostic accuracy of lumbar facet joint nerve blocks. Pain Physician 2012;15: E869–907.
5. Long DM, BenDebba M, Torgerson WS. Persistent back pain and sciatica in the United States: patient characteristics. J Spinal Disord 1996;9:40–58.
6. Kalichman L, Kim DH, Li L, et al. Computed tomography-evaluated features of spinal degeneration: prevalence, intercorrelation, and association with self-reported low back pain. Spine J 2010;10(3):200–8.
7. Atluri S, Datta S, Falco FJE, et al. Systematic review of diagnostic utility and therapeutic effectiveness of thoracic facet joint interventions. Pain Physician 2008;11: 611–29.
8. Manchikanti KN, Atluri S, Singh V, et al. An update of evaluation of therapeutic thoracic facet joint interventions. Pain Physician 2012;15(4):E463–81.
9. Joshi A, Amrhein TJ, Holmes MA, et al. The Source and the Course of the Articular Branches to the T4-T8 Zygapophysial Joints. Pain Med 2019;20(12). https://doi.org/10.1093/pm/pnz116.
10. Bogduk N. The innervation of the lumbar spine. Spine (Phila Pa 1976) 1983;8(3): 286–93.
11. Lord SM, McDonald GJ, Bogduk N. Percutaneous Radiofrequency Neurotomy of the Cervical Medial Branches. Neurosurg Q 1998;8(4). https://doi.org/10.1097/00013414-199812000-00004.
12. Rees W. Multiple bilateral subcutaneous rhizolysis of segmental nerves in the treatment of the intervertebral disc syndrome. Ann Gen Prac 1971;26:126–7.
13. Shealy CN. Percutaneous radiofrequency denervation of spinal facets. treatment for chronic back pain and sciatica. J Neurosurg 1975;43:448–51.
14. Starr JB, Gold L, McCormick Z, et al. Trends in lumbar radiofrequency ablation utilization from 2007 to 2016. Spine J 2019;19(6). https://doi.org/10.1016/j.spinee.2019.01.001.
15. Cosman ER, Dolensky JR, Hoffman RA. Factors That Affect Radiofrequency Heat Lesion Size. Pain Med 2014;15:2020–36.
16. International Spine Intervention Society. Principles of Thermal Radiofrequency. In: Bogduk N, editor. Practice Guidelines for Spinal Diagnostic and Treatment Procedures. 2nd edn. San Francisco: International Spine Intervention Society; 2013. p. 15–25.
17. Juch JNS, Maas ET, Ostelo RWJG, et al. Effect of Radiofrequency Denervation on Pain Intensity Among Patients With Chronic Low Back Pain. JAMA 2017;318(1). https://doi.org/10.1001/jama.2017.7918.

18. McCormick ZL, Vorobeychik Y, Gill JS, et al. Guidelines for composing and assessing a paper on the treatment of pain: A practical application of evidence-based medicine principles to the mint randomized clinical trials. Pain Med (United States) 2018;19(11). https://doi.org/10.1093/pm/pny046.

19. Cohen SP, Raja SN. Pathogenesis, diagnosis, and treatment of lumbar Zygapophysial (facet) joint pain. Anesthesiology 2007;106(3):591–614.

20. Won HS, Yang M, Kim YD. Facet joint injections for management of low back pain: a clinically focused review. Anesth Pain Med 2020;15(1):8–18. https://doi.org/10.17085/apm.2020.15.1.8.

21. Boswell MV, Manchikanti L, Kaye AD. A best-evidence systematic appraisal of the diagnostic accuracy and utility of facet (zygapophysial) joint injections in chronic spinal pain. Pain Physician 2015;18(4):E497–533.

22. Smith C, Defrancesch F, Patel J. Spine intervention society factfinders for patient safety radiofrequency neurotomy for facet joint pain in patients with permanent pacemakers and defibrillators. Pain Med 2019;20(2):411–2.

23. Horlocker TT, Vandermeulen E, Kopp SL, et al. Regional Anesthesia in the Patient Receiving Antithrombotic or Thrombolytic Therapy: American Society of Regional Anesthesia and Pain Medicine Evidence-Based Guidelines (Fourth Edition). Reg Anesth Pain Med 2018;43(3):263–309.

24. Cohen SP, Bajwa ZH, Kraemer JJ, et al. Factors Predicting Success and Failure for Cervical Facet Radiofrequency Denervation. Reg Anesth Pain Med 2007; 32(6). https://doi.org/10.1097/00115550-200711000-00007.

25. Depalma MJ, Ketchum JM, Trussell BS, et al. Does the Location of Low Back Pain Predict Its Source? PM R 2011;3(1):33–9.

26. Lewinnek GE, Warfield CA. Facet joint degeneration as a cause of low back pain. Clin Orthop Relat Res 1986;213:216–22.

27. Laslett M, Öberg B, Aprill CN, et al. Zygapophysial joint blocks in chronic low back pain: a test of Revel's model as a screening test. BMC Musculoskelet Disord 2004;5(1). https://doi.org/10.1186/1471-2474-5-43.

28. Revel ME, Listrat VM, Chevalier XJ. Facet joint block for low back pain: identifying predictors of a good response. Arch Phys Med Rehabil 1992;73(9):824–8.

29. Jackson RP, Jacobs RR, Montesano PX. Facet joint injection in low-back pain: A prospective statistical study. Spine (Phila Pa 1976) 1988;13(9):966–71.

30. Helbig T, Lee CK. The Lumbar Facet Syndrome. Spine 1988;13(1). https://doi.org/10.1097/00007632-198801000-00015.

31. Cohen SP, Bhaskar A, Bhatia A, et al. Consensus practice guidelines on interventions for lumbar facet joint pain from a multispecialty, international working group. Reg Anesth Pain Med 2020;45(6):424–67.

32. Manchikanti L, Pampati V, Fellows B, et al. The inability of the clinical picture to characterize pain from facet joints. Pain Physician 2000;3(2):158–66.

33. Cohen SP, Doshi TL, Kurihara C, et al. Waddell (Nonorganic) Signs and Their Association with Interventional Treatment Outcomes for Low Back Pain. Anesth Analg 2021;639–51.

34. Perolat R, Kastler A, Nicot B, et al. Facet joint syndrome: from diagnosis to interventional management. Insights into Imaging 2018;9(5):773–89.

35. Dolan A, Ryan P, Arden N. The value of SPECT scans in identifying back pain likely to benefit from facet joint injection. Rheumatology 1996;35(12). https://doi.org/10.1093/rheumatology/35.12.1269.

36. Holder LE, Machin JL, Asdourian PL, et al. Planar and high-resolution SPECT bone imaging in the diagnosis of facet syndrome. J Nucl Med 1995;36(1):37–44.

37. Conger A, Burnham T, Speckman RA, et al. The Accuracy of SPECT/CT for Diagnosing Lumbar Zygapophyseal Joint Pain: a Systematic Review. Curr Phys Med Rehabil Rep 2019;7(4). https://doi.org/10.1007/s40141-019-00237-4.
38. DePalma MJ, Ketchum JM, Saullo T. What Is the Source of Chronic Low Back Pain and Does Age Play a Role? Pain Med 2011;12(2). https://doi.org/10.1111/j.1526-4637.2010.01045.x.
39. Manchukonda R, Manchikanti K, Cash K, et al. Facet joint pain in chronic spinal pain: An evaluation of prevalence and false-positive rate of diagnostic blocks. J Spinal Disord Tech 2007;20(7):539–45.
40. Cohen SP, Stojanovic MP, Crooks M, et al. Lumbar zygapophysial (facet) joint radiofrequency denervation success as a function of pain relief during diagnostic medial branch blocks: a multicenter analysis. Spine J 2008;8(3):498–504.
41. Stojanovic MP, Sethee J, Mohiuddin M, et al. MRI Analysis of the Lumbar Spine: Can It Predict Response to Diagnostic and Therapeutic Facet Procedures? Clin J Pain 2010;26(2). https://doi.org/10.1097/AJP.0b013e3181b8cd4d.
42. Kornick C, Scott Kramarich S, Lamer TJ, et al. Complications of Lumbar Facet Radiofrequency Denervation. Spine 2004;29(12). https://doi.org/10.1097/01.BRS.0000128263.67291.A0.
43. Jeon HY, Shin JW, Kim DH, et al. Spinal cord stimulator malfunction caused by radiofrequency neuroablation. Korean J Anesthesiol 2010;59:226–8.
44. Bautista A, Dadabayev A, Rosenquist E. Bipolar radiofrequency neurotomy to treat neck and back pain in patients with automatic implantable cardioverter defibrillator. Pain Physician 2016;19:E505–9.
45. American Society of Anesthesiologists. Practice Advisory for the Perioperative Management of Patients with Cardiac Implantable Electronic Devices: Pacemakers and Implantable Cardioverter-Defibrillators: An Updated Report by the American Society of Anesthesiologists Task Force on Perioperative Management of Patients with Cardiac Implantable Electronic Devices. Anesthesiology 2011;114(2):247–61.
46. Barbieri M, Bellini M. Radiofrequency neurotomy for the treatment of chronic pain: interference with implantable medical devices. Anestezjologia Intensywna Terapia 2014;46(3). https://doi.org/10.5603/AIT.2014.0029.
47. Friedrich J, Itano EM, Lynn RR. Management of Cardiac Implantable Electrical Devices in Patients Undergoing Radiofrequency Ablation for Spine Pain: Physician Survey and Review of Guidelines. Pain Physician 2020;23(4):E335–42.
48. Smith C, DeFrancesch F, Patel J. Radiofrequency Neurotomy for Facet Joint Pain in Patients with Permanent Pacemakers and Defibrillators. Pain Med 2019;20(2). https://doi.org/10.1093/pm/pny213.
49. Burnham T, Hilgenhurst G, McCormick ZL. Second-degree Skin Burn from a Radiofrequency Grounding Pad: A Case Report and Review of Risk-Mitigation Strategies. PM R 2019;11(10):1139–42.
50. Onyima C, Chinn M, Chin M. Epidural abscess after lumbar medial branch blocks in a patient on disease-modifying anti-rheumatic drug and corticosteroid. Reg Anesth Pain Med 2021;46(10). https://doi.org/10.1136/rapm-2021-102656.
51. Carr CM, Plastaras CT, Pingree MJ, et al. Immediate Adverse Events in Interventional Pain Procedures: A Multi-Institutional Study. Pain Med 2016;17(12). https://doi.org/10.1093/pm/pnw051.
52. Endres S, Hefti K, Schlimgen E, et al. Update of a Study of Not Ceasing Anticoagulants for Patients Undergoing Injection Procedures for Spinal Pain. Pain Med 2020;21(5). https://doi.org/10.1093/pm/pnz354.

53. Narouze S, Benzon HT, Provenzano D, et al. Interventional spine and pain procedures in patients on antiplatelet and anticoagulant medications (Second Edition): Guidelines from the American Society of regional Anesthesia and pain medicine, the European Society of regional Anaesthesia and pain Therapy, the American Academy of pain medicine, the International neuromodulation Society, the North American Neuromodulation Society, and the World Institute of Pain. Reg Anesth Pain Med 2018;43(3):225–62.

54. Kaye AD, Manchikanti L, Novitch MB. Responsible, safe, and effective use of antithrombotics and anticoagulants in patients undergoing interventional techniques: American Society of interventional pain physicians (ASIPP) guidelines. Pain Physician 2019;22:S75–128.

55. Smith CC, Schneider B, McCormick ZL, et al. Risks and Benefits of Ceasing or Continuing Anticoagulant Medication for Image-Guided Procedures for Spine Pain: A Systematic Review. Pain Med 2018;19(3). https://doi.org/10.1093/pm/pnx152.

56. Endres S, Shufelt A, Bogduk N. The Risks of Continuing or Discontinuing Anticoagulants for Patients Undergoing Common Interventional Pain Procedures. Pain Med 2016. https://doi.org/10.1093/pm/pnw108.

57. Lord SM, Barnsley L, Wallis BJ, et al. Percutaneous Radio-Frequency Neurotomy for Chronic Cervical Zygapophyseal-Joint Pain. N Engl J Med 1996;335(23). https://doi.org/10.1056/NEJM199612053352302.

58. McDonald GJ, Lord SM, Bogduk N. Long-term follow-up of patients treated with cervical radiofrequency neurotomy for chronic neck pain. Neurosurgery 1999;45(1):61–7.

59. Sapir DA, Gorup JM. Radiofrequency medial branch neurotomy in litigant and nonlitigant patients with cervical whiplash: A prospective study. Spine 2001;26(12):E268–73.

60. Barnsley L. Percutaneous radiofrequency neurotomy for chronic neck pain: Outcomes in a series of consecutive patients. Pain Med 2005;6(4):282–6.

61. Shin WR, Kim HI, Shin DG, et al. Radiofrequency neuro- tomy of cervical medial branches for chronic cervicobrachialgia. J Korean Med Sci 2006;21(1):119–25.

62. Speldewinde GC. Outcomes of percutaneous zygapophysial and sacroiliac joint neurotomy in a community setting. Pain Med 2011;12(2):209–18.

63. MacVicar J, Borowczyk JM, Borowczyk JM, et al. Cervical medial branch radiofrequency neurotomy in New Zealand. Pain Med 2012;13(5):647–54.

64. Burnham T, Conger A, Salazar F, et al. The Effectiveness of Cervical Medial Branch Radiofrequency Ablation for Chronic Facet Joint Syndrome in Patients Selected by a Practical Medial Branch Block Paradigm. Pain Med (United States) 2020;21(10):2071–6.

65. Engel A, King W, Schneider BJ, et al. The effectiveness of cervical medial branch thermal radiofrequency neurotomy stratified by Selection Criteria: A systematic review of the Literature. Pain Med (United States) 2020;21(11):2726–37.

66. Seghal N, Dunbar EE, Shah RV, et al. Systematic review of diagnostic utility of facet (zygapophysial) joint injections in chronic spinal pain: An update. Pain Physician 2007;10:213–28.

67. Boswell MV, Colson JD, Sehgal N, et al. A systematic review of therapeutic facet joint interventions in chronic spinal pain. Pain Physician 2007;10:229–54.

68. Lee DG, Ahn SH, Cho YW, et al. Comparison of intraarticular thoracic facet joint steroid injection and thoracic medial branch block for the management of thoracic facet joint pain. Spine 2018;43:76–80.

69. Gungor S, Candan B. The efficacy and safety of cooled-radiofrequency neurotomy in the treatment of chronic thoracic facet (zygapophyseal) joint pain: A retrospective study. Medicine (United States) 2020;99(14). https://doi.org/10.1097/MD.0000000000019711.

70. Speldewinde GC. Thoracic Zygapophysial Joint Thermal Neurotomy: A Cohort Revealing Additional Outcomes by Specific Joint Groupings. Pain Med 2021; 22(2). https://doi.org/10.1093/pm/pnaa304.

71. Rohof O, Chen CK. The response to radiofrequency neurotomy of medial branches including a bipolar system for thoracic facet joints. Scand J Pain 2018;18(4). https://doi.org/10.1515/sjpain-2018-0048.

72. Joo YC, Park JY, Kim KH. Comparison of alcohol ablation with repeated thermal radiofrequency ablation in medial branch neurotomy for the treatment of recurrent thoracolumbar facet joint pain. J Anesth 2013;27(3). https://doi.org/10.1007/s00540-012-1525-0.

73. MacVicar J, Borowczyk JM, MacVicar AM, et al. Lumbar Medial Branch Radiofrequency Neurotomy in New Zealand. Pain Med 2013;14(5). https://doi.org/10.1111/pme.12000.

74. Dreyfuss P, Halbrook B, Pauza K, et al. Efficacy and Validity of Radiofrequency Neurotomy for Chronic Lumbar Zygapophysial Joint Pain. Spine 2000;25(10). https://doi.org/10.1097/00007632-200005150-00012.

75. Cohen SP, Strassels SA, Kurihara C, et al. Establishing an Optimal "Cutoff" Threshold for Diagnostic Lumbar Facet Blocks A Prospective Correlational Study. Clin J Pain 2013;29(5):382–91.

76. McCormick ZL, Marshall B, Walker J, et al. Long-Term Function, Pain and Medication Use Outcomes of Radiofrequency Ablation for Lumbar Facet Syndrome. Int J Anesthetics Anesthesiology 2015;2(2). https://doi.org/10.23937/2377-4630/2/2/1028.

77. Conger A, Burnham T, Salazar F, et al. The effectiveness of radiofrequency ablation of medial branch nerves for chronic lumbar facet joint syndrome in patients selected by guideline-concordant dual comparative medial branch blocks. Pain Med (United States) 2020;21(5):902–9.

78. McCormick ZL, Choi H, Reddy R, et al. Randomized prospective trial of cooled versus traditional radiofrequency ablation of the medial branch nerves for the treatment of lumbar facet joint pain. Reg Anesth Pain Med 2019;44(3):389–97.

79. Schneider BJ, Doan L, Maes MK, et al. Systematic Review of the Effectiveness of Lumbar Medial Branch Thermal Radiofrequency Neurotomy, Stratified for Diagnostic Methods and Procedural Technique. Pain Med 2020;21(6). https://doi.org/10.1093/pm/pnz349.

80. Lee CH, Chung CK, Kim CH. The efficacy of conventional radiofrequency denervation in patients with chronic low back pain originating from the facet joints: a meta-analysis of randomized controlled trials. The Spine J 2017;17(11). https://doi.org/10.1016/j.spinee.2017.05.006.

81. van Eerd M, de Meij N, Kessels A, et al. Efficacy and Long-term Effect of Radiofrequency Denervation in Patients with Clinically Diagnosed Cervical Facet Joint Pain. Spine 2021;46(5). https://doi.org/10.1097/BRS.0000000000003799.

Sacroiliac Joint Interventions

Aaron J. Yang, MD[a,b], Byron J. Schneider, MD[b,c], Scott Miller, MD[a,b],*

KEYWORDS

- Sacroiliac joint • Sacroiliac joint injections • Radiofrequency ablation
- Interventional spine procedures • Spine injections • Low back pain
- Sacral lateral branches

KEY POINTS

- Clinical suspicion alone, which can include patient history and physical examination maneuvers, in conjunction with imaging, has proved ineffective in accurately diagnosing sacroiliac joint (SIJ) pain.
- Historically, focus on the SIJ region has remained on the intraarticular portion of the SIJ complex, with intraarticular SIJ injection with anesthetic ± corticosteroid as the reference standard for diagnosis and treatment.
- Ongoing investigation into the anatomy and innervation of the entire sacroiliac joint complex has uncovered a better understanding of differentiating intraarticular and extraarticular portions of the SIJ complex, leading to other potential pain generators and targets of therapeutics.
- Outcomes for targeted SIJ injections remain mixed largely due to varied patient selection criteria, including block paradigms, and ongoing anatomic and pathophysiological understanding of this region.

INTRODUCTION

The sacroiliac joint complex (SIJC) is a common cause of nonradicular low back pain, with reported prevalence rates ranging between 15% and 30%.[1–3] The complex anatomy and pathophysiology must be considered in both the diagnosis and treatment of SIJ pain. Clinical suspicion alone or a "clinical diagnosis," which can include patient history and physical examination maneuvers, in conjunction with imaging, has proved ineffective in accurately diagnosing SIJ pain.[4–6] With these difficulties in making an accurate diagnosis due to a nonspecific clinical presentation, developing successful treatment approaches and algorithms has proved difficult. Therapeutic treatments include exercise, activity modification, oral and topical pharmacologic agents,

a Physical Medicine and Rehabilitation, Vanderbilt University Medical Center, 2201 Children's Way Suite 1318, Nashville, TN 37212, USA; b Vanderbilt Stallworth Rehabilitation Hospital, 2201 Children's Way Suite 1318, Nashville, TN 37212, USA; c Vanderbilt University Medical Center, 2201 Children's Way Suite 1318, Nashville, TN 37212, USA
* Corresponding author.
E-mail address: scott.miller@vumc.org

Phys Med Rehabil Clin N Am 33 (2022) 251–265
https://doi.org/10.1016/j.pmr.2022.01.002
1047-9651/22/© 2022 Elsevier Inc. All rights reserved.

therapy, and manipulation. However, the focus of this section is limited to image-guided interventional approaches targeting the SIJC.

There has been significant utilization of SIJ intraarticular (IA) injections over the past 20 years.[7] Importantly, these utilization rates do not capture utilization of other interventions that target the SIJC such as sacral lateral branch (SLB) nerve blocks, SLB radiofrequency ablation, and percutaneous SIJ fusion. Historically, focus on the SIJ region has remained on the IA portion of the SIJC, in part due to the reliance on IA SIJ injection with anesthetic ± corticosteroid as the reference standard for diagnosis and treatment. In expanding this focus, there has been continued investigation with regard to novel therapeutic injectate options, imaging guidance, as well as patient selection criteria for IA injections. However, there is also ongoing investigation into the anatomy and innervation of the entire SIJC. Stemming from this is a better understanding of differentiating IA and extraarticular portions of the sacroiliac joint complex, and this will guide diagnostic and therapeutic options in the future, with a possible shift in variety and utilization of procedures targeting both aspects of the SIJC. Expanding the approach to SIJC pain will hopefully result in improved outcomes and patient satisfaction. Thus, as we move toward precision medicine in interventional spine care, it is imperative to investigate more targeted diagnostic and therapeutic approaches for all interventional approaches, including the SIJC.

PATIENT SELECTION CRITERIA

In order to appropriately select patients for SIJ interventions, an understanding of relevant anatomy is imperative. A true diarthrodial joint, the SIJ is a weight-bearing structure that transmits forces between the upper and lower body. It has a fibrous capsule and synovial fluid. The articular portion of the joint consists of bone, articular cartilage, and joint capsule. The superior portion of the joint is mainly ligamentous, whereas the inferior portion of this joint contains articular cartilage. The posterior extraarticular structures include the overlying dorsal ligaments, regional muscles, and tendons. The entire SIJC is likely innervated both anteriorly and posteriorly. The SIJ itself receives anterior via the lumbosacral trunks, obturator nerve, and gluteal nerves. Posteriorly, the posterior joint capsule and other extraarticular structures are primarily innervated by the posterior sacral network, made up of the S1-S3 dorsal rami and fibers of the L5 dorsal ramus.[8–10] Importantly, anatomic studies performed in both cadavers and healthy individuals, as can be highlighted in **Fig. 1**, have shown variability in the innervation patterns of the SIJC.[11,12]

This research suggests an important distinction between the IA portion of the joint, which is primarily innervated anteriorly with some posterior contribution, and the posterior ligamentous component of the SIJC, which is exclusively innervated posteriorly.

Accordingly, patient selection and subsequent interventional diagnostic and treatment options for suspected SIJ pain can be conceptualized in **Table 1**.

Not only does the SIJC anatomy guide our interventional approach, but considerations of the pathophysiologic mechanisms of SIJC pain also allow us to form concept validity and determine injectate utility for targeted structures and mechanisms. The most common pathophysiologic mechanism responsible for SIJ pain remains degenerative osteoarthritis, leading to hypomobility from IA joint calcifications.[13,14] With mechanistic inhibition of the inflammatory cascade suspected in the IA space, glucocorticoid injections have remained the cornerstone of SIJ injections. However, other pain generators include a hypermobile joint resulting from pregnancy or childbirth, extraarticular ligamentous structures, apparent leg length discrepancy, and inflammatory arthritis.[3] Given the difference in these underlying processes, different injectates,

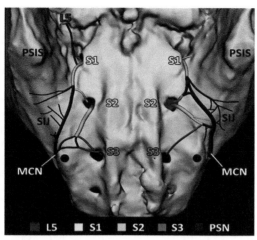

Fig. 1. Three-dimensional view of SIJ innervation from a digitized cadaveric specimen. *(Adapted from* Loh and colleagues "sacroiliac Joint Diagnostic Block and Radiofrequency Ablation Techniques", with permission. Originally from BMJ Publishing Group Limited, Regional Anesthesia & Pain Medicine, Roberts SL et al.,[11,75] with permission.)

treatment considerations, or interventional approaches may be warranted once patient selection has occurred.

Diagnosis

In 1994, the International Association for the Study of Pain (IASP) defined 3 criteria for diagnosing SIJ pain: localized pain in the sacroiliac region, pain that is produced by tension with several maneuvers, and pain that decreases with local infiltration of anesthetics to the articulation.[15] Unsurprisingly, the utility in each of these in identifying SIJ pain and appropriately selecting patients for intervention has been the focus of multiple research efforts.

History and physical examination

Pain referral patterns have shown limited utility in the diagnosis of SIJ pathology. Multiple studies have shown limited evidence of any specific pain referral pattern isolated to a certain region that responds to a diagnostic IA injection, as can be seen in **Fig. 2**.[16] These studies vary in pain referral patterns with suspected SIJ pathology, between responders and nonresponders, as well as significant overlap with pain referral patterns of other lumbosacral and IA pain, limiting its sensitivity and specificity.[2,16–18] Beyond pain referral patterns, other patient history details are similarly not accurate or reliable in

Table 1
Sacroiliac Joint Interventional Procedures

Anatomic Target	Diagnostic Injection	Therapeutic Injectate
Intraarticular SIJ	*Image-guided anesthetic injection*	*Corticosteroid prolotherapy (with hypertonic saline and dextrose) platelet-rich plasma*
Posterior SIJ complex	*Sacral lateral branch block*	*Corticosteroid prolotherapy (with hypertonic saline and dextrose) platelet-rich plasma*

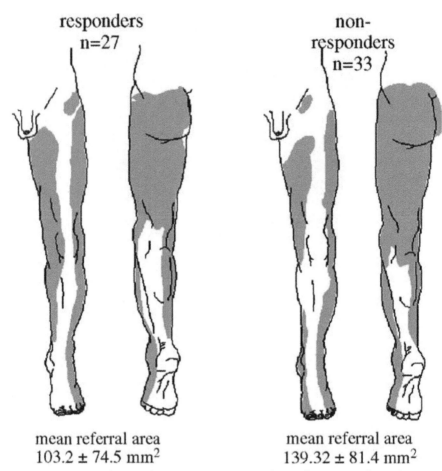

Fig. 2. Distribution of pain referral patterns to responders and nonresponders to intraarticular SIJ injections. (*Adapted from* van der Wurff and colleagues "Intensity mapping of pain referral areas in sacroiliac joint pain patients", with permission.)

diagnosing SIJC pain as detailed in a recent systematic review.[19] Physical examination findings have not been consistently shown to be reliable in the diagnosis of SIJC pain. Early studies looking at the predictive value of a single or combination of physical examination maneuvers compared with both single or dual SIJ blocks did not show evidence of any diagnostic utility.[4,20] More recent studies suggested that with increasing numbers of positive provocative maneuvers, the diagnosis of SIJ pathology is more likely and absence of any maneuvers, more unlikely.[20] However, these findings were refuted in the most recent research by Schneider and colleagues,[6] which was more consistent with early research failing to find an association between single or multiple positive physical examination maneuvers and a positive diagnostic response to an IA injection. With these studies using an IA SIJ as the diagnostic reference standard, this carries the assumption that SIJ pain sources are limited only to being IA in origin.

Imaging

Correlations between SIJC pain and imaging findings remains poor except for certain isolated circumstances such as rheumatologic disease and trauma. In cases of sacroiliitis, common to spondyloarthropathies, plain radiographs and MRI findings will show sclerosis, erosions, and ankylosis. In cases of trauma, fractures or joint disruption may be visible.[21,22] In the absence of these conditions, radiographic modalities have poor sensitivity, specificity, and diagnostic utility; up to 40% of asymptomatic patients may demonstrate positive imaging findings and more often many patients with SIJC pain will have normal imaging.[21,23,24] However, it is worth noting that SIJ abnormalities on MRI and a possible association with SIJ pain as referenced against a diagnostic injection has not been studied to date.[24] The diagnostic utility of radionucleotide bone scintigraphy in SIJ pathology referenced against a diagnostic block has been shown to have 100% specificity but 12.9% sensitivity.[25,26] However, radionucleotide bone scintigraphy exposes a patient to significant radiation, so in the context of such low-sensitivity routine clinical use is likely not warranted.[25,26] In essence, there are no imaging modalities that meaningfully aide in the diagnosis of SIJC pain in the absence of inflammatory disease or trauma.

Diagnostic block

The third criterion of the IASP diagnosis of SIJ pain, image-guided IA injection of anesthetic, has been adopted as the reference standard for the past 30+ years. There is good concept and construct validity to this, as it has been proved that in asymptomatic volunteers the injection of contrast medium leading to capsular distension results in pain and that in symptomatic patients IA SIJ anesthetic injections result in analgesia.[27–30] Multiple studies have attempted to quantify the diagnostic utility of an anesthetic IA injection. Firstly, technical factors may affect the validity of a fluoroscopic guided IA SIJ injection. As detailed by Kennedy and colleagues, an IA injection can only be confirmed on fluoroscopy if an arthrogram is achieved as evidenced by linear streaks of contrast medium between joint margins, absence of escape contrast medium into or onto structures surrounding the joint including ventral capsule tears, and confirmation of intravascular injection not having occurred. Quantitatively, Maigne and colleagues[19] reported a false-positive rate of 47% for a single IA anesthetic injection using the most rigorous of standards via dual blocks and a 75% pain relief as the positive threshold.[31] The false-negative rate of an IA anesthetic injection has not reliably been reported. Presumably, less rigorous criteria for diagnosis such as a single-block paradigm or thresholds of a positive block being lessened to 50% relief will inherently diminish the specificity of this diagnostic modality.

Using an IA injection as the reference standard carries with it some inherent limitation, most notably as this is based on the assumption that all SIJC pain is IA in origin. Research now demonstrates this assumption may be incorrect, as there may be extra-articular sources of potential pain. Specifically, Dreyfuss and colleagues[27,28] experimentally demonstrated that probing of the posterior sacral ligaments and posterior joint capsule can induce pain in asymptomatic volunteers and that injection of local anesthetic on the SLBs reliably anesthetizes these same structures. This same study found that the IA portion of the joint remained sensate even when the posterior SLBs were anesthetized. This research introduced the idea of SLB blocks (SLBBs) as a means to diagnose posterior SIJC complex pain. Just as importantly, this study found the SLBB will not be diagnostic for IA SIJC pain. Further research on SLBBs in symptomatic patients and in describing the population prevalence of posterior SIJC pain is still needed. Nonetheless, it is apparent that limiting our scope of the SIJC to only the IA joint has potentially excluded various pathologies and targets for treatment. Even more, this may have, although not necessarily, clouded prior research on prevalence, history, and physical examination findings.

Ultimately, appropriate patient selection for SIJ procedures is multifaceted. One study suggested the importance of using multiple components when selecting patients. This study showed that by using a positive approach to diagnostic block with the addition of 3 positive physical examination maneuvers, therapeutic relief of greater than 50% from IA injection improved to 50% at months versus only 29% using positive diagnostic response alone.[32] Each aspect of this approach in isolation, as discussed earlier, may have limited utility; however, when used in combination, this may provide more accurate and appropriate selection of patients for appropriate procedures.

Risks and Contraindications

Any interventional procedure bears inherent risk. To that point, care must be taken in properly selecting patients for a diagnostic or therapeutic SIJC injection.

There are 2 absolute contraindications to any fluoroscopic guided procedure, including those targeting the SIJ:[33]

- Pregnancy
- Systemic or localized infection near or at the procedural location.

Understanding that certain risks that are inherent to fluoroscopically all guided interventional procedures, SIJ procedures are otherwise historically very safe. Certain components to the procedure itself will bear inherent risks, whereas others exist secondary to the type of injectate used and regional anatomy. The following risks are not specifically isolated to SIJ procedures alone but remain consistent with other fluoroscopically guided interventional procedures:

- Radiation exposure: studies have shown limited radiation exposure with single diagnostic or therapeutic SIJ injections.[34] The cumulative radiation exposure has not been validated for repeat procedures in the SIJ region.
- Needle-based technique:
  o Soreness/worsening pain at the injection site[35]
  o Vasovagal reaction[36]
  o Bleeding: per Spine Intervention Society and American Society of Regional Anesthesia and Pain Medicine consensus guidelines, if patient stratification occurs appropriately and benefits of the procedure is expected, the seriousness of the risks of stopping anticoagulation for this extraspinal procedure greatly outweigh the increased risk of bleeding if anticoagulation/antiplatelet medication is continued.[33,37]
- Injectate
  o Contrast: allergy to contrast media may warrant special consideration by the provider regarding additional steps and precautions to ensure safety.
  o Anesthetic: the main risk regarding local anesthetic involves temporary sciatic nerve block, as will be discussed later.[31,38]
  o Corticosteroid:
    ▪ Facial flushing/sweating
    ▪ With IA corticosteroid use, there remains the unlikely but possible systemic absorption and the following side effects, not at all specific to SIJ injection: hyperglycemia, decreased bone mineral density and increased fracture risk, temporary hypothalamic-pituitary-adrenal suppression, Cushing syndrome, and immunosuppression with increased risk of infection.[39,40]

Anatomically, the lumbosacral plexus passes ventrally to the SIJ capsule. There is a known ventral capsular defect, reported in up to 61% of patients in a single study.[41] Accordingly, there are rare reports of temporary sciatic nerve block following an IA

SIJ injection with anesthetic. This uncommon complication can occur with low anesthetic volumes; however, it is usually precipitated by too anterior placement of the needle in the joint and a corresponding ventral capsular defect.[31,38] Of note, such a complication should be visible on fluoroscopy and thus the risk of such can be mitigated.

Lastly, there are 2 case reports of pyogenic sacroiliitis[42] and spinal epidural abscess with resulting endocarditis and meningitis[43] following SIJ injection. Notably, the latter occurred in an immunocompromised patient.

Outcome Data

As discussed, variability in multiple aspects of SIJC-targeted interventional approaches exists. These differences include imaging used, injectate, criteria of block, and targets of procedure. This variability and subsequent outcome studies are further discussed later and summarized in **Table 2**.

Image guidance for sacroiliac joint complex procedures

There are numerous imaging options for the performance of SIJ procedures including fluoroscopy, ultrasound (US), and computed tomography. Each option carries unique considerations, although fluoroscopy is the most common imaging technique. Regardless, image guidance is necessary, as studies have shown that without any image guidance, IA needle placement successfully occurs in only 8% to 22% of cases.[44,45] There has been recent increased usage of US for SIJ IA injections due to reported benefits including ease of use, clinical availability, ability to visual soft tissue structures, and lack of ionizing radiation. However, US image guidance also has certain limitations that may affect its usage. Ultrasound is unable to visualize vascular flow within the joint as compared with fluoroscopy, which can detect vascular uptake in the SIJ region between 5% and 62%.[46,47] If vascular uptake is significant and

Table 2
Sacroiliac joint interventional outcome data

Anatomic Target	Injectate	Study	Level of Evidence	"Relief" Criteria	% Patients w/ "Relief"	Follow-up Duration
Intraarticular SIJ	Corticosteroid	Kennedy et al Systematic review	Moderate	—	—	—
	Corticosteroid	Maugars et al	—	>70%	80%	1 mo
	Corticosteroid	Lilianh et al	—	>50%	67%	6 wk
	PRP	Burnham et al Systematic review	Very low	—	—	—
	PRP	Singla et al	—	>50%	90%	3 mo
	Prolotherapy	Kim et al	—	>50%	63%	6 mo
Posterior SIJ complex	Sacral lateral branch RFA	Yang et al Comprehensive review	Limited by variability in patient selection technique and technology use	—	—	—
	Sacral lateral branch RFA	Cohen et al	—	>50%	47%	33 mo
	Sacral lateral branch RFA	Patel et al	—	>50%	79	1 mo

undetected, there is potential failure of the injectate to reach target structures. In the case of a diagnostic injection, this can potentially lead to a false-negative test result.[47] Research has also shown significant variability in the ability of US to successfully achieve IA access, ranging from 5% to 96%.[48,49] Given this broad range, there are clearly numerous variables to consider, including the operator-dependent nature of US and how IA position is assessed in these studies.[48–51] It is important to note, however, that successful deposition of injectate exclusively into the IA space does not occur 100% of the time with US or fluoroscopy and that this miss rate is likely somewhat higher with US.[47,51]

Sacroiliac intraarticular joint injection

The effectiveness of therapeutic IA SIJ injections is best categorized by the type of injectate used. There are certain variables, however, that uniformly affect the outcomes literature. As detailed earlier, there are inherent challenges in accurately selecting patients with true and known SIJ pain for clinical trials, limiting our ability to determine true effectiveness of SIJ IA injections for this specific diagnosis. Even more specifically, each injectate may theoretically treat a different subtype of SIJ pathology, which may also need to be considered. For example, there is strong concept validity for why corticosteroid would be an ideal injectate for an underlying inflammatory sacroiliitis and perhaps less so for an SIJ thought be osteoarthritic. As detailed earlier, the imaging modality used may affect how often the treatment medication is successfully deposited at the target. And lastly, the volume of injectate used in a study must be considered, as the joint itself has a maximum capacity of approximately 2.5 mL.[52] Exceeding this volume of injectate results in losing target specificity, given likely extraarticular overflow of the injectate to adjacent.[29,30]

- Injectate:
  o Corticosteroid
    - A 2015 systematic review concluded that evidence for therapeutic SIJ corticosteroid joint injections was moderate.[19] Effectiveness is notably varied based on differences in patient selection patterns and "pain relief" cutoffs. Of the highest reported "pain improvement," Maugars and colleagues,[53,54] reported, in 2 separate studies, relief in approximately 80% of patients. However, for one study using a double-block paradigm, meaning only patients who achieved greater than 75% relief from both diagnostic blocks ultimately received the therapeutic injection, and 67% of patients experienced greater than 50% pain relief from baseline at 6-week follow-up.[55] As a whole, these results seem both variable and marginal. This likely is reflective, at least in part, of most studies including a very heterogenous patient population. This is highlighted in one recent study, which overall found the success rates of IA SIJ corticosteroid injection to be that 29% of patients achieve at least 50% pain relief at 6 months. As previously mentioned in discussing patient selection criteria, when patients were retrospectively analyzed and only those who had both a positive anesthetic response and at least 3 positive examination maneuvers preinjection that also normalized postinjection, success rates were much higher with 50% achieving 50% relief at 6 months. This study suggests that ultimately improving patient selection for IA SIJ steroid injections beyond clinical diagnosis would likely greatly improve outcomes seen with this procedure.[32]
  o Platelet-rich plasma (PRP)
    - A 2020 systematic review concluded that the evidence for PRP injection for suspected SIJ complex pain was very low.[56] Early preliminary studies have

suggested positive results; however, there is such limited research as a whole, making it difficult to draw conclusions and larger cohort and randomized controlled trials (RCTs) need to be performed. Only 1 RCT and 2 case series were identified that met criteria, all for which SIJ IA injections were performed in these studies.[57–59] In the included RCT, US-guided PRP versus corticosteroid injection were compared. Of note, this study used US guidance and only enrolled patients with 3 or more positive examination maneuvers and imaging findings that suggest sacroiliitis. This study found higher percentage of patients getting greater than 50% pain relief at 3 months in the PRP group at 90% versus 25% in the steroid group.[59] Very low-quality evidence does not mean that intervention with this injectate is ineffective but simply that it is impossible to draw conclusion on the efficacy on this injectate without more research to further this investigation.

o Prolotherapy w/o hypertonic saline/dextrose

■ The understood pathophysiologic mechanism of prolotherapy via high-concentrate dextrose is via acting as an irritant to the painful and degenerative tissue that promotes normal cell/tissue growth and healing ensues.[60,61] Ligamentous laxity is a potential subcategory of SIJC pain, which in theory may benefit from prolotherapy. Kim and colleagues[62] suggested improved effectiveness of prolotherapy with greater than 50% pain reduction at 6 months with prolotherapy in 63% of patients versus 27% in the steroid group. There is minimal outcomes research on this otherwise, and significantly more research is needed to further investigate this potential injectate.

Sacral lateral branch radiofrequency ablation

Once the posterior innervation of the SIJC was described, the SLBs garnered increased attention as a potentially new target to therapeutically target. This new target was seen as a potential means to close the gap on why only 10% to 30% of the patients suspected to have SIJC pain respond to IA-targeted procedures.[20,31,63,64] However, SLB radiofrequency ablation (RFA) is challenging due to the anatomic variability of the SLBs. In order to successfully capture all potential locations of the nerves, the nerves must be targeted at multiple sites and at multiple depths.[27,28] Initial studies for SLB RFA procedures noted a responder rate of approximately 50% for greater than 50% pain reduction at 3 months, which is lower than cervical and lumbar RFA outcomes.[65,66] The most common theme across all these studies were that most of the patients were selected based on a single IA joint injection, whereas no studies to date have used dual controlled multisite multidepth blocks[67]; this is problematic in that diagnostic IA SIJ injections do not target the posterior SIJC.

A 2021 comprehensive review concluded that current evidence for therapeutic SLB RFN is limited by wide variability in patient selection criteria, nerve branches targeted, procedural approach, and technology used.[68] Although some of these early studies have shown favorable results with positive response to SLB RFA of 32% to 89%, there has been wide variability in outcomes, and it is difficult to draw conclusions based on this varied research to date.[67] Two separate sham controlled trials to date, both using cooled RFA technology, have shown promising results, albeit with different block criteria but expressing greater than 50% relief in pain compared with sham at 3 months in 47% versus 12% in one study and 79% versus 14% in another study at 1 month.[69,70] With these positive results, there is hope that additional research can reproduce these findings and improve our ability to effectively target posterior, extraarticular sources of SIJC complex pain. First, well-done studies using multisite, multidepth SLB blocks as a means of rigorous patient selection are needed. It is also important to further investigate variable techniques and technology in addition to conventional multielec-trode RFA probes such as palisade bipolar techniques and cooled RF, all designed to account for the variable anatomy of the posterior SLBs.[71–74]

DISCUSSION

Ultimately, the SIJC is a commonly investigated and diagnosed cause of nonradicular low back and buttock pain. From an interventional perspective, there is only a small portion of patients in whom there is a clinical diagnosis of such who actually have SIJ or SIJC complex pain as diagnosed by either IA or lateral branch anesthetic injec-tion. This challenge in diagnosis is at least in part the reason that there are highly var-iable outcomes reported when investigating therapeutic SIJC injections. As detailed earlier, there is limited utility of history, physical examination, and imaging in diag-nosing SIJC pain when referenced against diagnostic injection. This is further compli-cated by evidence that the SIJC is in fact composed of an IA capsular joint with predominantly anterior innervation and the posterior capsule and ligamentous struc-tures that are exclusively posteriorly innervated. Diagnostic research that focused on IA pain as a reference may not necessarily be applicable to SIJC pain as a whole. IA-based treatments that were evaluated on clinical diagnosis alone assuredly included patients who did not have true IA SIJ pain; however, some of those without IA pain who were destined to fail an IA treatment may in fact still respond to a treat-ment targeting the posterior structures. Lastly, early research focused on SLB RFN likely had suboptimal inclusion criteria by using an IA block, and future research should aim to use the diagnosis of posterior SIJC pain via SLBB to select patients for this procedure. In addition to SLBRFN, advancements in other types of injectates such as PRP, which in theory could be applied to either the IA joint or to the posterior SIJC elements, may lead to additional interventional treatments.

Understanding these nuisances, our ability to accurately identify, diagnose, and therapeutically target these pain generators will allow for not only improved knowledge of this region but subsequently and more importantly, improved ability of interventional physicians to provide patients with relief. Rigorous and accurate patient selection criteria, as for any interventional procedure, is paramount to future research. As new technologies and techniques are unveiled and investigated, it is also important to understand the face and construct validity of these new interventions. Finally, hav-ing a strong understanding of the current available and growing body of research is necessary for the appropriate utilization of these procedures moving forward.

SUMMARY

In summary, the SIJC is composed of complex anatomy of numerous potential pain generators that demonstrate varying pathophysiology and differing innervations. This heterogeneity has been a challenge to advancing research and clinical care. Mov-ing forward, individualized approaches taking these factors into account may be a path forward to improved outcomes. Thus, as we move toward precision medicine in interventional spine care, it is imperative to investigate more targeted diagnostic and therapeutic approaches for SIJC.

CLINICS CARE POINTS

- Clinical suspicion alone, which can include patient history and physical examination maneuvers, in conjunction with imaging, has proved ineffective in accurately diagnosing SIJ pain.

- Historically, focus on the SIJ region has remained on the IA portion of the SIJC, with IA SIJ injection with anesthetic ± corticosteroid as the reference standard for diagnosis and treatment.
- Ongoing investigation into the anatomy and innervation of the entire sacroiliac joint complex has uncovered a better understanding of differentiating IA and extraarticular portions of the SIJC, leading to other potential pain generators and targets of therapeutics.
- Outcomes for targeted SIJ injections remain mixed largely due to varied patient selection criteria, including block paradigms and ongoing anatomic and pathophysiological understanding of this region.

DISCLOSURE

The authors have nothing to disclose.

REFERENCES

1. DePalma MJ, Ketchum JM, Saullo T. What is the source of chronic low back pain and does age play a role? Pain Med 2011;12(2):224–33.
2. Schwarzer AC, Aprill CN, Bogduk N. The sacroiliac joint in chronic low back pain. Spine (Phila Pa 1976 1995;20(1):31–7.
3. Cohen SP, Chen Y, Neufeld NJ. Sacroiliac joint pain: a comprehensive review of epidemiology, diagnosis and treatment. Expert Rev Neurother 2013;13(1):99–116.
4. Dreyfuss P, Michaelsen M, Pauza K, et al. The value of medical history and physical examination in diagnosing sacroiliac joint pain. Spine (Phila Pa 1976 1996;21(22):2594–602.
5. Dreyfuss P, Dryer S, Griffin J, et al. Positive sacroiliac screening tests in asymptomatic adults. Spine (Phila Pa 1976) 1994;19(10):1138–43.
6. Schneider BJ, Ehsanian R, Rosati R, et al. Validity of physical exam maneuvers in the diagnosis of sacroiliac joint pathology. Pain Med 2020;21(2):255–60.
7. Manchikanti L, Manchikanti MV, Vanaparthy R, et al. Utilization patterns of sacroiliac joint injections from 2000 to 2018 in fee-for-service medicare population. Pain Physician 2020;23(5):439–50.
8. Solonen KA. The sacroiliac joint in the light of anatomical, roentgenological and clinical studies. Acta Orthop Scand Suppl 1957;27:1–127.
9. Ikeda R. [Innervation of the sacroiliac joint. Macroscopical and histological studies]. Nihon Ika Daigaku Zasshi 1991;58(5):587–96.
10. Grob KR, Neuhuber WL, Kissling RO. [Innervation of the sacroiliac joint of the human]. Z Rheumatol 1995;54(2):117–22.
11. Roberts SL, Burnham RS, Ravichandiran K, et al. Cadaveric study of sacroiliac joint innervation: implications for diagnostic blocks and radiofrequency ablation. Reg Anesth Pain Med 2014;39(6):456–64.
12. Cox RC, Fortin JD. The anatomy of the lateral branches of the sacral dorsal rami: implications for radiofrequency ablation. Pain Physician 2014;17(5):459–64.
13. Eno JJT, Boone CR, Bellino MJ, et al. The prevalence of sacroiliac joint degeneration in asymptomatic adults. J Bone Joint Surg Am 2015;97(11):932–6.
14. Buchanan BK, Varacallo M. Sacroiliitis. In: StatPearls. StatPearls publishing; 2021. Available at: http://www.ncbi.nlm.nih.gov/books/NBK448141/. Accessed November 14, 2021.

15. Merskey H, Bogduk N. International association for the study of pain. In: Classification of chronic pain: Descriptions of chronic pain Syndromes and Definitions of pain terms. End. IASP Press; 1994.

16. van der Wurff P, Buijs EJ, Groen GJ. Intensity mapping of pain referral areas in sacroiliac joint pain patients. J Manipulative Physiol Ther 2006;29(3):190–5.

17. Slipman CW, Jackson HB, Lipetz JS, et al. Sacroiliac joint pain referral zones. Arch Phys Med Rehabil 2000;81(3):334–8.

18. Lesher JM, Dreyfuss P, Hager N, et al. Hip joint pain referral patterns: a descriptive study. Pain Med 2008;9(1):22–5.

19. Kennedy DJ, Engel A, Kreiner DS, et al. Fluoroscopically guided diagnostic and therapeutic intra-articular sacroiliac joint injections: a systematic review. Pain Med 2015;16(8):1500–18.

20. Laslett M, Aprill CN, McDonald B, et al. Diagnosis of sacroiliac joint pain: Validity of individual provocation tests and composites of tests. Man Ther 2005;10(3):207–18.

21. Montandon C, Costa MAB, Carvalho TN, Júnior MEM, Teixeira KISS. SACROILIITIS: IMAGING EVALUATION. :8.

22. Puhakka KB, Jurik AG, Schiottz-Christensen B, et al. Magnetic resonance imaging of sacroiliitis in early seronegative spondylarthropathy. Abnormalities correlated to clinical and laboratory findings. Rheumatology (Oxford) 2004;43(2):234–7.

23. Elgafy H, Semaan HB, Ebraheim NA, et al. Computed tomography findings in patients with sacroiliac pain. Clin Orthop Relat Res 2001;382:112–8.

24. Varkas G, de Hooge M, Renson T, et al. Effect of mechanical stress on magnetic resonance imaging of the sacroiliac joints: assessment of military recruits by magnetic resonance imaging study. Rheumatology (Oxford) 2018;57(3):508–13.

25. Slipman CW, Sterenfeld EB, Chou LH, et al. The value of radionuclide imaging in the diagnosis of sacroiliac joint syndrome. Spine (Phila Pa 1976 1996;21(19):2251–4.

26. Maigne JY, Boulahdour H, Chatellier G. Value of quantitative radionuclide bone scanning in the diagnosis of sacroiliac joint syndrome in 32 patients with low back pain. Eur Spine J 1998;7(4):328–31.

27. Dreyfuss P, Henning T, Malladi N, et al. The ability of multi-site, multi-depth sacral lateral branch blocks to anesthetize the sacroiliac joint complex. Pain Med 2009;10(4):679–88.

28. Dreyfuss P, Snyder BD, Park K, et al. The ability of single site, single depth sacral lateral branch blocks to anesthetize the sacroiliac joint complex. Pain Med 2008;9(7):844–50.

29. Fortin JD, Dwyer AP, West S, et al. Sacroiliac joint: pain referral maps upon applying a new injection/arthrography technique. Part I: Asymptomatic volunteers. Spine (Phila Pa 1976) 1994;19(13):1475–82.

30. Fortin JD, Aprill CN, Ponthieux B, et al. Sacroiliac joint: pain referral maps upon applying a new injection/arthrography technique. Part II: Clinical evaluation. Spine (Phila Pa 1976) 1994;19(13):1483–9.

31. Maigne JY, Aivaliklis A, Pfefer F. Results of sacroiliac joint double block and value of sacroiliac pain provocation tests in 54 patients with low back pain. Spine (Phila Pa 1976 1996;21(16):1889–92.

32. Schneider BJ, Ehsanian R, Huynh L, et al. Pain and functional outcomes after sacroiliac joint injection with anesthetic and corticosteroid at six months, stratified by anesthetic response and physical exam maneuvers. Pain Med 2020;21(1):32–40.

33. Bogduk N. Practice Guidelines for Spinal Diagnostic & Treatment Procedures - 2nd Edition. 2nd ed.

34. Cushman D, Flis A, Jensen B, et al. The effect of body mass index on fluoroscopic time and radiation dose during sacroiliac joint injections. PM R. 2016;8(8):767–72.

35. Plastaras CT, Joshi AB, Garvan C, et al. Adverse events associated with fluoroscopically guided sacroiliac joint injections. PM R 2012;4(7):473–8.

36. Kennedy DJ, Schneider B, Casey E, et al. Vasovagal rates in flouroscopically guided interventional procedures: a study of over 8,000 injections. Pain Med 2013;14(12):1854–9.

37. Narouze S, Benzon HT, Provenzano D, et al. Interventional Spine and Pain Procedures in Patients on Antiplatelet and Anticoagulant Medications (Second Edition): Guidelines From the American Society of Regional Anesthesia and Pain Medicine, the European Society of Regional Anaesthesia and Pain Therapy, the American Academy of Pain Medicine, the International Neuromodulation Society, the North American Neuromodulation Society, and the World Institute of Pain. Reg Anesth Pain Med 2018;43(3):225–62.

38. van der Wurff P, Buijs EJ, Groen GJ. A multitest regimen of pain provocation tests as an aid to reduce unnecessary minimally invasive sacroiliac joint procedures. Arch Phys Med Rehabil 2006;87(1):10–4.

39. Friedly JL, Comstock BA, Heagerty PJ, et al. Systemic effects of epidural steroid injections for spinal stenosis. Pain 2018;159(5):876–83.

40. Younes M, Neffati F, Touzi M, et al. Systemic effects of epidural and intra-articular glucocorticoid injections in diabetic and non-diabetic patients. Joint Bone Spine 2007;74(5):472–6.

41. Fortin JD, Kissling RO, O'Connor BL, et al. Sacroiliac joint innervation and pain. Am J Orthop (Belle Mead NJ) 1999;28(12):687–90.

42. Lee MH, Byon HJ, Jung HJ, et al. Pyomyositis of the iliacus muscle and pyogenic sacroiliitis after sacroiliac joint block -A case report-. Korean J Anesthesiol 2013;64(5):464–8.

43. Nagpal G, Flaherty JP, Benzon HT. Diskitis, osteomyelitis, spinal epidural abscess, meningitis, and endocarditis following sacroiliac joint injection for the treatment of low-back pain in a patient on therapy for hepatitis C Virus. Reg Anesth Pain Med 2017;42(4):517–20.

44. Rosenberg JM, Quint TJ, de Rosayro AM. Computerized tomographic localization of clinically-guided sacroiliac joint injections. Clin J Pain 2000;16(1):18–21.

45. Hansen HC. Is fluoroscopy necessary for sacroiliac joint injections? Pain Physician 2003;6(2):155–8.

46. Sullivan WJ, Willick SE, Chira-Adisai W, et al. Incidence of intravascular uptake in lumbar spinal injection procedures. Spine (Phila Pa 1976 2000;25(4):481–6.

47. Jee H, Lee JH, Park KD, et al. Ultrasound-guided versus fluoroscopy-guided sacroiliac joint intra-articular injections in the noninflammatory sacroiliac joint dysfunction: a prospective, randomized, single-blinded study. Arch Phys Med Rehabil 2014;95(2):330–7.

48. Stelzer W, Stelzer D, Stelzer E, et al. Success rate of intra-articular sacroiliac joint injection: fluoroscopy vs ultrasound guidance—a cadaveric study. Pain Med 2019;20(10):1890–7.

49. De Luigi AJ, Saini V, Mathur R, et al. Assessing the accuracy of ultrasound-guided needle placement in sacroiliac joint injections. Am J Phys Med Rehabil 2019;98(8):666–70.

50. Perry JM, Colberg RE, Dault SL, et al. A cadaveric study assessing the accuracy of ultrasound-guided sacroiliac joint injections. PM R 2016;8(12):1168–72.

51. Soneji N, Bhatia A, Seib R, et al. Comparison of fluoroscopy and ultrasound guidance for sacroiliac joint injection in patients with chronic low back pain. Pain Pract 2016;16(5):537–44.

52. Lee JM, Kim DH. Measurement of Sacroiliac Joint Volume Using Live Fluoroscopy. :7.

53. Maugars Y, Mathis C, Berthelot JM, et al. Assessment of the efficacy of sacroiliac corticosteroid injections in spondylarthropathies: a double-blind study. Br J Rheumatol 1996;35(8):767–70.

54. Maugars Y, Mathis C, Vilon P, et al. Corticosteroid injection of the sacroiliac joint in patients with seronegative spondylarthropathy. Arthritis Rheum 1992;35(5):564–8.

55. Liliang PC, Lu K, Weng HC, et al. The therapeutic efficacy of sacroiliac joint blocks with triamcinolone acetonide in the treatment of sacroiliac joint dysfunction without spondyloarthropathy. Spine (Phila Pa 1976 2009;34(9):896–900.

56. Burnham T, Sampson J, Speckman RA, et al. The effectiveness of platelet-rich plasma injection for the treatment of suspected sacroiliac joint complex pain; a systematic review. Pain Med 2020;21(10):2518–28.

57. Navani A, Gupta D. Role of intra-articular platelet-rich plasma in sacroiliac joint pain. Tech Reg Anesth Pain Management 2015;19(1):54–9.

58. Ko GD, Mindra S, Lawson GE, et al. Case series of ultrasound-guided platelet-rich plasma injections for sacroiliac joint dysfunction. J Back Musculoskelet Rehabil 2017;30(2):363–70.

59. Singla V, Batra YK, Bharti N, et al. Steroid vs. Platelet-rich plasma in ultrasound-guided sacroiliac joint injection for chronic low back pain. Pain Pract 2017;17(6):782–91.

60. Linetsky FS, Manchikanti L. Regenerative injection therapy for axial pain. Tech Reg Anesth Pain Management 2005;9(1):40–9.

61. Stem cell prolotherapy in regenerative medicine: background, theory and protocols. J Prolotherapy 2012;. https://journalofprolotherapy.com/stem-cell-prolotherapy-in-regenerative-medicine-background-theory-and-protocols/. [Accessed 19 July 2021]. Accessed.

62. Kim WM, Lee HG, Jeong CW, et al. A randomized controlled trial of intra-articular prolotherapy versus steroid injection for sacroiliac joint pain. J Altern Complement Med 2010;16(12):1285–90.

63. Manchikanti L, Singh V, Pampati V, et al. Evaluation of the relative contributions of various structures in chronic low back pain. Pain Physician 2001;4(4):308–16.

64. Laslett M, Young SB, Aprill CN, et al. Diagnosing painful sacroiliac joints: a validity study of a McKenzie evaluation and sacroiliac provocation tests. Aust J Physiother 2003;49(2):89–97.

65. Burnham T, Conger A, Salazar F, et al. The effectiveness of cervical medial branch radiofrequency ablation for chronic facet joint syndrome in patients selected by a practical medial branch block paradigm. Pain Med 2020;21(10):2071–6.

66. Schneider BJ, Doan L, Maes MK, et al. Systematic review of the effectiveness of lumbar medial branch thermal radiofrequency neurotomy, stratified for diagnostic methods and procedural technique. Pain Med 2020;21(6):1122–41. Accessed July 19, 2021. https://www.google.com/search?q=Schneider+BJ%2C+Doan+L%2C+Maes+MK%2C+et+al.+Systematic+Review+of+the+Effectiveness+of+Lumbar+Medial+Branch+Thermal+Radiofrequency+Neurotomy%

2C+Stratified+for+Diagnostic+Methods+and+Procedural+Technique.+′′′
Pain+medicine.+2020%3B21(6)%3A1122-1141.&oq=Schneider+BJ%2C+
Doan+L%2C+Maes+MK%2C+et+al.+Systematic+Review+of+the+
Effectiveness+of+Lumbar+Medial+Branch+Thermal+Radiofrequency+Neur-
otomy%2C+Stratified+for+Diagnostic+Methods+and+Procedural+Techni-
que.+Pain+medicine.+2020%3B21(6)%
3A1122-1141.&aqs=chrome..69i57.828j0j7&sourceid=chrome&ie=UTF-8.

67. Yang AJ, McCormick ZL, Zheng PZ, et al. Radiofrequency ablation for posterior
    sacroiliac joint complex pain: a narrative review. PM R 2019;11(Suppl 1):
    S105–13.

68. Yang AJ, Wagner G, Burnham T, et al. Radiofrequency ablation for chronic pos-
    terior sacroiliac joint complex pain: a comprehensive review. Pain Med 2021;
    22(Suppl 1):S9–13.

69. Cohen SP, Hurley RW, Buckenmaier CC, et al. Randomized placebo-controlled
    study evaluating lateral branch radiofrequency denervation for sacroiliac joint
    pain. Anesthesiology 2008;109(2):279–88.

70. Patel N, Gross A, Brown L, et al. A randomized, placebo-controlled study to
    assess the efficacy of lateral branch neurotomy for chronic sacroiliac joint pain.
    Pain Med 2012;13(3):383–98.

71. Tinnirello A, Barbieri S, Todeschini M, et al. Conventional (Simplicity III) and
    cooled (SInergy) radiofrequency for sacroiliac joint denervation: one-year retro-
    spective study comparing two devices. Pain Med 2017;18(9):1731–44.

72. Bayerl SH, Finger T, Heiden P, et al. Radiofrequency denervation for treatment of
    sacroiliac joint pain-comparison of two different ablation techniques. Neurosurg
    Rev 2020;43(1):101–7.

73. Dutta K, Dey S, Bhattacharyya P, et al. Comparison of efficacy of lateral branch
    pulsed radiofrequency denervation and intraarticular depot methylprednisolone
    injection for sacroiliac joint pain. Pain Physician 2018;21(5):489–96.

74. Speldewinde GC. Successful thermal neurotomy of the painful sacroiliac liga-
    ment/joint complex-a comparison of two techniques. Pain Med 2020;21(3):561–9.

75. Loh E, Burnham TR, Burnham RS. Sacroiliac joint diagnostic block and radiofre-
    quency ablation techniques. Phys Med Rehabil Clin N Am 2021;32(4):725–44.

Peripheral Joint Injections

Austin Marcolina, DO[a],*, Kevin Vu, MD[b], George Chang Chien, DO[c]

KEYWORDS

- Peripheral joint injection • Joint pain • Landmark guidance • Image guidance
- Corticosteroid • Hyaluronic acid • Platelet-rich plasma • Mesenchymal stromal cells

KEY POINTS

- Peripheral joint pain is a common cause of debility with a prevalence of approximately 68%.
- Peripheral joint injection is a common interventional treatment for patients with underlying joint pathology that is not responsive to conservative management.
- Serious complications associated with peripheral joint injections are rare, although special precaution should be taken in settings of repeat corticosteroid injections.
- Corticosteroid injections have the most robust collection of data supporting its use in peripheral joint injections, although the efficacy is limited to short-term follow-up in most peripheral joint targets.
- Image guidance with either ultrasound or fluoroscopy provides superior accuracy and superior efficacy in comparison with landmark guidance, pending the injectate used and the target.

INTRODUCTION

Peripheral joint injections are a common interventional treatment of peripheral joint–mediated pain, including arthritis, tendinopathy, and bursitis that are not responsive to conservative management. Degenerative changes of articular joints are often related to these symptoms through chronic inflammatory changes, which typically arise due to repetitive trauma, autoimmune disease, or metabolic abnormalities.[1] The primary diagnosis for degenerative disease in the peripheral joints is osteoarthritis but can also include rheumatoid arthritis, gout, and other less common etiologies. Chronic inflammatory damage to the articular surfaces and joint capsules can lead to pain and functional decline. As such, the use of peripheral joint injections after the failure of typical conservative treatment, including physical therapy and oral medications, is common.[2] Although these injections are typically not curative in nature,

---

[a] Department of Physical Medicine and Rehabilitation, University of Texas Southwestern Medical Center, 5161 Harry Hines Boulevard, Dallas, TX 75219, USA; [b] Department of Physical Medicine and Rehabilitation, Spaulding Rehabilitation Hospital, 300 1st Avenue, Charlestown, MA 02129, USA; [c] Department of Physical Medicine and Rehabilitation, Ventura County Medical Center, 300 Hillmont Avenue, Ventura, CA 93003, USA
* Corresponding author.
E-mail address: austin.marcolina14@gmail.com

Phys Med Rehabil Clin N Am 33 (2022) 267–306
https://doi.org/10.1016/j.pmr.2022.01.005
1047-9651/22/© 2022 Elsevier Inc. All rights reserved.

their primary objective is to decrease pain to allow functional improvement concurrently with physical and pharmaceutical modalities. Common injectates used for peripheral joint injections include local anesthetic, corticosteroid, hyaluronic acid (HA), platelet-rich plasma (PRP), and mesenchymal stromal cells (MSCs).

PATIENT SELECTION CRITERIA

Peripheral joint injections are often used in the treatment of chronic inflammatory and degenerative diseases of the shoulder, elbow, wrist, hand, hip, knee, ankle, and foot. Although osteoarthritis related to advancing age or previous trauma is a common indication, other indications may include bursitis, rheumatoid arthritis, and tendinopathy.[3–5] Patients undergoing peripheral joint injections have often previously attempted conservative medical treatment, including oral and topical medications, physical therapy, and lifestyle modification without significant improvement.Additionally, patients with late-stage disease may also consider peripheral joint injections, primarily using corticosteroid as an injectate, as a bridge measure before considering surgical management.[6]

RISKS AND CONTRAINDICATIONS

Common contraindications for peripheral joint injections include septic arthritis, periarticular cellulitis, bacteremia, acute fractures, osteomyelitis, joint prostheses, uncontrolled bleeding or clotting disorders, and a history of allergy or anaphylaxis to the injectate.[2,7] Additionally, corticosteroid injections are contraindicated in the setting of osteoporosis, joint instability, uncontrolled hypertension, uncontrolled diabetes mellitus, and intratendinous injection.[6,8]

Complications related to peripheral joint injections are rare but require consideration. Iatrogenic joint infection is a potential concern; however, the estimated incidence is 0.0001%.[9] Other complications include bleeding, swelling, acute pain, and erythema of the injection site. More concerning are complications related to injectates, with corticosteroids being the most rigorously studied and reported on. Sequelae following corticosteroid injections include tendinous and ligamentous rupture with chronic and frequent injections, seizures, anaphylaxis, and stroke related to particulate use of steroids.[6,10,11] Furthermore, repeat corticosteroid injections, especially when used with minimal time between injections, seem to increase the risk of complications.[10,12] In vitro data have demonstrated that local anesthetics and corticosteroids are harmful to chondrocytes and tenocytes and may reduce the cartilage and meniscus health over time.[13–16] Reported complications with HA, PRP, and MSCs have been minimal, with isolated reports of postinjection erythema, swelling, and worsening pain.

OUTCOMES DATA AND DISCUSSION
Shoulder Injections

There are three common anatomic targets that are used for shoulder injections: the glenohumeral joint, subacromial subdeltoid bursa, and acromioclavicular joints (ACJs).

Glenohumeral joint
The glenohumeral joint (GHJ) is a complex, dynamic articulation between the glenoid of the scapula and the proximal humerus and requires stabilization from soft tissue structures, including the rotator cuff muscles.[17] Common indications for GHJ injections include adhesive capsulitis, primary or secondary osteoarthritis, and rheumatoid arthritis (**Tables 1** and **2**).[18]

Table 1	
Glenohumeral joint injectate outcomes	
Injectates	**Summary of Outcomes**
Corticosteroid	• Corticosteroid is effective at significantly improving pain, ROM, and function at short- and intermediate- term follow-up.[19–21] • The greatest efficacy of corticosteroid is noted within the first 6–12 wk postinjection.[21] • Corticosteroid has a B level of evidence for adhesive capsulitis and C level of evidence for GHJ OA.[19] • There is no difference in improvement in pain, ROM, or function between 20 mg and 40 mg triamcinolone injections for adhesive capsulitis at 3-wk follow-up.[22]
Hyaluronic acid	• HA has been shown to be efficacious in pain and functional outcomes on intermediate- and long-term follow-up for both OA and adhesive capsulitis.[19,23] • In comparison with corticosteroids, HA provides similar, significant improvement in pain and function for adhesive capsulitis at 1-mo follow-up but statistically superior results at 6-mo follow-up.[23] • HA has a C level of evidence for both adhesive capsulitis and GHJ OA.[19]
Platelet-rich plasma	• Based on several case reports and a cohort study, PRP provides an improvement in pain and functional measures for both adhesive capsulitis and GHJ OA.[24–26] • PRP has shown more significant improvement in pain and function at 12-wk follow-up when compared to a single corticosteroid injection for adhesive capsulitis.[26]
Mesenchymal stromal cells	• A single case series showed improvement in pain and function following a single dose of MSCs for GHJ OA.[27] • There have been no published studies comparing BMAC to other injectates in the GHJ.

Abbreviations: BMAC, bone marrow aspirate concentrate; ROM, range of motion.

Subacromial subdeltoid bursa

The subacromial subdeltoid (SASD) bursa is a synovial cavity that is located deep to the deltoid muscle and extends from below the acromion medially to beyond the greater tubercle of the humerus (**Fig. 1**). Notably, the bursa is just superficial to the supraspinatus tendon.[37] Common indications for SASD bursa injections include subacromial impingement syndrome, rotator cuff tendinopathy, and partial-thickness or full-thickness rotator cuff tears. The most commonly affected rotator cuff muscle is the supraspinatus (**Tables 3 and 4**).[38]

Acromioclavicular joint

The ACJ is a planar, diarthrodial articulation between the acromion and the clavicle and contains a fibrous disk that is prone to degeneration.[49] The most common indication for ACJ injection is pain secondary to osteoarthritis that has failed other conservative measures (**Tables 5 and 6**).[18]

Shoulder Injection Discussion

Peripheral joint injections into the three shoulder targets described previously are efficacious in providing at least short-term improvement in pain and function. It should be noted that while there are theoretic pathologic indications for each injection target (eg,

Table 2
Outcomes for forms of guidance for glenohumeral joint injections

Forms of Guidance	Accuracy (%)	Summary of Outcomes
Landmark	37.6–76[28,29]	• Landmark guidance produces statistically significant improvement in pain control and function at 6-wk follow-up when corticosteroid is used for GHJ OA.[20]
Ultrasound	92–100[28–32]	• US guidance exhibits statistically significant improvement in pain control and function at up to 9-wk follow-up when corticosteroid is used for GHJ OA (6-wk) and adhesive capsulitis (9-wk).[20,33] • US guidance has greater efficacy in improving pain control at 6-wk follow-up when compared to landmark guidance although functional outcomes are not significantly different with corticosteroid for GHJ OA.[20] • There is a significantly longer therapeutic effect, and fewer injections per year are required when using US guidance in comparison with landmark guidance when using corticosteroid for GHJ OA.[34]
Fluoroscopy	68–100[30–32,35]	• Fluoroscopic guidance produces statistically significant improvement in pain, ROM, and function at 1-wk to 12-mo follow-up, pending on the study cited. The greatest improvement was noted following corticosteroid injections for adhesive capsulitis.[33,36] • There is no statistically significant difference in pain, ROM, or function between fluoroscopic and US guidance at 1-wk, 5-wk, and 9-wk follow-up with corticosteroid injections for GHJ OA.[33]

Abbreviation: US, ultrasound.

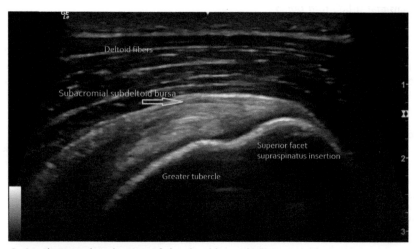

Fig. 1. An ultrasound evaluation of the shoulder with the supraspinatus in long axis that could be used for a SASD bursa injection.

Table 3
Subacromial subdeltoid bursa injectate outcomes

Injectates	Summary of Outcomes
Corticosteroid	• Corticosteroid delivers a significant improvement in pain and function at 6-wk follow-up, although this improvement is not maintained at 12-mo follow-up for most patients with subacromial impingement and rotator cuff tendinopathy.[39–41]
Hyaluronic acid	• HA demonstrates no significant improvement in pain or function, with no significant difference when compared to placebo for subacromial impingement.[41]
Platelet-rich plasma	• PRP provides a significant improvement in pain, shoulder external rotation, and function for rotator cuff tendinopathy at 3-mo and 6-mo follow-up.[42–44] • PRP also has a statistically significant advantage in pain, external rotation, and function at 3-mo and 6-mo follow-up when compared to corticosteroid for rotator cuff tendinopathy.[42,43]
Mesenchymal stromal cells	• A single case series showed an improvement in pain and function following MSC administration for partial- or full-thickness rotator cuff tears.[27] • MSCs show similar improvements in pain and function when compared to PRP at 3-mo follow-up for patients with a partial tear of the rotator cuff tendon.[44]

SASD injection for impingement syndrome), the shoulder joint can exhibit continuity between separate spaces, which may allow for efficacious treatment through use of an alternate target.[58,59] Additionally, the above analysis of the literature evaluated single-target injections when evaluating for efficacy, but other studies have shown pain and functional superiority following multisite injections, especially in the case of adhesive capsulitis.[60–62]

Table 4
Outcomes for forms of guidance for subacromial subdeltoid bursa injections

Forms of Guidance	Accuracy (%)	Summary of Outcomes
Landmark	42.8–93[40,45,46]	• Landmark guidance produces a significant improvement in pain and function in comparison with baseline when corticosteroid is used for rotator cuff tendinopathy.[40]
Ultrasound	100[32,40]	• US guidance with a corticosteroid injectate exhibits a significant improvement in pain, ROM, and function in comparison with baseline.[28,40,47] • There are contrasting data on the superiority of US guidance in comparison with landmark guidance, with one meta-analysis finding statistical superiority in pain, ROM, and function at 6-wk follow-up whereas another prospective, RCT showed no statistical or clinical difference between the two forms of guidance at 3-mo follow-up when corticosteroid was used.[40,47]
Fluoroscopy	No published rates of accuracy	• Fluoroscopic guidance with a corticosteroid injectate produces a significant improvement in pain and function in 83% of patients treated with a mean duration of 6 mo postinjection.[48]

Abbreviation: RCT, randomized control trial.

Table 5
Acromioclavicular joint injectate outcomes

Injectates	Summary of Outcomes
Corticosteroid	• Contrasting evidence exists regarding the efficacy of corticosteroids for ACJ injections. • Multiple studies have shown statistically significant improvement in pain and ROM at short-term follow-up,[50,51] with one study describing statistically significant improvement up to 6-mo follow-up for ACJ OA.[51] • In contrast, per a large systematic review, there is no clear evidence to support whether corticosteroids into ACJ for OA are effective or ineffective.[52]
Hyaluronic acid	• There are no published studies directly evaluating the outcomes of pain and function following HA for ACJ injections.
Platelet-rich plasma	• In a single, prospective RCT, PRP has shown statistically significant improvement in Constant score at 1-mo and 3-mo follow-up for ACJ OA.[53]
Mesenchymal stromal cells	• A single case report describes pain and functional improvement up to 18-mo follow-up following adipose-derived MSC injection with a reduction of subchondral cysts, synovitis, and subchondral edema on imaging at 12-mo follow-up.[54]

Imaging

Image guidance provides superior accuracy for all three shoulder injection targets, with ultrasound (US) having the greatest collection of data to support its use. This is especially evident when noting the significant variability in published accuracy rates for landmark guidance that is noted in the **tables 2**, **4**, and **6**. Additionally, US has been shown to provide superior efficacy in the form of pain, range of motion (ROM), or function for all three shoulder injection targets; however, it should be noted that studies describing no significant difference in comparison with landmark guidance have also been published. The evaluation of fluoroscopic guidance for shoulder injections is limited compared with that of US guidance as there are few published studies describing its efficacy in pain and functional outcomes following shoulder injections.

Although it was not directly evaluated in the studies summarized, image guidance may also be beneficial in cases of challenging anatomy or large patient body habitus

Table 6
Outcomes for forms of guidance for acromioclavicular joint injections

Forms of Guidance	Accuracy (%)	Summary of Outcomes
Landmark	24–72[28,51,55]	• Landmark guidance with a corticosteroid injectate for ACJ OA produces nonclinically significant improvement in pain and function at 1-wk, 3-wk, 1-mo, 3-mo, and 6-mo follow-up.[51,56]
Ultrasound	95–100[28,51]	• Based on retrospective analysis, US guidance exhibits statistical superiority in comparison with landmark guidance for pain and function at 6-mo follow-up when corticosteroid is used for ACJ OA.[51]
Fluoroscopy	100[57]	• There are no published studies directly evaluating the outcomes of pain and function following fluoroscopically guided ACJ injections.

to ensure accurate placement of the injectate. Moreover, as the studies describing no significant differences between image and landmark guidance used corticosteroid as the injectate, further research is required to evaluate the importance of image guidance for injections using noncorticosteroid injectates. Overall, image guidance allows for superior accuracy and potentially superior efficacy in pain and functional outcomes in comparison with landmark guidance.

Injectates
Corticosteroids have the most data supporting their use in all three shoulder injection targets summarized, especially in cases of GHJ osteoarthritis (OA), adhesive capsulitis, and subacromial impingement. As noted by several of the summarized studies, corticosteroids have the greatest efficacy in short and intermediate time points (6–12 weeks postinjection), with limited efficacy at long-term follow-up (12 months postinjection). Unlike GHJ and SASD bursa, there is contrasting evidence regarding the efficacy of corticosteroids for ACJ injections, with Chaudhury and colleagues describing no clear evidence to support whether corticosteroid is effective for ACJ OA.[52] Further evaluation of corticosteroids for adhesive capsulitis illustrated similar outcomes for both 20 mg and 40 mg doses of triamcinolone, which may limit some of the complications seen with larger dosages of steroids, although this has not been directly studied.[22,63]

Meanwhile, HA provides superior efficacy to corticosteroid at 6-month follow-up for adhesive capsulitis and GHJ osteoarthritis, but there remains a paucity of evidence to support its use in either SASD bursa or ACJ injections. Orthobiologic therapies, including PRP and MSCs, have the strongest support for their use in rotator cuff tendinopathy and partial-thickness and full-thickness rotator cuff tears, with PRP having a more robust collection of data and exhibiting superior efficacy to corticosteroid at 6-month follow-up. Studies describing the efficacy of PRP and MSCs for GHJ and ACJ OA and adhesive capsulitis are limited to case reports, case series, cohort studies, and small prospective studies. As such, further investigation is required before their widespread implementation for shoulder injections.

Elbow Injections

There are three common anatomic targets for elbow injections: the intra-articular elbow joint (IAEJ), medial epicondyle, and lateral epicondyle.

Intra-articular elbow joint
The IAEJ is a synovial hinge joint that contains three separate aspects of the joint—the radiocapitellar (RC) joint, the ulnotrochlear joint, and the proximal radioulnar joint (**Fig. 2**). The most common area for injection within the IAEJ is from a lateral aspect into the RC joint. Common indications for IAEJ injection are osteoarthritis, rheumatoid arthritis, and juvenile idiopathic arthritis (**Tables 7** and **8**).[64].

Lateral epicondyle
The lateral epicondyle is an anatomic landmark at the lateral aspect of the distal humerus that serves as an attachment site for the radial collateral ligament and the common extensor tendon (**Fig. 3**). The most common indication for lateral epicondyle injection is common extensor tendinopathy, also known as lateral epicondylitis or tennis elbow.[71] Common extensor tendinopathy is a common musculoskeletal pathology that affects 1% to 3% of adults annually.[72] As such, there has been a significant amount of research into the efficacy of lateral epicondyle injections for its management (**Tables 9** and **10**).

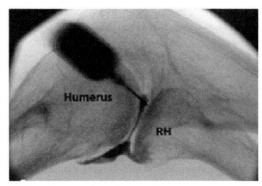

Fig. 2. A fluoroscopically guided intra-articular elbow injection with a lateral-to-medial approach.

Medial epicondyle

The medial epicondyle is an anatomic landmark at the medial aspect of the humerus that serves as an attachment site for the ulnar collateral ligament, the pronator teres, and the common flexor tendons (**Fig. 4**). The most common indication for medial epicondyle injection is common flexor tendinopathy, also known as medial epicondylitis or golfer's elbow (**Tables 11** and **12**).[92]

Elbow Injection Discussion

Peripheral joint injections into the three elbow region targets presented previously provide at least short-term efficacy for pain and functional improvement.

Imaging

Image guidance offers superior accuracy for both IAEJ and lateral epicondyle injections when compared to landmark guidance. However, in direct comparison between US and landmark guidance for IAEJ OA, IAEJ rheumatoid arthritis (RA), and lateral epicondylitis, there were no significant differences in outcomes for pain or function. As

Table 7	
Intra-articular elbow joint injectate outcomes	
Injectates	**Outcomes**
Corticosteroid	• On prospective analysis, corticosteroid provides statistically significant improvement in pain at rest, during movement, and in relation to morning stiffness at 1-wk and 4-wk follow-up for IAEJ in RA.[65]
	• Per a separate retrospective review, up to 96% of corticosteroid injections for AIEJ in OA and RA demonstrate improved pain from baseline, although the duration of relief was not presented.[66]
Hyaluronic acid	• Based on a small, prospective trial, HA produces limited, nonsignificant pain relief at 3-mo follow-up and no benefit at 6-mo follow-up in posttraumatic elbow OA.[67]
Platelet-rich plasma	• There are no published studies directly evaluating the outcomes of pain and function following PRP for IAEJ injections.
Mesenchymal stromal cells	• There are no published studies directly evaluating the outcomes of pain and function following MSC for IAEJ injections in human participants.

Table 8
Outcomes for forms of guidance for intra-articular elbow joint injections

Form of Guidance	Accuracy (%)	Efficacy
Landmark	64–100[65,68]	• Landmark guidance exhibits a significant improvement in pain scores at 2-, 4-, and 6-wk follow-up when corticosteroid is used for IAEJ OA and RA.[65,68]
Ultrasound	91[68]	• US guidance is effective at providing a significant improvement in pain scores at 2- and 6-wk follow-up for inflammatory arthritis.[68] • While the differences in outcomes between US- and landmark-guided injections did not meet statistical significance, accurate injections were found to be superior to inaccurate injections in functional outcomes at 6-wk follow-up.[68]
Fluoroscopy	100[69,70]	• There are no published studies directly evaluating the outcomes of pain and function following fluoroscopically guided IAEJ injections.

fluoroscopically guided IAEJ injections have primarily been used for intra-articular joint arthrography, there is limited data discussing the outcomes associated with fluoroscopic guidance. Furthermore, the evaluation of forms of guidance for medial epicondyle injections is limited by a paucity of literature describing accuracy rates and outcomes. Although no significant outcomes differences were found between landmark and US guidance for corticosteroid injectates in the elbow region, the orthobiologic injectate data presented all used US guidance. As such, image guidance should be used in cases of noncorticosteroid injectates in the elbow region and more data support the use of US, rather than fluoroscopy, in cases in which image guidance is preferred.

Injectates

Corticosteroid has the greatest body of evidence to support its use for injections in the elbow region, especially for short-term (<6 week) outcomes. Interestingly, although pmc_1231_gr8_3c.tif - corticosteroid has robust data to support its use for short-term outcomes in the elbow region, Olausson and colleagues described negative outcomes at 26-week follow-up after corticosteroid injection for lateral epicondylitis when

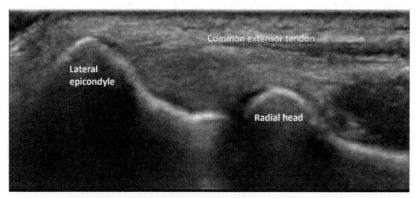

Fig. 3. A long-axis US evaluation of the lateral aspect of the elbow, including the lateral epicondyle, common extensor tendon, and radial head.

Table 9
Lateral epicondyle injectate outcomes

Injectates	Outcomes
Corticosteroid	• Corticosteroid demonstrates improvement in pain and function at short-term (<6-wk) follow-up for lateral epicondylitis, based on multiple systematic reviews.[73,74] • A systematic review also noted improved pain and grip strength at 4-wk and 12-wk follow-up; however, a negative overall improvement was found at 26-wk follow-up in comparison with stretching and exercise.[73] • Multiple other studies have shown inconclusive results or worse outcomes when compared with placebo or shock-wave therapy at long-term follow-up for lateral epicondylitis.[75–77]
Hyaluronic acid	• HA provides a significantly greater improvement in pain and grip strength at 1-wk, 2-wk, 1-mo, 3-mo, and 12-mo follow-up in comparison with saline for lateral epicondylitis.[78] • Hypertonic dextrose prolotherapy exhibits superior efficacy to HA in pain and grip strength at 12-wk follow-up, although both groups had significant improvement in comparison with baseline for lateral epicondylitis.[79]
Platelet-rich plasma	• Based on multiple prospective studies, PRP produces improvement in pain and function at long-term follow-up (between 8 wk and 2 y) that is superior to corticosteroid for lateral epicondylitis.[80–82] • Retrospective review also found PRP to reduce the need for surgical intervention for lateral epicondylitis.[83] • Contradictory evidence also exists, noting no significant difference between PRP and saline.[84]
Mesenchymal stromal cells	• Both BMAC and adipose-derived MSC injections have led to improved pain and function at long-term follow-up (up to 2 y) for lateral epicondylitis in small, prospective studies.[85–87] • There are no published studies directly comparing MSCs with other injectates for lateral epicondyle injections and the outcomes of pain and function.

Table 10
Outcomes for forms of guidance for lateral epicondyle injections

Form of Guidance	Accuracy (%)	Efficacy
Landmark	30[88]	• Landmark guidance with corticosteroid exhibits improvement in pain and function at short-term follow-up for lateral epicondylitis.[74]
Ultrasound	100[89]	• US guidance demonstrates improvement in pain and function when corticosteroids, PRP, and MSCs are used as injectates for lateral epicondylitis.[80–82,85–87] • However, in direct comparison of landmark with US guidance for corticosteroid injections, there is no significant difference in pain or function at 6-wk or 6-mo follow-up.[90,91]
Fluoroscopy	No published rates of accuracy	• There are no published studies directly evaluating the outcomes of pain and function following fluoroscopically guided lateral epicondyle injections.

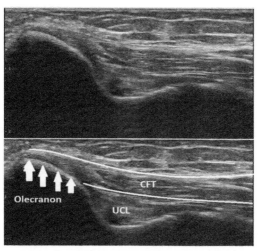

Fig. 4. A long-axis US evaluation of the medial aspect of the elbow, including the common flexor tendon (CFT), ulnar collateral ligament (UCL), and olecranon.

compared to stretching and exercise. Other studies have also found limited improvement in pain and function for corticosteroid use in elbow targets for peripheral joint injections after short-term follow-up. Additionally, corticosteroid has been shown to cause common extensor tendon rupture following lateral epicondyle injections.[96]

PRP and MSCs, meanwhile, offer long-term efficacy for lateral epicondylitis and may be a valuable option in those seeking long-term benefits although the studies describing said findings are fewer and smaller in power. HA has shown benefit in comparison with saline for lateral epicondylitis, but its use in IAEJ and medial epicondyle injections is not supported by the available data. Additionally, the use of PRP and MSCs for IAEJ and medial epicondyle injections requires further investigation before regular use.

Table 11	
Medial epicondyle injectate outcomes	
Injectates	**Outcomes**
Corticosteroid	• Based on prospective analysis, corticosteroids have shown a significant improvement in pain and function when compared to saline at 6-wk follow-up for medial epicondylitis, but there are no significant differences at 3-mo and 1-y follow-up between the injectates.[93]
Hyaluronic acid	• There are no published studies directly evaluating the outcomes of pain and function following HA for medial epicondyle injections.
Platelet-rich plasma	• PRP produces similar, statistically significant improvement in time to full ROM and time to pain-free status when compared to surgical intervention for type 1 medial epicondylitis.[94] • A separate study demonstrated similar, clinically significant improvements in pain and function for medial epicondylitis when compared to the Tenex procedure.[95]
Mesenchymal stromal cells	• There are no published studies directly evaluating the outcomes of pain and function following MSCs for medial epicondyle injections in humans.

Table 12
Outcomes for forms of guidance for medial epicondyle injections

Form of Guidance	Accuracy (%)	Efficacy
Landmark	No published rates of accuracy	• Landmark guidance demonstrates improvement in pain and function when corticosteroid is used as an injectate for medial epicondylitis.[93] • There are no published studies directly comparing the efficacy of landmark vs image guidance.
Ultrasound	No published rates of accuracy	• US guidance exhibits improvement in pain and function using PRP as an injectate for medial epicondylitis.[94,95] • There are no published studies directly comparing the efficacy of ultrasound vs other forms of guidance.
Fluoroscopy	No published rates of accuracy	• There are no published studies directly evaluating the outcomes of pain and function following fluoroscopically guided medial epicondyle injections.

Wrist/Hand Injections

There are three common anatomic targets for wrist/hand injections: the distal radioulnar joint (DRUJ), first carpometacarpal joint (1st CMCJ), and first dorsal wrist extensor compartment (FDWEC).

Distal radioulnar joint

The DRUJ is the articulation at the sigmoid notch of the radius and the ulnar head. It plays a key role in facilitating forearm protonation and supination, as well as the stabilization of the ulnar side of the wrist, along with other soft tissue structures.[97] Common indications for DRUJ injection are rheumatoid arthritis, osteoarthritis, and posttraumatic arthritis (**Tables 13 and 14**).[98]

First carpometacarpal joint

The first carpometacarpal joint (1st CMCJ) is a biconcave-convex saddle joint and serves as the articulation between the trapezium and the first metacarpal of the thumb

Table 13
Distal radioulnar joint injectate outcomes

Injectates	Outcomes
Corticosteroid	• Based on a randomized, prospective, single-blinded trial, corticosteroid was shown to produce improvement in pain and function at 1-, 3-, and 6-mo follow-up for DRUJ OA and RA.[99] • A separate prospective study exhibited efficacious results for pain and functional improvement at both 20 mg and 40 mg doses of triamcinolone for DRUJ RA.[100] • Furthermore, corticosteroid is useful as a prophylactic measure in decreasing the severity of wrist pain in acute distal radius fractures although this was no longer significant at 6-mo follow-up.[101]
Hyaluronic acid	• There are no published studies directly evaluating the outcomes of pain and function following HA for DRUJ injections.
Platelet-rich plasma	• PRP provides a significant improvement in pain and function at 3-mo follow-up in cases of distal radius fracture based on a single prospective study.[102]
Mesenchymal stromal cells	• There are no published studies directly evaluating the outcomes of pain and function following MSCs for DRUJ injections.

Table 14
Outcomes for forms of guidance for distal radioulnar joint injections

Form of Guidance	Accuracy (%)	Efficacy
Landmark	75.8–97[65,99]	• Landmark guidance demonstrates significant improvement in pain and function when corticosteroid was used as an injectate.[99]
Ultrasound	100[103]	• US guidance exhibits significant improvement in pain and function when using corticosteroid as an injectate.[99] • However, it has not been shown to have significantly different outcomes when compared to landmark guidance for corticosteroid injections for wrist pain in acute distal radius fractures.[101]
Fluoroscopy	82–100[104,105]	• Fluoroscopic guidance demonstrates improvement in pain and function when PRP is used as an injectate following distal radius fracture.[102] • There are no published studies directly comparing the efficacy of fluoroscopy vs other forms of guidance.

(**Fig. 5**).[106] As it lacks bony stability, it requires stabilization through several ligaments, including the anterior oblique, posterior oblique, radial collateral, ulnar collateral, and intermetacarpal ligaments.[106,107] Common indications for 1st CMCJ injections include osteoarthritis, rheumatoid arthritis, and posttraumatic arthritis (**Tables 15** and **16**).

First dorsal wrist extensor compartment
The FDWEC is located at the radial aspect of the wrist and contains the tendons of the abductor pollicis longus and the extensor pollicis brevis.[127] The most common indication for FDWEC injection is de Quervain's tenosynovitis (**Tables 17** and **18**).

Wrist and Hand Injection Discussion

Although the wrist and hand are less common targets for peripheral joint injections, the outcomes show similar potential benefits when compared to the shoulder and elbow.

Imaging
Similar to the shoulder and elbow, the use of image guidance provides superior accuracy when compared to landmark guidance for all three wrist and hand injection

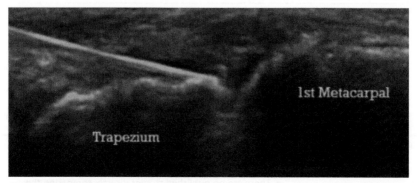

Fig. 5. A proximal-to-distal approach for US-guided 1st CMC joint injection. Both the first metacarpal and trapezium are visualized.

Table 15
First carpometacarpal joint injectate outcomes

Injectates	Outcomes
Corticosteroid	• Multiple studies have shown significant improvement in pain at short-term (1-mo) follow-up with corticosteroid, but the improvement is not sustained at 3-, 6-, or 12-mo follow-up for 1st CMCJ OA.[108,109] • In contrast, one study found no significant difference between corticosteroid and saline at 4- and 12-wk follow-up for 1st CMCJ OA.[110]
Hyaluronic acid	• HA has provided significant improvement in pain and function at 1-, 3-, and 6-mo follow-up for 1st CMCJ OA.[111–115] • Contrasting evidence exists for whether HA is superior to corticosteroid for pain and functional outcomes, with several studies showing superior outcomes for HA at longer term follow-up (>1-mo) and in cases of more severe symptoms associated with 1st CMCJ OA.[112–116]
Platelet-rich plasma	• PRP exhibits statistically significant improvement in pain and function at 3-, 6-, and 12-mo follow-up for 1st CMCJ OA.[117–119] • Moreover, PRP has superior efficacy in pain and functional outcomes compared to corticosteroid at 3- and 12-mo follow-up for 1st CMCJ OA.[119]
Mesenchymal stromal cells	• Both BMAC and adipose-derived MSCs provide statistically significant improvement in pain and function at 12-mo follow-up for 1st CMCJ OA.[120–123]

targets. When examining FDWEC, even though landmark guidance has been reported to have 100% accuracy in entering the compartment, it has been shown to be less efficacious in identifying and successfully injecting multiple septated compartments.[138] This is a pertinent finding, as a separate cadaveric study identified multiple septae in the FDWEC in 77.5% of cadaver wrists studied, lending further support to the

Table 16
Outcomes for forms of guidance for first carpometacarpal joint injections

Form of Guidance	Accuracy (%)	Efficacy
Landmark	63–98[108,124,125]	• Landmark guidance demonstrates statistically significant improvement in pain when using corticosteroid and HA for 1st CMCJ OA.[113,116]
Ultrasound	88[125]	• US guidance produces statistically significant improvement in pain when corticosteroid, HA, PRP, and MSCs are used for 1st CMCJ OA.[112,117,120] • Based on a large retrospective review, there is no significant difference in time between injections or progression to surgery between US-guided and landmark-guided injections when corticosteroid is used for 1st CMCJ OA.[126]
Fluoroscopy	100%[124]	• Fluoroscopic guidance exhibits improvement in pain and function when MSCs are used as an injectate for 1st CMCJ OA.[121] • There are no published studies directly comparing the efficacy of fluoroscopy vs other forms of guidance.

Table 17
First dorsal wrist extensor compartment injectate outcomes

Injectates	Outcomes
Corticosteroid	• Several studies report a significant improvement in pain and function in up to 88% of patients at 6-mo follow-up with sustained improvement in a subset of patients at 12-mo follow-up for de Quervain's tenosynovitis.[128–131] • A series of two corticosteroid injections has been shown to exhibit no further need for intervention in 73.4% of patients, whereas a similar outcome is only seen in 51.8% of patients who receive a single corticosteroid injection for de Quervain's tenosynovitis.[129]
Hyaluronic acid	• HA provides a significant improvement in pain and function, as well as a reduction in the risk of recurrence when used as a supplemental injectate with corticosteroid at 6-mo follow-up for de Quervain's tenosynovitis.[132] • However, HA does not demonstrate significantly superior outcomes in pain or function when compared to corticosteroid.[132]
Platelet-rich plasma	• PRP has shown a significant improvement in pain and function at 6-mo follow-up for de Quervain's tenosynovitis.[133,134] • Furthermore, PRP demonstrates statistical superiority in comparison with corticosteroid for pain, function, and tendon thickness under ultrasound at 6-mo follow-up.[134]
Mesenchymal stromal cells	• There are no published studies directly evaluating the outcomes of pain and function following MSCs for FDWEC injections.

use of US guidance.[139] Ultrasound guidance has also exhibited superior outcomes in pain and function when compared to landmark guidance for FDWEC injections. However, its use in DRUJ and 1st CMCJ injections was not found to be significantly different in comparison with landmark guidance when evaluating pain and functional outcomes.

Although there are case reports and small studies supporting the use of fluoroscopic guidance for orthobiologic treatments, there is limited data comparing its

Table 18
Outcomes for forms of guidance for first dorsal wrist extensor compartment injections

Form of Guidance	Accuracy (%)	Efficacy
Landmark	100% into at least one compartment; however, only 33% (2/6) were successfully injected into multiple, septated compartments	• Landmark guidance exhibits efficacy in pain and functional improvement when corticosteroid is used as an injectate in 83%–88% of patients.[130,135]
Ultrasound	100% into at least one compartment; however, only 75% (six out of eight) were successfully injected into multiple, septated compartments	• US guidance is efficacious in improving pain and function when corticosteroid is used as an injectate in 94.1%–97% of patients with de Quervain's tenosynovitis.[136,137]
Fluoroscopy	No published rates of accuracy	• There are no published studies directly evaluating the outcomes of pain and function following fluoroscopically guided FDWEC injections.

efficacy with that of US or landmark guidance. Like the previous sections, the studies that used orthobiologic injectates all had image guidance. As such, image guidance should be used in cases of noncorticosteroid injectates in the wrist/hand region. Additionally, more data support the use of US, rather than fluoroscopy, in cases where image guidance is preferred.

Injectate

Corticosteroid is the primary injectate in the wrist/hand and produces short-term improvement for pain and function in DRUJ OA, DRUJ RA, distal radius fracture, and 1st CMCJ OA. Notably, the use of corticosteroid in de Quervain's tenosynovitis has shown more sustained improvement in comparison with the other injection targets described, which could potentially negate the concerns of repeat steroid use. HA has the most robust data for its use as a solo injectate in 1st CMCJ injections, although contrasting evidence exists regarding its superiority to corticosteroid. HA has also been shown to be efficacious as a supplemental injectate with corticosteroid for de Quervain's tenosynovitis, but data to support its application as a solo injectate are limited.

Both PRP and MSCs produce pain and functional improvement in 1st CMCJ OA while PRP also provides significant improvement as an injectate for de Quervain's tenosynovitis. Furthermore, PRP has shown superior long-term outcomes in comparison with corticosteroid for both 1st CMC OA and de Quervain's tenosynovitis, which may be of interest in patients interested in longer term improvement without surgical intervention. However, as described previously, well-designed, larger power studies are needed before the widespread application of noncorticosteroid injectates for wrist/hand targets.

Hip Injections

There are two common anatomic targets that are used for hip injections: the intra-articular hip joint, also known as the femoral-acetabular joint, and the greater trochanteric bursa.

Intra-articular hip joint

The hip is composed of a ball-and-socket joint comprising the femoral head nestled within the cartilage of the pelvic acetabulum and associated labrum (**Fig. 6**). A true

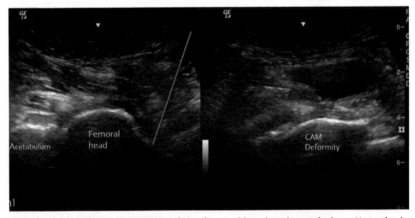

Fig. 6. Left image: Ultrasound image of the femoral head and acetabulum. Note the integrity of the acetabulum and smoothness of the femoral head. The orange line indicates a possible needle trajectory into the intra-articular space. Right image: Nonspherical femoral head consistent with a cam deformity of the hip joint, visualized on ultrasound.

joint, the hip has a synovial capsule with which the articulating cartilage and synovial fluid within the capsule provide cushioning and lubrication for movement of the joint **(Fig. 7)**.[140] Nociceptors within the hip are often concentrated alongside vascular structures at the labral base of the joint.[141] As described above, chronic inflammation related to this capsule leads to clinical symptoms of pain, loss of ROM, and reduced function for patients **(Tables 19** and **20)**.

Greater trochanteric bursa

The trochanteric bursa is located lateral to the lateral greater trochanter of the femur, deep to the gluteus maximus, and adjacent to other hip girdle muscles that attach to the greater trochanter. Greater trochanteric bursitis often presents as lateral thigh pain which may be confused with hip pain. This inflammation may arise from overuse injury or chronic trauma to the greater trochanter. Injections into the trochanteric bursa can often serve as diagnostic and therapeutic options for greater trochanteric bursitis **(Tables 21** and **22)**.

Hip Injection Discussion

Imaging

When considering the use of imaging in intra-articular hip and greater trochanteric bursa injections, there is strong evidence for the use of US or fluoroscopy to allow accurate injection. The American Medical Society for Sports Medicine's guidelines state that there is "strong evidence for ultrasound guided injections in [hip joints]," with level 1 evidence for improved accuracy in hip joints and level 3 evidence for increased

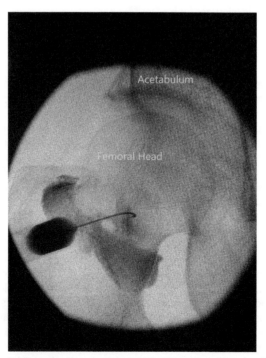

Fig. 7. A fluoroscopically guided intra-articular hip injection with a confirmation of placement with radiopaque contrast.

Injectates	Summary of Outcomes
Table 19	
Intra-articular hip joint injectate outcomes	
Corticosteroid	• Meta-analysis found that corticosteroids had a short-lived but significant effect on pain and function, with typical length of effect peaking at 1 wk and lasting for 3–4 wk for hip OA.[142,143] • There is weaker evidence that these injections additionally improve ROM.[143]
Hyaluronic acid	• HA concurrently with physical therapy is significantly effective in reducing pain during activity and at rest, as well as improving functional outcome scores for hip OA.[144] • HA was also noted to reduce NSAID usage by 48.2% at the 3 mo postinjection mark for hip OA.[145] • Conversely, other studies have noted minimal improvement when compared to placebo or normal saline for hip OA.[146,147] • HA did not demonstrate significant improvements in WOMAC pain or function scores when compared to corticosteroids, and single injection of HA was no more effective than placebo in changing VAS or functional outcomes for hip OA.[148–150]
Platelet-rich plasma	• PRP has shown persistent improvement in pain up to 6-mo follow-up for hip OA.[151] • Meta-analysis of PRP vs HA studies also noted significantly lower VAS for the PRP group at 2-mo follow-up.[151]
Mesenchymal stromal cells	• Limited conclusions can be drawn because of a lack of currently available evidence. • Literature review comprised of case studies noted improvement in WOMAC scores and VAS scores at 6-mo follow-up across patients with MSC hip injections for hip OA.[152]

Abbreviations: NSAID, nonsteroidal anti-inflammatory drug; VAS, visual analog scale; WOMAC, Western Ontario and McMaster Universities Osteoarthritis Index.

efficacy of hip joints with US guidance.[28,156–158] Fluoroscopy is often used as the gold standard to confirm placement of injection needles in studies, but published rates of accuracy are not available in the literature.

In contrast, the greater trochanter bursa has classically been done with landmark guidance. Cohen and colleagues noted that when comparing fluoroscopic versus blind landmark injection of the trochanteric bursa, there was no significant difference in outcomes in a multicenter trial. Furthermore, the additional cost of fluoroscopy and delay in care may be detrimental to patients.[173] US-guided injections may be of limited use, with a cadaveric study noting that although US had a higher rate of accuracy compared to landmark guided, there was no significant difference in pain or functional outcomes.[168]

Injectates
Ongoing evaluation of injectates for the hip has shown the difficulty of effectively treating degenerative and inflammatory disease of this area. Corticosteroids continue to be the mainstay of short- to-medium-term treatment for both injection sites with consistent reduction of pain and improvement of functional symptoms. Although they have been proven to demonstrate benefits in the intra-articular joint, side effects and consequences of chronic use of corticosteroids injections should be considered, as patient's run the risk of further degeneration of their articular surfaces. HA, although initially returning positive outcomes, is suspected to be less efficacious compared

Table 20
Outcomes for forms of guidance for intra-articular hip joint injections

Forms of Guidance	Accuracy (%)	Summary of Outcomes
Landmark	66.7–77.5[153–155]	• Multiple studies have noted the poor accuracy of hip joint injection based on landmark guidance.[154,156] • Per retrospective review, 82% of patients responded positively and experienced >50% pain relief when using corticosteroid for hip OA.
Ultrasound	97–100[28]	• The American Medical Society for Sports Medicine's guidelines state that there is "strong evidence for ultrasound guided injections in [hip joints]," with level 1 evidence for improved accuracy in hip joints and level 3 evidence for increased efficacy of hip joints with US guidance.[157] • Several other meta-analyses and studies have shown that US significantly improves accuracy and efficacy related to increased function and decreased pain at 1-mo, 3-mo, and 6-mo follow-up for hip OA when using corticosteroid.[28,148,158] • One prospective study noted that intra-articular injection by fluoroscopy or US significantly improved pain and function scores at 4-wk follow-up for hip OA, but there was no significant difference between the two modalities in measured outcomes.[159]
Fluoroscopy	No published rate of accuracy	• Patients tend to prefer the convenience of US over fluoroscopy although the study did not note the efficacy of either modality.[160] • Fluoroscopic-guided injections of corticosteroids noted significant decrease in pain scores at 6–8 wk follow-up for hip OA.[161,162]

Table 21
Greater trochanteric bursa injectate outcomes

Injectates	Summary of Outcomes
Corticosteroid	• A multicenter, randomized trial found significant effect on resolution of symptoms at 3-mo follow-up for greater trochanteric bursitis, but this effect became nonsignificant at 12-mo follow-up.[163,164] • Response ranges to corticosteroids have been described as 60%–100%, with nonresponse likely indicating other differentials of lateral hip pain than greater trochanteric bursitis.[165]
Platelet-rich plasma	• PRP and corticosteroid injections were significantly efficacious up to 12-wk follow-up for greater trochanteric bursitis, although PRP was also noted to have continued efficacy up to 24-wk follow-up.[164] • Meta-analyses noted that PRP was effective in reducing pain and increasing functional outcomes up to 3-mo follow-up with a residual effect seen at 12-mo follow-up; however, there were inconclusive findings regarding its superiority to corticosteroid for greater trochanteric bursitis.[166]
Mesenchymal stromal cells	• A case report on bone marrow–derived MSC injection into the bursa showed significant improvement in pain and function up to 1 y[167]

Table 22
Outcomes for forms of guidance for greater trochanteric bursa injections

Forms of Guidance	Accuracy (%)	Summary of Outcomes
Landmark	45–67[168,169]	• 45% of first needle placements for the greater trochanteric bursa were confirmed via bursagram, followed by 23% for the second and third attempts.[170] • 55% of patients reported significant recovery of pain symptoms at 3-mo follow-up when corticosteroid was used.[163] • A separate study noted landmark-guided injections with corticosteroid significantly decreased pain scores at 2-wk and 6-mo follow-up.[171]
Ultrasound	92[168]	• A cadaveric study noted a nonsignificant difference in US compared to landmark-guided rates of accuracy with 92% and 67% accuracy, respectively.[168] • Conversely, a different study noted that US guidance shows a significantly greater improvement in pain at 6-mo follow-up when compared to landmark guidance when each used corticosteroid, but there was no difference between the two forms of guidance for the duration of therapy or time-to-next intervention.[171]
Fluoroscopy	Confirmatory test for placement in multiple studies but no published specific rate of accuracy[172]	• A multicenter, double-blinded RCT found that there was no significant difference in pain outcomes between fluoroscopy and US when corticosteroid was used as an injectate.[173]

to corticosteroids as demonstrated in the above literature. Orthobiologic injectates have continued to show potential as a possible treatment for both hip targets with sustained reduction of symptoms in small prospective and case report studies. The heterogeneity of these regenerative studies, particularly related to size, risk of bias, study design, and preparation and methodology of these new injectates, limits the conclusions that can be drawn from them.

Knee Injections

There are two common anatomic targets that are used for knee injections: the intra-articular knee joint and the pes anserinus bursa.

Intra-articular knee joint

The knee is composed of a hinge joint comprising the tibial plateau articulating with the distal femur. Intra-articular menisci and collateral ligaments provide cushioning and stability of the joint, surrounded by synovial tissue and fluid to provide lubrication, similar to that of the hip (**Fig. 8**). Auricular nerves innervate the knee joint and capsule, with additional nonspecific muscular nerve branches. Histologic examination has shown that 45% to 80% of nerve fibers in the human knee are nociceptors, with a significant number of receptors in the surrounding fat pads.[141] Common pathologic conditions requiring intra-articular knee injections include osteoarthritis, inflammatory arthritis, and rheumatoid arthritis (**Tables 23** and **24**).

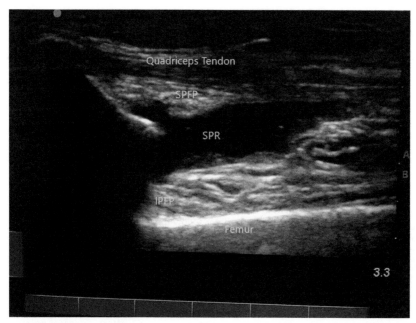

Fig. 8. An enlarged suprapatellar recess (SPR) noted in a long-axis US evaluation of the knee. Other notable structures on the image include the quadriceps tendon, suprapatellar fat pad (SPFP), and the femur.

Pes anserine bursa

The pes anserine bursa is located over the medial epicondyle of the knee superficial to the medial collateral ligament (MCL) and underlies the semimembranosus, gracilis, and semitendinosus tendons. It serves as lubrication for these tendons over underlying tissue and can become inflamed as a result of overuse injury or stress on the bursa, particularly in athletes. Common symptoms of pes anserinus bursitis include pain over the medial epicondyle of the knee exacerbated by activity. The most common indications for injection are typically bursitis and tendinopathy (**Tables 25** and **26**).

Knee Injection Discussion

Imaging

There is strong evidence for the use of US, but not fluoroscopy, in intra-articular knee joint injections. Level 1 evidence points to US significantly increasing the accuracy and efficacy of intra-articular injections.[32,157,192] Knee injections via previously used landmarks have shown a "wide margin of accuracy with respect to landmark-guided injection, ranging from 55% to 100%," with US improving accuracy and therapeutic duration of knee injections.[28]

Although there is limited literature describing other imaging modalities in pes anserinus bursitis, one study evaluated the use of US to localize these injections in cadavers. Despite the superficial location of the pes anserine bursa, 17% of landmark-guided injections were determined to be accurate whereas US-guided injections were significantly more accurate at 92%.[200] Similarly, another study found US-guided injections were both more accurate and efficacious in actual patients at 4-week follow-up.[201]

Table 23
Intra-articular knee joint injectate outcomes

Injectates	Summary of Outcomes
Corticosteroid	• A Cochrane review for corticosteroids for knee OA showed a small improvement in physical function and moderate improvement in pain at 1-mo follow-up.[174] • Corticosteroid use over time has been associated with severe meniscal damage, a higher Kellgren–Lawrence osteoarthritis grades, and a decreased likelihood of long-term response to repeat corticosteroid injections.[175,176]
Hyaluronic acid	• A meta-analysis noted statistically significant improvement in pain at 3-mo follow-up for knee OA, although this was not found to be clinically significant.[177] • In a longitudinal 5-y study for knee OA, HA provided a significant improvement in functional scores up to 24-mo follow-up, but scores returned to baseline in later follow-ups.[178,179]
Platelet-rich plasma	• Based on a prospective, double-blinded, RCT, PRP has shown a significant improvement in pain and function in both single- and double-injection series groups compared to placebo for knee OA.[180] • PRP demonstrated significant improvement in functional scores for up to 24-mo follow-up and had a greater functional improvement when compared to HA for knee OA.[178,179] • Significant patient satisfaction and pain reduction with average onset of therapeutic effects around 18 d postinjection.[181,182] • A meta-analysis showed leukocyte-poor PRP produces the greatest improvement in WOMAC functional scores when compared to leukocyte-rich PRP, HA, or placebo for knee OA.[183] • Comparatively, PRP noted to be similarly effective as corticosteroids in improving pain and function for knee OA but with further significant improvement at the 15-wk, 6-mo, and 1-y mark.[184,185]
Mesenchymal stromal cells	• Based on a RCT meta-analysis, MSCs demonstrate a significant improvement in VAS, pain, and functional scores compared to baseline, estimating the length of effect up to 24–48 mo. However, this is limited by a high risk of bias and the use of level 3 evidence because of the low availability of studies.[186] • There is no significant difference in pain or function scores at 12 mo between PRP and PRP + MSC treatment.[187] • There are contrasting conclusions regarding improvements in cartilage quality and nonsignificant findings in terms of cartilage volume increase.[188–190]

Injectates

Corticosteroids have demonstrated their efficacy for the treatment of degenerative joint disease of the knee and are particularly useful for acute flares of inflammatory knee pain. Similarly, corticosteroids are also the primary treatment for pes anserinus bursitis. Combined with other conservative measures, they can be a useful tool for management of knee pain and decreased function but may be limited in their long-term applicability. Chronic use in the intra-articular space is recommended with caution because of reports of cartilage degeneration. HA has minimal improvement in symptoms in large-scale meta-analyses as above but may be recommended as a supplementary treatment. Orthobiologic treatments, including PRP and MSCs, have shown increasing promise, with many small studies reporting significantly improved pain and functional scores with some lasting efficacy at both knee targets. The recent

Table 24
Outcomes for forms of guidance for intra-articular knee joint injections

Forms of Guidance	Accuracy (%)	Summary of Outcomes
Landmark	39–100[28]	• The most accurate approaches are the lateral midpatellar approach at 76%–93% and the anterolateral approach at 85%.[28] • Between the three typical approaches (superolateral, anteromedial, and anterolateral), there is no significant difference in efficacy as measured by WOMAC scores as all demonstrate decreases at 1-wk and 4-wk follow-up.[191]
Ultrasound	75–100[192,193]	• Level 1 evidence points to US significantly increasing the accuracy and efficacy of intra-articular injections.[32,157,192] • US-guided corticosteroid injections for knee OA provide significant reductions in pain scores, response rate, and therapeutic duration when compared to landmark-guided injections.[194]
Fluoroscopy	Commonly used as a confirmatory test for placement but no published specific rate of accuracy[32]	• There have been no published studies directly evaluating the efficacy of fluoroscopic-guided intra-articular knee joint injections.

Table 25
Pes anserine bursa joint injectate outcomes

Injectates	Summary of Outcomes
Corticosteroid	• Corticosteroid is well tolerated and is typically used for refractory pain following conservative management in pes anserine bursitis.[195] • Corticosteroid injections are comparable to physical therapy in efficacy, as both significantly decrease VAS and WOMAC scores at 8-wk follow-up in pes anserine bursitis.[196,197]
Platelet-rich plasma	• PRP has shown significantly improved function and pain at 6-mo follow-up with a one-time injection for pes anserine bursitis.[198] • Leukocyte-rich PRP was found to provide significant improvement in pain and function in comparison with baseline for both one and two injection series for pes anserine bursitis.[199]
Mesenchymal stromal cells	• A case report involving a patient with chronic pes anserine bursitis reported significant improvement with a one-time injection of bone marrow–derived MSCs up to 12-mo follow-up.[167]

Table 26
Outcomes for forms of guidance for pes anserine bursa joint injections

Forms of Guidance	Accuracy (%)	Summary of Outcomes
Landmark	17[200]	• Landmark-guided injections were efficacious in lowering VAS pain scores in patients at 1-wk and 4-wk follow-up for pes anserine bursitis.[201]
Ultrasound	92[201]	• US-guided injections were more accurate and produced a greater decrease in VAS at 1 wk and 4 wk when compared to blind landmark injections for pes anserine bursitis.[201]
Fluoroscopy	No published rate of accuracy	• There have been no published studies directly evaluating the efficacy of fluoroscopic-guided pes anserinus bursa injections.

Table 27
Tibiotalar joint injectate outcomes

Injectates	Summary of Outcomes
Corticosteroid	• Corticosteroids exhibit significant improvements in pain and swelling at 4-wk follow-up for tibiotalar OA.[203]
Hyaluronic acid	• A RCT of repeated HA injections with up to a 5-injection regimen did show significant improvement in pain and function for tibiotalar OA.[169] • However, contradictory evidence also exists, noting no significant differences between HA and normal saline for tibiotalar OA.[204]
Platelet-rich plasma	• PRP provides a significant improvement in VAS and Japanese Society for Sugery of the Foot Scale (JSSF) up to 12-wk follow-up without significant adverse events for tibiotalar OA.[205] • Initial small sample studies on PRP noted positive effects improvement in pain for talus osteochondral lesions.[206]
Mesenchymal stromal cells	• A small-scale study noted ankle OA did benefit from MSC injection, with improved walking distances and WOMAC scores.[207]

Table 28
Outcomes for forms of guidance for tibiotalar joint injections

Forms of Guidance	Accuracy (%)	Summary of Outcomes
Landmark	24–85[28,157]	• There are mixed studies with different estimates of accuracy; however, landmark guidance produces accuracy lower than that of image-guided techniques.[193]
Ultrasound	64–100[28,157]	• US guidance with a corticosteroid injectate is efficacious in improving pain and function at 3-mo follow-up for tibiotalar RA.[208]
Fluoroscopy	No published rate of accuracy	• There have been no published studies directly evaluating the efficacy of fluoroscopic-guided tibiotalar injections.

introduction of PRP and MSC injections highlights the need for larger well-designed studies given the significant heterogeneity in preparation, constitution, and frequency of these treatments. Although these treatments show potential, they should be discussed thoroughly with patients before treatment.

Foot and Ankle Joint Injections

Two of the major targets for injection in the foot and ankle are the tibiotalar joint and the plantar fascia.

Tibiotalar joint

The ankle joint is another hinged joint in the lower extremity, comprising the tibia, fibula, and talus of the foot. Surrounded by synovium and articular cartilage of the talus, the ankle joint has been found to have multiple innervations from the tibial, sural, deep peroneal, and saphenous nerves (**Tables 27** and **28**).[202]

Plantar fascia

The plantar fascia consists of a collagen aponeurosis, originating over the medial tubercle of the calcaneus to the metatarsal heads. As part of the longitudinal arch of the foot, the plantar fascia is a common overuse injury complaint, often originating at its insertion point at the medial tubercle.[209] Typically described as a mixed inflammatory and degenerative process, plantar fasciitis is often described as a medial heel pain

Table 29 Plantar fascia injectate outcomes	
Injectates	**Summary of Outcomes**
Corticosteroid	• A Cochrane review noted that corticosteroids "may slightly reduce heel pain for up to 1 month after treatment," but did not have significant effect beyond 6-mo follow-up in either VAS or other functional outcomes for plantar fasciitis.[210] • Adverse outcomes to corticosteroid injections were rare but included plantar fascia rupture (estimated incidence rate 2.2% after 2.67 injections) and infection.[210,211] • One meta-analysis found that corticosteroid injections were more effective than autologous blood products for reducing pain scores at 1-mo follow-up but that PRP was more effective at 1-y follow-up for plantar fasciitis.[212]
Hyaluronic acid	• Both HA and corticosteroids are efficacious in significantly improving pain and functional measures at 24-wk follow-up for plantar fasciitis.[213] • A multicenter, double-blinded RCT found that high-dose HA injection for plantar fasciopathy significantly improved VAS scores from baseline to 5-wk follow up and improved significantly when compared to the control group.[214]
Platelet-rich plasma	• Based on a meta-analysis, PRP is statistically superior to corticosteroid in the measures of pain at 3-mo, 6-mo, and 12-mo follow-up and functional outcomes at 6-mo and 12-mo follow-up. However, the meta-analysis was limited by a high risk of bias and low-quality studies.[215] • A separate meta-analysis similarly described significant improvements in favor of PRP over corticosteroid for functional outcomes at 6-mo and 12-mo follow-up and pain at 3-mo, 6-mo, and 12-mo follow-up for chronic plantar fasciitis.[216]
Mesenchymal stromal cells	• There are no published studies directly evaluating the outcomes of pain and function following MSC for PF injections.

Table 30		
Outcomes for forms of guidance for plantar fascia injections		
Forms of Guidance	Accuracy (%)	Summary of Outcomes
Landmark	No published rate of accuracy	• Landmark-guided corticosteroid injections for PF produce significant improvements in VAS, plantar fascia thickness, and fat pad thickness at 24-mo follow-up.[217] • No significant difference was found in the above measures when landmark guidance was compared to scintigraphy and ultrasound guidance.[217]
Ultrasound	No published rate of accuracy	• US guidance with a corticosteroid injectate significantly improves VAS, tenderness threshold, response rate, and plantar fascia thickness.[218]
Fluoroscopy	No published rate of accuracy	• There have been no published studies directly evaluating the efficacy of fluoroscopic guided plantar fascia injections.

often worse in the morning and progressively improving throughout the day (**Tables 29** and **30**).

Foot and Ankle Injection Discussion

Imaging

Similar to the above joints, there is strong evidence for the use of US to provide accurate and efficacious injection. Level 2 evidence exists for tibiotalar joint injection accuracy with US, with reported rates of US accuracy at 100% versus tibiotalar landmark-guided injections success rates around 58% to 85%. Similar studies found more conservative estimates of accuracy to be 64% with US-guided injections versus 25% for landmark guided.[28,157] Although there are no available studies on the accuracy rate of plantar fascia regarding the use of imaging- versus landmark-guided injection, there is significant evidence for the overall improved pain and functional outcomes when US guidance is used for PF injections.

Injectates

Foot and ankle injections are less commonly targeted for significant intra-articular pathologic conditions, but injectates can provide some relief in patients who are symptomatic. Corticosteroids, as in the above joints, are the first-line treatment of degenerative and inflammatory conditions of the ankle and plantar fascia, with significant improvements in pain and functional scores. HA may also provide symptomatic relief in both ankle and plantar fascia, although not without controversy as to a causal relationship related to treatment effects. Orthobiologic treatments are limited by the availability of literature, but small-scale studies show improvements in pain and function in both PRP and MSC injections with minimal side effects. The plantar fascia may be a significant target for orthobiologic injections, with PRP being a modality that has shown long-term improvement when compared to corticosteroids across multiple meta-analyses.

SUMMARY

The available injectates, targets, and methods for the peripheral joint injections discussed are many and varied. Although this review is not comprehensive in nature, it highlights the major points of research and current state of the literature on the available injectates and image guidance.

The core of injectates currently are corticosteroids, HA, PRP, and MSCs with varying degrees of efficacy. Corticosteroids have proved their short-term effectiveness in the control of pain and improvement in function but should be used with caution because of potential long-term side effects, especially in cases of repeat injections. HA may have utility as an alternative injectate in the shoulder, elbow, knee, and ankle, but clinical improvement may be limited. Although functional outcomes related to orthobiologic treatments are tentatively positive, many obstacles stand in the way before widespread adoption. Literature regarding orthobiologic treatments continues to remain heterogeneous with variable degrees of bias. Larger scale studies continue to emerge, but the literature will need further substantiation with increasingly well-designed studies with decreased bias. One technical concern about PRP, HA, and MSCs continues to be the preparation, as a multitude of protocols exist. Controversy also exists in the frequency, amount, and constitution of these injectates. HA has many animal and nonanimal sources, as well as differing density, concentration, and volumes of the injectate. PRP also has differing formulation recommendations for centrifuge protocol and the inclusion of leukocytes in its preparation. MSCs continue to need further investigation in large-scale trials, and despite initial findings being positive, it too suffers from the same heterogeneity in procurement as PRP.[219]

The three forms of guidance used on peripheral joint injections continue to be landmark, US, and fluoroscopic guidance. Although accuracy and efficacy have been demonstrated in all three forms of guidance, the use of image guidance allows for superior accuracy and potentially superior efficacy, especially when using noncorticosteroid injectates. Between US and fluoroscopic guidance, US has a more robust collection of data to support its accuracy and efficacy for peripheral joint injections. However, it should be noted that the individual administering the injection should be proficient in their use of the image-guided technique before widespread implementation, and image-guided procedures require significant training and equipment to administer.

Ultimately, the use of injectate and form of guidance should be led by patient pathology, preferences, and goal of treatment. A key concept in the use of peripheral extremity injections is that none of the injectates are inherently not curative. Therefore, practitioners should aim for restored function and possible stabilization of the pathologic process and encourage the use of adjunct conservative treatment, such as physical therapy, for optimal benefits.

CLINICS CARE POINTS

- Image guidance provides superior accuracy and efficacy when compared to landmark guidance for peripheral joint injections, especially when using ultrasound guidance and noncorticosteroid injectates.

- Corticosteroids remain the typical first-line injections for a wide variety of peripheral joint ailments, but increasing attention to the long-term consequences of this injectate may limit their overall utility.

- Hyaluronic acid remains a controversial injectate, with some limited utility in larger, weight-bearing joints and upper extremity joints.

- Although platelet-rich plasma does show some initial trends in efficacy, further evidence on a likely multifaceted mechanism of action and standardization of procurement is required before a definitive recommendation can be made.

- Further evidence for mesenchymal stromal cell injections is required before any significant conclusions can be drawn about their use in peripheral joint injections.
- Patient education and a holistic view of their pathologic conditions and preferences should be discussed before the use of any injectate, especially those defined as orthobiologic in nature.

DISCLOSURE

None of the authors have any financial conflicts of interest to disclose.

REFERENCES

1. Zhao Z, Ma JX, Ma XL. Different Intra-articular Injections as Therapy for Hip Osteoarthritis: A Systematic Review and Network Meta-analysis. Arthroscopy 2020;36(5):1452–1464 e1452.
2. Millard RS, Dillingham MF. Peripheral joint injections: lower extremity. Phys Med Rehabil Clin N America 1995;6(4):841–9.
3. Hart L. Corticosteroid and other injections in the management of tendinopathies: a review. Clin J Sport Med 2011;21(6):540–1.
4. Ostergaard M, Halberg P. Intra-articular corticosteroids in arthritic disease: a guide to treatment. BioDrugs 1998;9(2):95–103.
5. Pekarek B, Osher L, Buck S, et al. Intra-articular corticosteroid injections: a critical literature review with up-to-date findings. Foot (Edinb). 2011;21(2):66–70.
6. Kompel AJ, Roemer FW, Murakami AM, et al. Intra-articular corticosteroid injections in the hip and knee: perhaps not as safe as we thought? Radiology 2019; 293(3):656–63.
7. Cardone DA, Tallia AF. Joint and soft tissue injection. Am Fam Physician 2002; 66(2):283–8.
8. Halpern AA, Horowitz BG, Nagel DA. Tendon ruptures associated with corticosteroid therapy. West J Med 1977;127(5):378–82.
9. Pfenninger JL. Injections of joints and soft tissue: Part I. General guidelines. Am Fam Physician 1991;44(4):1196–202.
10. Honcharuk E, Monica J. Complications Associated with Intra-Articular and Extra-Articular Corticosteroid Injections. JBJS Rev 2016;4(12).
11. Sethi P, Treece J, Onweni C, et al. Antidote or Poison: A Case of Anaphylactic Shock After Intra-Articular Corticosteroid Injection. Cureus 2017;9(8):e1625.
12. Holland C, Jaeger L, Smentkowski U, et al. Septic and aseptic complications of corticosteroid injections: an assessment of 278 cases reviewed by expert commissions and mediation boards from 2005 to 2009. Dtsch Arztebl Int 2012; 109(24):425–30.
13. Kreuz PC, Steinwachs M, Angele P. Single-dose local anesthetics exhibit a type-, dose-, and time-dependent chondrotoxic effect on chondrocytes and cartilage: a systematic review of the current literature. Knee Surg Sports Traumatol Arthrosc 2018;26(3):819–30.
14. Zhang AZ, Ficklscherer A, Gülecyüz MF, et al. Cell Toxicity in Fibroblasts, Tenocytes, and Human Mesenchymal Stem Cells-A Comparison of Necrosis and Apoptosis-Inducing Ability in Ropivacaine, Bupivacaine, and Triamcinolone. Arthroscopy 2017;33(4):840–8.
15. Pelletier J-P, Raynauld J-P, Abram F, et al. Intra-articular corticosteroid knee injection induces a reduction in meniscal thickness with no treatment effect on cartilage volume: a case–control study. Scientific Rep 2020;10(1):13789.

16. Carofino B, Chowaniec DM, McCarthy MB, et al. Corticosteroids and local anesthetics decrease positive effects of platelet-rich plasma: an in vitro study on human tendon cells. Arthroscopy 2012;28(5):711–9.

17. Chang LR, Anand P, Varacallo M. Anatomy, Shoulder and Upper Limb, Glenohumeral Joint. In: StatPearls. Treasure Island: FL; 2021.

18. Berger JS, Dangaria HT. Joint Injections & Procedures. In: Maitin IB, Cruz E, editors. CURRENT diagnosis & treatment: physical medicine & Rehabilitation. New York, NY: McGraw-Hill Education; 2015.

19. Gross C, Dhawan A, Harwood D, et al. Glenohumeral joint injections: a review. Sports Health 2013;5(2):153–9.

20. Sage W, Pickup L, Smith TO, et al. The clinical and functional outcomes of ultrasound-guided vs landmark-guided injections for adults with shoulder pathology–a systematic review and meta-analysis. Rheumatology (Oxford) 2013; 52(4):743–51.

21. Song A, Higgins LD, Newman J, et al. Glenohumeral corticosteroid injections in adhesive capsulitis: a systematic search and review. Pm r 2014;6(12):1143–56.

22. Kim KH, Park JW, Kim SJ. High- vs Low-Dose Corticosteroid Injection in the Treatment of Adhesive Capsulitis with Severe Pain: A Randomized Controlled Double-Blind Study. Pain Med 2018;19(4):735–41.

23. Merolla G, Sperling JW, Paladini P, et al. Efficacy of Hylan G-F 20 versus 6-methylprednisolone acetate in painful shoulder osteoarthritis: a retrospective controlled trial. Musculoskelet Surg 2011;95(3):215–24.

24. Aslani H, Nourbakhsh ST, Zafarani Z, et al. Platelet-Rich Plasma for Frozen Shoulder: A Case Report. Arch Bone Jt Surg 2016;4(1):90–3.

25. Freitag JB, Barnard A. To evaluate the effect of combining photo-activation therapy with platelet-rich plasma injections for the novel treatment of osteoarthritis. BMJ Case Rep 2013;2013.

26. Barman A, Mukherjee S, Sahoo J, et al. Single Intra-articular Platelet-Rich Plasma Versus Corticosteroid Injections in the Treatment of Adhesive Capsulitis of the Shoulder: A Cohort Study. Am J Phys Med Rehabil 2019;98(7):549–57.

27. Centeno CJ, Al-Sayegh H, Bashir J, et al. A prospective multi-site registry study of a specific protocol of autologous bone marrow concentrate for the treatment of shoulder rotator cuff tears and osteoarthritis. J Pain Res 2015;8:269–76.

28. Daniels EW, Cole D, Jacobs B, et al. Existing Evidence on Ultrasound-Guided Injections in Sports Medicine. Orthop J Sports Med 2018;6(2). 2325967118756576.

29. Mattie R, Kennedy DJ. Importance of Image Guidance in Glenohumeral Joint Injections: Comparing Rates of Needle Accuracy Based on Approach and Physician Level of Training. Am J Phys Med Rehabil 2016;95(1):57–61.

30. Rutten MJCM, Collins JMP, Maresch BJ, et al. Glenohumeral joint injection: a comparative study of ultrasound and fluoroscopically guided techniques before MR arthrography. Eur Radiol 2009;19(3):722–30.

31. Amber KT, Landy DC, Amber I, et al. Comparing the accuracy of ultrasound versus fluoroscopy in glenohumeral injections: a systematic review and meta-analysis. J Clin Ultrasound 2014;42(7):411–6.

32. Daley EL, Bajaj S, Bisson LJ, et al. Improving injection accuracy of the elbow, knee, and shoulder: does injection site and imaging make a difference? A systematic review. Am J Sports Med 2011;39(3):656–62.

33. Bae JH, Park YS, Chang HJ, et al. Randomized controlled trial for efficacy of capsular distension for adhesive capsulitis: fluoroscopy-guided anterior versus

ultrasonography-guided posterolateral approach. Ann Rehabil Med 2014;38(3): 360–8.

34. Moore TS, Paffett CL, Sibbitt WL, et al. Glenohumeral Injection Using Anatomic Landmark Versus Sonographic Needle Guidance. bioRxiv 2018;395293.

35. Farmer KD, Hughes PM. MR Arthrography of the Shoulder. Am J Roentgenology 2002;178(2):433–4.

36. Lorbach O, Kieb M, Scherf C, et al. Good results after fluoroscopic-guided intra-articular injections in the treatment of adhesive capsulitis of the shoulder. Knee Surg Sports Traumatol Arthrosc 2010;18(10):1435–41.

37. Kennedy MS, Nicholson HD, Woodley SJ. Clinical anatomy of the subacromial and related shoulder bursae: A review of the literature. Clin Anat 2017;30(2): 213–26.

38. Varacallo M, El Bitar Y, Mair SD. Rotator Cuff Syndrome. Treasure Island (FL): StatPearls; 2021.

39. Fawcett R, Grainger A, Robinson P, et al. Ultrasound-guided subacromial-subdeltoid bursa corticosteroid injections: a study of short- and long-term outcomes. Clin Radiol 2018;73(8). 760.e767-760.e712.

40. Bhayana H, Mishra P, Tandon A, et al. Ultrasound guided versus landmark guided corticosteroid injection in patients with rotator cuff syndrome: Randomised controlled trial. J Clin Orthop Trauma 2018;9(Suppl 1):S80–5.

41. Penning LI, de Bie RA, Walenkamp GH. The effectiveness of injections of hyaluronic acid or corticosteroid in patients with subacromial impingement: a three-arm randomised controlled trial. J Bone Joint Surg Br 2012;94(9):1246–52.

42. Dadgostar H, Fahimipour F, Pahlevan Sabagh A, et al. Corticosteroids or platelet-rich plasma injections for rotator cuff tendinopathy: a randomized clinical trial study. J Orthopaedic Surg Res 2021;16(1):333.

43. Jo CH, Lee SY, Yoon KS, et al. Allogeneic Platelet-Rich Plasma Versus Corticosteroid Injection for the Treatment of Rotator Cuff Disease: A Randomized Controlled Trial. J Bone Joint Surg Am 2020;102(24):2129–37.

44. Kim SJ, Kim EK, Kim SJ, et al. Effects of bone marrow aspirate concentrate and platelet-rich plasma on patients with partial tear of the rotator cuff tendon. J Orthop Surg Res 2018;13(1):1.

45. Hee CK, Ju GS, Jin LH, et al. Comparision of Blind Technique and Ultrasonography Guided Technique of Subacromial Subdeltoid Bursa Injection. J Korean Acad Rehabil Med 2010;34(2):209–13.

46. Mathews PV, Glousman RE. Accuracy of subacromial injection: anterolateral versus posterior approach. J Shoulder Elbow Surg 2005;14(2):145–8.

47. Wu T, Song HX, Dong Y, et al. Ultrasound-guided versus blind subacromial-subdeltoid bursa injection in adults with shoulder pain: A systematic review and meta-analysis. Semin Arthritis Rheum 2015;45(3):374–8.

48. Hambly N, Fitzpatrick P, MacMahon P, et al. Rotator cuff impingement: correlation between findings on MRI and outcome after fluoroscopically guided subacromial bursography and steroid injection. AJR Am J Roentgenol 2007;189(5): 1179–84.

49. Flores DV, Goes PK, Gomez CM, et al. Imaging of the Acromioclavicular Joint: Anatomy, Function, Pathologic Features, and Treatment. Radiographics 2020; 40(5):1355–82.

50. Kurta I, Datir S, Dove M, et al. The short term effects of a single corticosteroid injection on the range of motion of the shoulder in patients with isolated acromioclavicular joint arthropathy. Acta Orthop Belg 2005;71(6):656–61.

51. Park KD, Kim TK, Lee J, et al. Palpation Versus Ultrasound-Guided Acromiocla-vicular Joint Intra-articular Corticosteroid Injections: A Retrospective Compara-tive Clinical Study. Pain Physician 2015;18(4):333–41.

52. Chaudhury S, Bavan L, Rupani N, et al. Managing acromio-clavicular joint pain: a scoping review. Shoulder Elbow 2018;10(1):4–14.

53. Ramesh Raja C, Sudhakar T, Jambukeswaran PST, et al. PRP in acromio-clavicular joint arthritis – A prospective analysis. IP Int J Orthopaedic Rheumatol 2021;6:80–3.

54. Freitag J, Wickham J, Shah K, et al. Effect of autologous adipose-derived mesenchymal stem cell therapy in the treatment of acromioclavicular joint oste-oarthritis. BMJ Case Rep 2019;12(2):e227865.

55. Scillia A, Issa K, McInerney VK, et al. Accuracy of in vivo palpation-guided acro-mioclavicular joint injection assessed with contrast material and fluoroscopic evaluations. Skeletal Radiol 2015;44(8):1135–9.

56. Sabeti-Aschraf M, Stotter C, Thaler C, et al. Intra-articular versus periarticular acromioclavicular joint injection: a multicenter, prospective, randomized, controlled trial. Arthroscopy 2013;29(12):1903–10.

57. Javed S, Sadozai Z, Javed A, et al. Should all acromioclavicular joint injections be performed under image guidance? J Orthop Surg (Hong Kong) 2017;25(3). 2309499017731633.

58. Gofeld M, Hurdle MF, Agur A. Biceps Tendon Sheath Injection: An Anatomical Conundrum. Pain Med 2019;20(1):138–42.

59. Sun Y, Liu S, Chen S, et al. The Effect of Corticosteroid Injection Into Rotator In-terval for Early Frozen Shoulder: A Randomized Controlled Trial. Am J Sports Med 2018;46(3):663–70.

60. Koraman E, Turkmen I, Uygur E, et al. A Multisite Injection Is More Effective Than a Single Glenohumeral Injection of Corticosteroid in the Treatment of Primary Frozen Shoulder: A Randomized Controlled Trial. Arthroscopy 2021;37(7): 2031–40.

61. Yektas A, Tug A, Gumus F, et al. [Effects of triple shoulder injection accompa-nied by fluoroscopy on pain experienced by patients with chronic shoulder pain]. Agri 2014;26(4):165–70.

62. Cuce I, Sencan S, Demir FU, et al. Efficacy of fluoroscopy-guided triple shoulder injection for older patients with nonspecific shoulder pain. Eur Geriatr Med 2019; 10(4):595–602.

63. Koh KH. Corticosteroid injection for adhesive capsulitis in primary care: a sys-tematic review of randomised clinical trials. Singapore Med J 2016;57(12): 646–57.

64. Cardone DA, Tallia AF. Diagnostic and therapeutic injection of the elbow region. Am Fam Physician 2002;66(11):2097–100.

65. Lopes RV, Furtado RNV, Parmigiani L, et al. Accuracy of intra-articular injections in peripheral joints performed blindly in patients with rheumatoid arthritis. Rheu-matology 2008;47(12):1792–4.

66. Brown EM Jr, Frain JB, Udell L, et al. Locally administered hydrocortisone in the rheumatic diseases; a summary of its use in 547 patients. Am J Med 1953;15(5): 656–65.

67. van Brakel RW, Eygendaal D. Intra-Articular Injection of Hyaluronic Acid Is Not Effective for the Treatment of Post-traumatic Osteoarthritis of the Elbow. Arthrosc The J Arthroscopic Relat Surg 2006;22(11):1199–203.

68. Cunnington J, Marshall N, Hide G, et al. A randomized, double-blind, controlled study of ultrasound-guided corticosteroid injection into the joint of patients with inflammatory arthritis. Arthritis Rheum 2010;62(7):1862–9.

69. Lohman M, Borrero C, Casagranda B, et al. The posterior transtriceps approach for elbow arthrography: a forgotten technique? Skeletal Radiol 2009;38(5):513–6.

70. van Wagenberg J-M, Turkenburg JL, Rahusen FTG, et al. The posterior transtriceps approach for intra-articular elbow diagnostics, definitely not forgotten. Skeletal Radiol 2013;42(1):55–9.

71. Vaquero-Picado A, Barco R, Antuña SA. Lateral epicondylitis of the elbow. EFORT Open Rev 2016;1(11):391–7.

72. Degen RM, Conti MS, Camp CL, et al. Epidemiology and Disease Burden of Lateral Epicondylitis in the USA: Analysis of 85,318 Patients. Hss j 2018;14(1):9–14.

73. Olaussen M, Holmedal O, Lindbaek M, et al. Treating lateral epicondylitis with corticosteroid injections or non-electrotherapeutical physiotherapy: a systematic review. BMJ Open 2013;3(10):e003564.

74. Smidt N, Assendelft WJ, van der Windt DA, et al. Corticosteroid injections for lateral epicondylitis: a systematic review. Pain 2002;96(1–2):23–40.

75. Coombes BK, Bisset L, Brooks P, et al. Effect of Corticosteroid Injection, Physiotherapy, or Both on Clinical Outcomes in Patients With Unilateral Lateral Epicondylalgia: A Randomized Controlled Trial. JAMA 2013;309(5):461–9.

76. Assendelft WJ, Hay EM, Adshead R, et al. Corticosteroid injections for lateral epicondylitis: a systematic overview. Br J Gen Pract 1996;46(405):209–16.

77. Xiong Y, Xue H, Zhou W, et al. Shock-wave therapy versus corticosteroid injection on lateral epicondylitis: a meta-analysis of randomized controlled trials. Phys Sportsmed 2019;47(3):284–9.

78. Petrella RJ, Cogliano A, Decaria J, et al. Management of Tennis Elbow with sodium hyaluronate periarticular injections. Sports Med Arthrosc Rehabil Ther Technol 2010;2:4.

79. Apaydin H, Bazancir Z, Altay Z. Injection Therapy in Patients with Lateral Epicondylalgia: Hyaluronic Acid or Dextrose Prolotherapy? A Single-Blind, Randomized Clinical Trial. J Altern Complement Med 2020;26(12):1169–75.

80. Kemp JA, Olson MA, Tao MA, et al. Platelet-Rich Plasma versus Corticosteroid Injection for the Treatment of Lateral Epicondylitis: A Systematic Review of Systematic Reviews. Int J Sports Phys Ther 2021;16(3):597–605.

81. Kwapisz A, Prabhakar S, Compagnoni R, et al. Platelet-Rich Plasma for Elbow Pathologies: a Descriptive Review of Current Literature. Curr Rev Musculoskelet Med 2018;11(4):598–606.

82. Mi B, Liu G, Zhou W, et al. Platelet rich plasma versus steroid on lateral epicondylitis: meta-analysis of randomized clinical trials. Phys Sportsmed 2017;45(2):97–104.

83. Hastie G, Soufi M, Wilson J, et al. Platelet rich plasma injections for lateral epicondylitis of the elbow reduce the need for surgical intervention. J Orthop 2018;15(1):239–41.

84. Simental-Mendía M, Vilchez-Cavazos F, Álvarez-Villalobos N, et al. Clinical efficacy of platelet-rich plasma in the treatment of lateral epicondylitis: a systematic review and meta-analysis of randomized placebo-controlled clinical trials. Clin Rheumatol 2020;39(8):2255–65.

85. Khoury M, Tabben M, Rolón AU, et al. Promising improvement of chronic lateral elbow tendinopathy by using adipose derived mesenchymal stromal cells: a pilot study. J Exp Orthop 2021;8(1):6.

86. Lee SY, Kim W, Lim C, et al. Treatment of Lateral Epicondylosis by Using Allogeneic Adipose-Derived Mesenchymal Stem Cells: A Pilot Study. Stem Cells 2015; 33(10):2995–3005.

87. Singh A, Gangwar DS, Singh S. Bone marrow injection: A novel treatment for tennis elbow. J Nat Sci Biol Med 2014;5(2):389–91.

88. Keijsers R, van den Bekerom M, Koenraadt K, et al. Injection of tennis elbow: Hit and miss? A cadaveric study of injection accuracy. Knee Surg Sports Traumatol Arthrosc 2016;25.

89. Evans JP, Metz J, Anaspure R, et al. The spread of Injectate after ultrasound-guided lateral elbow injection – a cadaveric study. J Exp Orthopaedics 2018; 5(1):27.

90. Gulabi D, Uysal MA, Akça A, et al. USG-guided injection of corticosteroid for lateral epicondylitis does not improve clinical outcomes: a prospective randomised study. Arch Orthop Trauma Surg 2017;137(5):601–6.

91. Malahias MA, Kaseta MK, Kazas ST, et al. Image-guided versus palpation-guided injections for the treatment of chronic lateral epicondylopathy: a randomized controlled clinical trial. Handchir Mikrochir Plast Chir 2018;50(5):348–52.

92. Zahn KV, Byerly DW. Medial Epicondyle Injection. In: StatPearls. Treasure Island: FL; 2021.

93. Stahl S, Kaufman T. The efficacy of an injection of steroids for medial epicondylitis. A prospective study of sixty elbows. J Bone Joint Surg Am 1997;79(11): 1648–52.

94. Bohlen HL, Schwartz ZE, Wu VJ, et al. Platelet-Rich Plasma Is an Equal Alternative to Surgery in the Treatment of Type 1 Medial Epicondylitis. Orthopaedic J Sports Med 2020;8(3). 2325967120908952.

95. Boden AL, Scott MT, Dalwadi PP, et al. Platelet-rich plasma versus Tenex in the treatment of medial and lateral epicondylitis. J Shoulder Elbow Surg 2019;28(1): 112–9.

96. Smith AG, Kosygan K, Williams H, et al. Common extensor tendon rupture following corticosteroid injection for lateral tendinosis of the elbow. Br J Sports Med 1999;33(6):423–4.

97. Murray PM, Adams JE, Lam J, et al. Disorders of the distal radioulnar joint. Instr Course Lect 2010;59:295–311.

98. Chidgey LK. The Distal Radioulnar Joint:Problems and Solutions. JAAOS - J Am Acad Orthopaedic Surgeons 1995;3(2):95–109.

99. Nam SH, Kim J, Lee JH, et al. Palpation versus ultrasound-guided corticosteroid injections and short-term effect in the distal radioulnar joint disorder: a randomized, prospective single-blinded study. Clin Rheumatol 2014;33(12):1807–14.

100. Fukui A, Yamada H, Yoshii T. Effect of Intraarticular Triamcinolone Acetonide Injection for Wrist Pain in Rheumatoid Arthritis Patients: A Statistical Investigation. J Hand Surg Asian Pac 2016;21(2):239–45.

101. Saied A, Heshmati A, Sadeghifar A, et al. Prophylactic corticosteroid injection in ulnar wrist pain in distal radius fracture. Indian J Orthop 2015;49(4):393–7.

102. Namazi H, Mehbudi A. Investigating the effect of intra-articular PRP injection on pain and function improvement in patients with distal radius fracture. Orthop Traumatol Surg Res 2016;102(1):47–52.

103. Smith J, Rizzo M, Sayeed YA, et al. Sonographically guided distal radioulnar joint injection: technique and validation in a cadaveric model. J Ultrasound Med 2011;30(11):1587–92.

104. Lomasney LM, Cooper RA. Distal radioulnar joint arthrography: simplified technique. Radiology 1996;199(1):278–9.

105. Gilula LA, Hardy DC, Totty WG. Distal radioulnar joint arthrography. AJR Am J Roentgenol 1988;150(4):864–6.

106. Gillis J, Calder K, Williams J. Review of thumb carpometacarpal arthritis classification, treatment and outcomes. Can J Plast Surg 2011;19(4):134–8.

107. Ladd AL, Weiss AP, Crisco JJ, et al. The thumb carpometacarpal joint: anatomy, hormones, and biomechanics. Instr Course Lect 2013;62:165–79.

108. Maarse W, Watts AC, Bain GI. Medium-term outcome following intra-articular corticosteroid injection in first CMC joint arthritis using fluoroscopy. Hand Surg 2009;14(2–3):99–104.

109. Joshi R. Intraarticular corticosteroid injection for first carpometacarpal osteoarthritis. J Rheumatol 2005;32(7):1305–6.

110. Meenagh GK, Patton J, Kynes C, et al. A randomised controlled trial of intra-articular corticosteroid injection of the carpometacarpal joint of the thumb in osteoarthritis. Ann Rheum Dis 2004;63(10):1260–3.

111. Di Sante L, Cacchio A, Scettri P, et al. Ultrasound-guided procedure for the treatment of trapeziometacarpal osteoarthritis. Clin Rheumatol 2011;30(9):1195–200.

112. Monfort J, Rotés-Sala D, Segalés N, et al. Comparative efficacy of intra-articular hyaluronic acid and corticoid injections in osteoarthritis of the first carpometacarpal joint: results of a 6-month single-masked randomized study. Joint Bone Spine 2015;82(2):116–21.

113. Stahl S, Karsh-Zafrir I, Ratzon N, et al. Comparison of intraarticular injection of depot corticosteroid and hyaluronic acid for treatment of degenerative trapeziometacarpal joints. J Clin Rheumatol 2005;11(6):299–302.

114. Fuchs S, Mönikes R, Wohlmeiner A, et al. Intra-articular hyaluronic acid compared with corticoid injections for the treatment of rhizarthrosis. Osteoarthritis Cartil 2006;14(1):82–8.

115. Tenti S, Pascarelli NA, Giannotti S, et al. Can hybrid hyaluronic acid represent a valid approach to treat rizoarthrosis? A retrospective comparative study. BMC Musculoskelet Disord 2017;18(1):444.

116. Heyworth BE, Lee JH, Kim PD, et al. Hylan versus corticosteroid versus placebo for treatment of basal joint arthritis: a prospective, randomized, double-blinded clinical trial. J Hand Surg Am 2008;33(1):40–8.

117. Loibl M, Lang S, Dendl LM, et al. Leukocyte-Reduced Platelet-Rich Plasma Treatment of Basal Thumb Arthritis: A Pilot Study. Biomed Res Int 2016;2016:9262909.

118. Medina-Porqueres I, Martin-Garcia P, Sanz-De Diego S, et al. Platelet-rich plasma for thumb carpometacarpal joint osteoarthritis in a professional pianist: case-based review. Rheumatol Int 2019;39(12):2167–75.

119. Malahias MA, Roumeliotis L, Nikolaou VS, et al. Platelet-Rich Plasma versus Corticosteroid Intra-Articular Injections for the Treatment of Trapeziometacarpal Arthritis: A Prospective Randomized Controlled Clinical Trial. Cartilage 2021;12(1):51–61.

120. Murphy MP, Buckley C, Sugrue C, et al. ASCOT: Autologous Bone Marrow Stem Cell Use for Osteoarthritis of the Thumb-First Carpometacarpal Joint. Plast Reconstr Surg Glob Open 2017;5(9):e1486.

121. Centeno CJ, Freeman MD. Percutaneous injection of autologous, culture-expanded mesenchymal stem cells into carpometacarpal hand joints: a case series with an untreated comparison group. Wien Med Wochenschr 2014; 164(5–6):83–7.

122. Erne HC, Cerny MK, Ehrl D, et al. Autologous Fat Injection versus Lundborg Resection Arthroplasty for the Treatment of Trapeziometacarpal Joint Osteoarthritis. Plast Reconstr Surg 2018;141(1):119–24.

123. Haas EM, Eisele A, Arnoldi A, et al. One-Year Outcomes of Intraarticular Fat Transplantation for Thumb Carpometacarpal Joint Osteoarthritis: Case Review of 99 Joints. Plast Reconstr Surg 2020;145(1):151–9.

124. Pollard MA, Cermak MB, Buck WR, et al. Accuracy of injection into the basal joint of the thumb. Am J Orthop (Belle Mead Nj) 2007;36(4):204–6.

125. To P, McClary KN, Sinclair MK, et al. The Accuracy of Common Hand Injections With and Without Ultrasound: An Anatomical Study. Hand (N Y). 2017;12(6): 591–6.

126. Gershkovich GE, Boyadjian H, Conti Mica M. The Effect of Image-Guided Corticosteroid Injections on Thumb Carpometacarpal Arthritis. Hand (N Y). 2021; 16(1):86–92.

127. Hazani R, Engineer NJ, Cooney D, et al. Anatomic landmarks for the first dorsal compartment. Eplasty 2008;8:e53.

128. Rowland P, Phelan N, Gardiner S, et al. The Effectiveness of Corticosteroid Injection for De Quervain's Stenosing Tenosynovitis (DQST): A Systematic Review and Meta-Analysis. Open Orthop J 2015;9:437–44.

129. Oh JK, Messing S, Hyrien O, et al. Effectiveness of Corticosteroid Injections for Treatment of de Quervain's Tenosynovitis. Hand (N Y) 2017;12(4):357–61.

130. Ippolito JA, Hauser S, Patel J, et al. Nonsurgical Treatment of De Quervain Tenosynovitis: A Prospective Randomized Trial. Hand (N Y). 2020;15(2):215–9.

131. Peters-Veluthamaningal C, Winters JC, Groenier KH, et al. Randomised controlled trial of local corticosteroid injections for de Quervain's tenosynovitis in general practice. BMC Musculoskelet Disord 2009;10(1):131.

132. Orlandi D, Corazza A, Fabbro E, et al. Ultrasound-guided percutaneous injection to treat de Quervain's disease using three different techniques: a randomized controlled trial. Eur Radiol 2015;25(5):1512–9.

133. Peck E, Ely E. Successful treatment of de Quervain tenosynovitis with ultrasound-guided percutaneous needle tenotomy and platelet-rich plasma injection: a case presentation. Pm r 2013;5(5):438–41.

134. El-Rahim MDE. The Role of Platelet Rich Plasma in Comparison with Corticosteroids in the Treatment of De Quervain Tenosynovitis. The Med J Cairo Univ 2020; 88:141–8.

135. Richie CA 3rd, Briner WW Jr. Corticosteroid injection for treatment of de Quervain's tenosynovitis: a pooled quantitative literature evaluation. J Am Board Fam Pract 2003;16(2):102–6.

136. McDermott JD, Ilyas AM, Nazarian LN, et al. Ultrasound-guided injections for de Quervain's tenosynovitis. Clin Orthop Relat Res 2012;470(7):1925–31.

137. Danda RS, Kamath J, Jayasheelan N, et al. Role of Guided Ultrasound in the Treatment of De Quervain Tenosynovitis by Local Steroid Infiltration. J Hand Microsurg 2016;8(1):34–7.

138. Kutsikovich J, Merrell G. Accuracy of Injection Into the First Dorsal Compartment: A Cadaveric Ultrasound Study. J Hand Surg Am 2018;43(8):777.e771–5.

139. Mahakkanukrauh P, Mahakkanukrauh C. Incidence of a septum in the first dorsal compartment and its effects on therapy of de Quervain's disease. Clin Anat 2000;13(3):195–8.

140. Byrne DP, Mulhall KJ, Baker JF. Anatomy & biomechanics of the hip. The open Sports Med J 2010;4(1).

141. Ross JA, Greenwood AC, Sasser P III, et al. Periarticular injections in knee and hip arthroplasty: where and what to inject. The J arthroplasty 2017;32(9): S77–80.

142. Zhao Z, Ma J-x, Ma X-l. Different intra-articular injections as therapy for hip osteoarthritis: a systematic review and network meta-analysis. Arthrosc The J Arthroscopic Relat Surg 2020;36(5):1452–64. e1452.

143. McCabe PS, Maricar N, Parkes MJ, et al. The efficacy of intra-articular steroids in hip osteoarthritis: a systematic review. Osteoarthritis and Cartilage 2016; 24(9):1509–17.

144. Mauro GL, Sanfilippo A, Scaturro D. The effectiveness of intra-articular injections of Hyalubrix® combined with exercise therapy in the treatment of hip osteoarthritis. Clin Cases Mineral Bone Metab 2017;14(2):146.

145. Migliore A, Granata M, Tormenta S, et al. Hip viscosupplementation under ultrasound guidance riduces NSAID consumption in symptomatic hip osteoarthritis patients in a long follow-up. Data from Italian registry. Eur Rev Med Pharmacol Sci 2011;15(1):25–34.

146. Chandrasekaran S, Lodhia P, Suarez-Ahedo C, et al. Symposium: evidence for the use of intra-articular cortisone or hyaluronic acid injection in the hip. J hip preservation Surg 2015;3(1):5–15.

147. Kolasinski SL, Neogi T, Hochberg MC, et al. 2019 American College of Rheumatology/Arthritis Foundation guideline for the management of osteoarthritis of the hand, hip, and knee. Arthritis Rheum 2020;72(2):220–33.

148. Atchia I, Kane D, Reed MR, et al. Efficacy of a single ultrasound-guided injection for the treatment of hip osteoarthritis. Ann Rheum Dis 2011;70(1):110–6.

149. Qvistgaard E, Christensen R, Torp-Pedersen S, et al. Intra-articular treatment of hip osteoarthritis: a randomized trial of hyaluronic acid, corticosteroid, and isotonic saline. Osteoarthritis and cartilage 2006;14(2):163–70.

150. Richette P, Ravaud P, Conrozier T, et al. Effect of hyaluronic acid in symptomatic hip osteoarthritis: A multicenter, randomized, placebo-controlled trial. Arthritis Rheum Official J Am Coll Rheumatol 2009;60(3):824–30.

151. Ye Y, Zhou X, Mao S, et al. Platelet rich plasma versus hyaluronic acid in patients with hip osteoarthritis: a meta-analysis of randomized controlled trials. Int J Of Surg 2018;53:279–87.

152. McInnis KC, Chen ET, Finnoff JT, et al. Orthobiologics for the hip region: a narrative review. PM&R. 2020;12(10):1045–54.

153. Ziv YB, Kardosh R, Debi R, et al. An inexpensive and accurate method for hip injections without the use of imaging. JCR: J Clin Rheumatol 2009;15(3):103–5.

154. Leopold SS, Battista V, Oliverio JA. Safety and efficacy of intraarticular hip injection using anatomic landmarks. Clin Orthopaedics Relat Research® 2001;391: 192–7.

155. Dıraçoğlu D, Alptekin K, Dikici F, et al. Evaluation of needle positioning during blind intra-articular hip injections for osteoarthritis: fluoroscopy versus arthrography. Arch Phys Med Rehabil 2009;90(12):2112–5.

156. Hoeber S, Aly A-R, Ashworth N, et al. Ultrasound-guided hip joint injections are more accurate than landmark-guided injections: a systematic review and meta-analysis. Br J Sports Med 2016;50(7):392–6.

157. Finnoff JT, Hall MM, Adams E, et al. American Medical Society for Sports Medicine position statement: interventional musculoskeletal ultrasound in sports medicine. Clin J Sport Med 2015;25(1):6–22.

158. Kane D, Koski J. Musculoskeletal interventional procedures: With or without imaging guidance? Best Pract Res Clin Rheumatol 2016;30(4):736–50.

159. Furtado RNV, Pereira DF, Luz KRd, et al. Effectiveness of imaging-guided intra-articular injection: a comparison study between fluoroscopy and ultrasound. Revista Brasileira de Reumatologia 2013;53:476–82.

160. Byrd JT, Potts EA, Allison RK, et al. Ultrasound-guided hip injections: a comparative study with fluoroscopy-guided injections. Arthrosc The J Arthroscopic Relat Surg 2014;30(1):42–6.

161. Subedi N, Chew N, Chandramohan M, et al. Effectiveness of fluoroscopy-guided intra-articular steroid injection for hip osteoarthritis. Clin Radiol 2015;70(11):1276–80.

162. Deshmukh AJ, Thakur RR, Goyal A, et al. Accuracy of diagnostic injection in differentiating source of atypical hip pain. The J arthroplasty 2010;25(6):129–33.

163. Brinks A, van Rijn RM, Willemsen SP, et al. Corticosteroid injections for greater trochanteric pain syndrome: a randomized controlled trial in primary care. The Ann Fam Med 2011;9(3):226–34.

164. Begkas D, Chatzopoulos S-T, Touzopoulos P, et al. Ultrasound-guided platelet-rich plasma application versus corticosteroid injections for the treatment of greater trochanteric pain syndrome: a prospective controlled randomized comparative clinical study. Cureus 2020;12(1).

165. Williams BS, Cohen SP. Greater trochanteric pain syndrome: a review of anatomy, diagnosis and treatment. Anesth Analg 2009;108(5):1662–70.

166. Ali M, Oderuth E, Atchia I, et al. The use of platelet-rich plasma in the treatment of greater trochanteric pain syndrome: a systematic literature review. J hip preservation Surg 2018;5(3):209–19.

167. Henderson RG, Colberg RE. Pure bone marrow aspirate injection for chronic greater trochanteric pain syndrome: a case report. Pain Manag 2018;8(4):271–5.

168. Mu A, Peng P, Agur A. Landmark-guided and ultrasound-guided approaches for trochanteric bursa injection: a cadaveric study. Anesth Analg 2017;124(3):966–71.

169. Cohen MM, Altman RD, Hollstrom R, et al. Safety and efficacy of intra-articular sodium hyaluronate (Hyalgan®) in a randomized, double-blind study for osteoarthritis of the ankle. Foot Ankle Int 2008;29(7):657–63.

170. Cohen S, Narvaez J, Lebovits A, et al. Corticosteroid injections for trochanteric bursitis: is fluoroscopy necessary? A pilot study. Br J Anaesth 2005;94(1):100–6.

171. Mitchell WG, Kettwich SC, Sibbitt WL, et al. Outcomes and cost-effectiveness of ultrasound-guided injection of the trochanteric bursa. Rheumatol Int 2018;38(3):393–401.

172. Kurup H, Ward P. Do we need radiological guidance for hip joint injections? Acta orthopaedica Belgica 2010;76(2):205.

173. Cohen SP, Strassels SA, Foster L, et al. Comparison of fluoroscopically guided and blind corticosteroid injections for greater trochanteric pain syndrome: multicentre randomised controlled trial. Bmj 2009;338.

174. Jüni P, Hari R, Rutjes AW, et al. Intra-articular corticosteroid for knee osteoarthritis. Cochrane Database Syst Rev 2015;(10).

175. Maricar N, Parkes MJ, Callaghan MJ, et al. Structural predictors of response to intra-articular steroid injection in symptomatic knee osteoarthritis. Arthritis Res Ther 2017;19(1):1–10.

176. Wernecke C, Braun HJ, Dragoo JL. The effect of intra-articular corticosteroids on articular cartilage: a systematic review. Orthopaedic J Sports Med 2015; 3(5). 2325967115581163.

177. Rutjes AW, Jüni P, da Costa BR, et al. Viscosupplementation for osteoarthritis of the knee: a systematic review and meta-analysis. Ann Intern Med 2012;157(3): 180–91.

178. Di Martino A, Di Matteo B, Papio T, et al. Platelet-Rich Plasma Versus Hyaluronic Acid Injections for the Treatment of Knee Osteoarthritis: Results at 5 Years of a Double-Blind, Randomized Controlled Trial. Am J Sports Med 2019;47(2): 347–54.

179. Raeissadat SA, Rayegani SM, Hassanabadi H, et al. Knee osteoarthritis injection choices: platelet-rich plasma (PRP) versus hyaluronic acid (a one-year randomized clinical trial). Clin Med Insights: Arthritis Musculoskelet Disord 2015;8. CMAMD. S17894.

180. Patel S, Dhillon MS, Aggarwal S, et al. Treatment with platelet-rich plasma is more effective than placebo for knee osteoarthritis: a prospective, double-blind, randomized trial. The Am J Sports Med 2013;41(2):356–64.

181. Sánchez M, Anitua E, Azofra J, et al. Intra-articular injection of an autologous preparation rich in growth factors for the treatment of knee OA: a retrospective cohort study. Clin Exp Rheumatol 2008;26(5):910–3.

182. Kon E, Mandelbaum B, Buda R, et al. Platelet-rich plasma intra-articular injection versus hyaluronic acid viscosupplementation as treatments for cartilage pathology: from early degeneration to osteoarthritis. Arthrosc The J Arthroscopic Relat Surg 2011;27(11):1490–501.

183. Riboh JC, Saltzman BM, Yanke AB, et al. Effect of leukocyte concentration on the efficacy of platelet-rich plasma in the treatment of knee osteoarthritis. The Am J Sports Med 2016;44(3):792–800.

184. Forogh B, Mianehsaz E, Shoaee S, et al. Effect of single injection of platelet-rich plasma in comparison with corticosteroid on knee osteoarthritis: a double-blind randomized clinical trial. J Sports Med Phys Fitness 2016;56(7–8):901–8.

185. Elksniņš-Finogejevs A, Vidal L, Peredistijs A. Intra-articular platelet-rich plasma vs corticosteroids in the treatment of moderate knee osteoarthritis: a single-center prospective randomized controlled study with a 1-year follow up. J orthopaedic Surg Res 2020;15(1):1–10.

186. Pas HI, Winters M, Haisma HJ, et al. Stem cell injections in knee osteoarthritis: a systematic review of the literature. Br J Sports Med 2017;51(15):1125–33.

187. Lamo-Espinosa JM, Blanco JF, Sánchez M, et al. Phase II multicenter randomized controlled clinical trial on the efficacy of intra-articular injection of autologous bone marrow mesenchymal stem cells with platelet rich plasma for the treatment of knee osteoarthritis. J translational Med 2020;18(1):1–9.

188. Iijima H, Isho T, Kuroki H, et al. Effectiveness of mesenchymal stem cells for treating patients with knee osteoarthritis: a meta-analysis toward the establishment of effective regenerative rehabilitation. NPJ Regenerative Med 2018; 3(1):1–13.

189. Rodríguez-Merchán EC. Intra-articular injections of mesenchymal stem cells for knee osteoarthritis. Am J Orthop (Belle Mead NJ). 2014 Dec;43(12):E282–91. PMID: 25490014.

190. Kim SH, Ha C-W, Park Y-B, et al. Intra-articular injection of mesenchymal stem cells for clinical outcomes and cartilage repair in osteoarthritis of the knee: a meta-analysis of randomized controlled trials. Arch orthopaedic Trauma Surg 2019;139(7):971–80.
191. Wagner BS, Howe AS, Dexter WW, et al. Tolerability and efficacy of 3 approaches to intra-articular corticosteroid injections of the knee for osteoarthritis: a randomized controlled trial. Orthopaedic J Sports Med 2015;3(8). 2325967115600687.
192. Berkoff DJ, Miller LE, Block JE. Clinical utility of ultrasound guidance for intra-articular knee injections: a review. Clin interventions Aging 2012;7:89.
193. Hall MM. The accuracy and efficacy of palpation versus image-guided peripheral injections in sports medicine. Curr Sports Med Rep 2013;12(5):296–303.
194. Sibbitt WL Jr, Band PA, Kettwich LG, et al. A randomized controlled trial evaluating the cost-effectiveness of sonographic guidance for intra-articular injection of the osteoarthritic knee. JCR: J Clin Rheumatol 2011;17(8):409–15.
195. Helfenstein M Jr, Kuromoto J. Anserine syndrome. Revista brasileira de reumatologia 2010;50:313–27.
196. Sarifakioglu B, Afsar SI, Yalbuzdag SA, et al. Comparison of the efficacy of physical therapy and corticosteroid injection in the treatment of pes anserine tendino-bursitis. J Phys Ther Sci 2016;28(7):1993–7.
197. Yoon HS, Kim SE, Suh YR, et al. Correlation between ultrasonographic findings and the response to corticosteroid injection in pes anserinus tendinobursitis syndrome in knee osteoarthritis patients. J Korean Med Sci 2005;20(1):109–12.
198. Rowicki K, Płomiński J, Bachta A. Evaluation of the effectiveness of platelet rich plasma in treatment of chronic pes anserinus pain syndrome. Ortopedia, traumatologia, rehabilitacja 2014;16(3):307–18.
199. Karabaş Ç, Çaliş HT, Topaloğlu US, et al. Effects of ultrasound guided leukocyte-rich platelet-rich plasma (LR-PRP) injection in patients with pes anserinus tendinobursitis. Transfus Apher Sci 2021;103048.
200. Finnoff JT, Nutz DJ, Henning PT, et al. Accuracy of ultrasound-guided versus unguided pes anserinus bursa injections. PM&R. 2010;2(8):732–9.
201. Lee JH, Lee JU, Yoo SW. Accuracy and efficacy of ultrasound-guided pes anserinus bursa injection. J Clin Ultrasound 2019;47(2):77–82.
202. Gardner E, Gray D. The innervation of the joints of the foot. The Anatomical Rec 1968;161(2):141–8.
203. Vannabouathong C, Del Fabbro G, Sales B, et al. Intra-articular injections in the treatment of symptoms from ankle arthritis: a systematic review. Foot Ankle Int 2018;39(10):1141–50.
204. DeGroot H III, Uzunishvili S, Weir R, et al. Intra-articular injection of hyaluronic acid is not superior to saline solution injection for ankle arthritis: a randomized, double-blind, placebo-controlled study. JBJS 2012;94(1):2–8.
205. Fukawa T, Yamaguchi S, Akatsu Y, et al. Safety and efficacy of intra-articular injection of platelet-rich plasma in patients with ankle osteoarthritis. Foot Ankle Int 2017;38(6):596–604.
206. Mei-Dan O, Carmont MR, Laver L, et al. Platelet-rich plasma or hyaluronate in the management of osteochondral lesions of the talus. The Am J Sports Med 2012;40(3):534–41.
207. Emadedin M, GHORBANI LM, Fazeli R, et al. Long-term follow-up of intra-articular injection of autologous mesenchymal stem cells in patients with knee, ankle, or hip osteoarthritis. 2015.

208. Goncalves B, Ambrosio C, Serra S, et al. US-guided interventional joint procedures in patients with rheumatic diseases—When and how we do it? Eur J Radiol 2011;79(3):407–14.

209. Dyck DD Jr, Boyajian-O'Neill LA. Plantar fasciitis. Clin J Sport Med 2004;14(5): 305–9.

210. David JA, Sankarapandian V, Christopher PR, et al. Injected corticosteroids for treating plantar heel pain in adults. Cochrane Database Syst Rev 2017;(6).

211. Kim C, Cashdollar MR, Mendicino RW, et al. Incidence of plantar fascia ruptures following corticosteroid injection. Foot & ankle specialist 2010;3(6):335–7.

212. Whittaker GA, Munteanu SE, Menz HB, et al. Corticosteroid injection for plantar heel pain: a systematic review and meta-analysis. BMC Musculoskelet Disord 2019;20(1):1–22.

213. Raeissadat SA, Nouri F, Darvish M, et al. Ultrasound-guided injection of high molecular weight hyaluronic acid versus corticosteroid in management of plantar fasciitis: A 24-week randomized clinical trial. J pain Res 2020;13:109.

214. Kumai T, Samoto N, Hasegawa A, et al. Short-term efficacy and safety of hyaluronic acid injection for plantar fasciopathy. Knee Surg Sports Traumatol Arthrosc 2018;26(3):903–11.

215. Hohmann E, Tetsworth K, Glatt V. Platelet-Rich Plasma Versus Corticosteroids for the Treatment of Plantar Fasciitis: A Systematic Review and Meta-analysis. The Am J Sports Med 2021;49(5):1381–93.

216. Hurley ET, Shimozono Y, Hannon CP, et al. Platelet-rich plasma versus corticosteroids for plantar fasciitis: a systematic review of randomized controlled trials. Orthopaedic J Sports Med 2020;8(4). 2325967120915704.

217. Yucel I, Yazici B, Degirmenci E, et al. Comparison of ultrasound-, palpation-, and scintigraphy-guided steroid injections in the treatment of plantar fasciitis. Arch Orthop Trauma Surg 2009;129(5):695–701.

218. Li Z, Xia C, Yu A, et al. Ultrasound-versus palpation-guided injection of corticosteroid for plantar fasciitis: a meta-analysis. PloS one 2014;9(3):e92671.

219. Mautner K, Malanga GA, Smith J, et al. A call for a standard classification system for future biologic research: the rationale for new PRP nomenclature. PM&R. 2015;7(4):S53–9.

Trigger Point Injections

Malathy Appasamy, MBBS[a], Christopher Lam, MD[b], John Alm, DO[c],
Andrea L. Chadwick, MD, MSc, FASA[d],*

KEYWORDS

- Myofascial pain • Piriformis syndrome • Trigger point injection • Botulinum toxin
- Corticosteroid • Local anesthetic

KEY POINTS

- Trigger points are localized painful areas of skeletal muscle containing taut bands that can be exquisitely sensitive to digital pressure.
- Conservative treatment of myofascial pain is recommended; however, if this fails to relieve pain, then trigger point injections can be considered.
- Trigger point injections should be part of a multidisciplinary treatment program that includes physical therapy.
- Trigger point injections are commonly done with local anesthetic with or without corticosteroid, botulinum toxin, or without injectate (dry needling).
- The growing accessibility of imaging, including ultrasound and fluoroscopy, has improved available options for safe injection technique to myofascial trigger points.

INTRODUCTION

Myofascial pain is a common cause of acute and chronic pain. The term "myofascial pain" encompasses many different painful conditions and can exist independently of other pain generators, known as primary myofascial pain. Common primary myofascial pain diagnoses include piriformis syndrome, iliopsoas-related pain, and pain related to compression of the brachial plexus by the scalene muscles (neurogenic thoracic outlet syndrome). Frequently, myofascial pain coexists with or is secondary to other acute and chronic painful musculoskeletal conditions including (1) head and neck disorders (temporomandibular disorders, cervical degenerative disc disease, cervical facet arthropathy, neck pain after whiplash injury, cervicobrachial syndrome, and cervicogenic or chronic tension-type headache); (2) thoracolumbar back

[a] Department of Physical Medicine & Rehabilitation, Main Line Health System, 600 Evergreen Drive, 2nd Floor, Glen Mills, PA 19342, USA; [b] Department of Anesthesiology, University of Kansas School of Medicine, 3901 Rainbow Boulevard, Kansas City, KS 66160, USA; [c] Department of Physical Medicine & Rehabilitation, University of Kansas School of Medicine, 3901 Rainbow Boulevard, Kansas City, KS 66160, USA; [d] Department of Anesthesiology, University of Kansas School of Medicine, 3901 Rainbow Boulevard, MailStop 1034, Kansas City, KS 66160, USA
* Corresponding author.
E-mail address: anicol@kumc.edu

Phys Med Rehabil Clin N Am 33 (2022) 307–333
https://doi.org/10.1016/j.pmr.2022.01.011
1047-9651/22/© 2022 Elsevier Inc. All rights reserved.
pmr.theclinics.com

disorders (degenerative disc disease, kyphosis, scoliosis, and lumbar facet arthropathy); (3) pelvic pain; and (4) upper and lower extremity pain disorders. Myofascial pain is most effectively treated with a multimodal treatment plan including injection therapy (known as trigger point injections [TPIs]), physical therapy, postural or ergonomic correction, and treatment of underlying musculoskeletal pain generators.

The objectives of this review are to describe the known pathophysiology of myofascial pain and trigger points (TrPs), discuss the clinical presentation of myofascial pain and piriformis syndrome, an extremely common primary myofascial pain disorder, describe best practices for TPI and piriformis muscle injection therapy, and outline the current data for TPI therapy with local anesthetic and/or steroids and botulinum toxin.

NATURE OF THE PROBLEM: THE PATHOPHYSIOLOGY OF MYOFASCIAL PAIN AND TrPs

Although much remains to be discovered about the pathophysiology of myofascial pain, several mechanistic theories have been advanced in recent years. Certainly, as with most chronic pain conditions, the biopsychosocial model of pain pathophysiology applies.[1] Underlying biomechanical and postural factors may interact with neurologic factors, psychological elements including depression and anxiety, and hormonal and nutritional imbalances. These factors, in total or in part, may lead to peripheral sensitization, autonomic dysregulation, and central sensitization, which then amplifies the pain experienced by patients with myofascial pain. Vasoactive mediators, pronociceptive neurotransmitters, and inflammatory mediators including bradykinin, norepinephrine, serotonin, calcitonin gene–related peptide, substance P, tumor necrosis factor α, and interleukin-1β have all been identified in the hypersensitive loci of TrPs.[2–4] These substances are pronociceptive and sensitize peripheral nociceptors. In a sensitized state, nociceptors spontaneously discharge with a lower threshold to painful stimulation and also exhibit discharge to nonpainful stimuli.[5] Over time, this heightened abnormal peripheral sensory input creates a state of central neuronal sensitization.[6] The hypothalamus-pituitary-adrenocortical and sympathetic-adrenal-medullary system responses to experimentally induced stress in patients with myofascial pain has shown that plasma concentrations of cortisol, epinephrine, and norepinephrine were found to be significantly increased in myofascial pain patients than in healthy controls.[7]

CLINICAL PRESENTATION AND DIAGNOSIS
Myofascial Pain

A careful history and physical examination remain the keystone of diagnosis. As discussed previously, TrPs are localized painful areas of skeletal muscle containing taut bands that can be exquisitely sensitive to digital pressure (**Fig. 1**). TrPs may be active or latent. Active TrPs are present in patients with painful regional conditions. Latent TrPs are asymptomatic but may be revealed by deep palpation on physical examination. Latent TrPs are very common and have been identified in the shoulder girdle muscles of 45% to 55% of healthy young adults.[8] TrPs are different from tender points, which are defined as a localized area of tenderness in a muscle, muscle-tendon junction, fat pad, or bursal region.[9] Myofascial pain may occur after an injury, with chronic strain from repetitive microtrauma, or without any clear precipitating event. Aberrant body mechanics or postural abnormality may initiate or further maintain the problem. The quality of pain tends to be a deep "aching" of variable intensity and the pain is generally confined to a specific anatomic region. Characteristic referred pain patterns are associated with specific muscles, although these referral

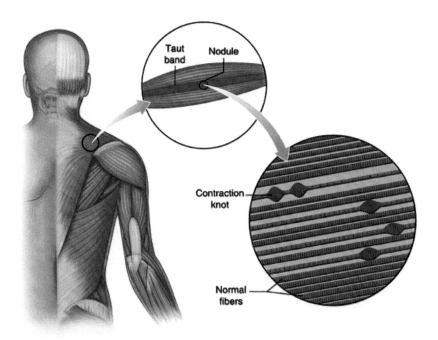

Trigger point complex

Fig. 1. Schematic of the anatomy of a taut band and trigger point.

patterns are often unreliable.[10] Commonly involved TrP musculature include the trapezius, splenii, cervical and lumbar paraspinal, piriformis, and quadratus lumborum.

Simons and colleagues have developed a set of diagnostic criteria that are often referenced when describing the features of TrPs including presence of taut band, tenderness from taut band, reproducibility of pain, local twitch response, restricted range of motion, autonomic symptoms, and referred pain.[11] Furthermore, palpation of an active TrP can cause referred pain through activation of the central nervous system along the distribution of the nerve innervating the muscle that is activated.[12]

It is essential to have hands-on training in the physical examination of myofascial pain and TrPs.[13] Musculoskeletal examination should be performed with the objective of identifying possible orthopedic or neurologic pathologies that could have a role in generating secondary myofascial pain and dysfunction. A distinct pattern of TrP findings may reveal itself in myofascial pain syndrome after a given insult.[14] These painful TrPs limit full range of passive motion in the afflicted muscle group. Although these findings have been suggested as diagnostic criteria,[15–17] investigators have found it problematic to demonstrate consistent agreement in the presence or absence of TrPs among examiners in blinded studies with control groups.[18–20] Discrepancies in diagnosis may be attributed in part to a lack of a standardized examination technique as well as variability in the interpretation of examination findings. Furthermore, variations in muscle anatomy, physical conditioning, and deconditioning can pose obstacles to proper diagnosis as well. The most reproducible diagnostic findings on physical examination include identification of a TrP in an affected muscle, referral of pain to a zone of reference, and reproduction of the patient's regular pain on physical examination.[21]

Differential diagnosis of myofascial pain should include (1) musculoskeletal and neuropathic disorders such as arthritis, degenerative disk disease, radiculopathy, bursitis, and tendonitis; (2) autoimmune or infectious etiologies; (3) metabolic and endocrine dysfunction; (4) psychiatric disorders including depression and anxiety; and (5) fibromyalgia or diffuse amplified musculoskeletal pain.

Imaging studies have only recently demonstrated anatomic changes associated with TrPs. Ultrasound (US) examination in combination with Doppler blood flow has been reported to allow visualization of TrPs, and US imaging can help direct muscle injection techniques. Recently developed techniques using magnetic resonance and US elastography purport to reveal changes in intramuscular signal consistent with TrPs, but the use of this technology in clinical practice has not yet been validated.[22,23]

Piriformis Syndrome

Piriformis syndrome consists of pain in the buttock with or without radiation in the distribution of the ipsilateral sciatic nerve. It is considered the principal pain generator in approximately 8% of patients presenting with the buttock as the origin of pain. The syndrome can be a consequence of an abnormal relationship between the sciatic nerve and the piriformis muscle that results in irritation of the sciatic nerve. A hypertrophic muscle, infection, or invasion of the muscle by tumor can cause pressure or irritation on the nerve.[24,25] In 78% to 84% of the population, the sciatic nerve passes in front of the muscle. In 12% to 21% of individuals, the divided nerve passes through or posterior to the piriformis and is exposed to muscle contractions, which trigger sciatic symptoms.[24]

There is no consensus set of diagnostic criteria and is often diagnosed from a history indicative of this condition with confirmatory physical examination with an often normal electrodiagnostic testing and imaging.[26] The syndrome should be considered in patients who have buttock pain, tenderness to palpation over the piriformis muscle, and possible symptoms of sciatic nerve pain. In addition, positive response to provocative maneuvers may indicate the diagnosis, including the following: specific confirmatory physical examination testing for piriformis syndrome includes the active piriformis test, the Beatty test, the FAIR test, and the Pace test.[26]

PATIENT SELECTION
Trigger Point Injection

TPI is a widely used invasive therapy wherein a needle is guided directly into a TrP that has been previously identified on physical examination. TPI is best used as part of a comprehensive multimodal treatment plan. This strategy can be particularly beneficial when TPI is initially used to reduce pain in patients otherwise intolerant of physical therapy or stretching, allowing the physical modalities to be more effective.[27] TPIs should be considered in patients once a thorough evaluation is completed to rule out other causes of back pain including muscle strain, axial back pain, structural causes of pain, discogenic back pain, vertebrogenic back pain, spinal stenosis, vertebral body disease (including fracture), and radicular back pain.

Piriformis Muscle Injection

As discussed previously, piriformis syndrome is a condition associated with low back pain where the traversing sciatic nerve is compressed by the sciatic nerve. Once diagnosed, patients can be treated with conservative management first, including pharmacologic therapy and physical therapy. If pain persists after conservative management, it is reasonable to trial a piriformis muscle injection.

Risks and Contraindications

The following conditions are contraindications to TPI and piriformis muscle injection: (1) infection, systemic or localized (absolute); (2) coagulopathy (relative); (3) distorted or complicated anatomy (relative); and (4) patient refusal (absolute).[28] According to the anticoagulation guidelines from the American Society of Regional Anesthesia and Pain Medicine, TPIs classify as a low-risk procedure.[28]

TPIs are commonly performed as an outpatient procedure. Although serious complications are rare, there have been case reports of complications particularly in the cervical and thoracic region.

The most commonly reported serious complication is pneumothorax.[29-31] A case series of 38 patients developed pneumothorax after acupuncture or acupoint insertion with one death from pneumothorax in the series.[32] Specific attention to TrP technique and use of ultrasound guidance can help avoid this complication in the cervical and thoracic injections.[33,34] Management of iatrogenic pneumothorax depends on size of the pneumothorax and symptoms and can range from observation, oxygen supplementation and close monitoring to ultrasound or CT-guided aspiration and tube thoracotomy.[35,36]

Rare possibility of intrathecal injection has been reported in a 28-year-old woman after superficial trapezius TPI.[37] This patient developed respiratory depression and pneumocephalus requiring emergency tracheal intubation and ventilatory support and fully recovered over the course of 24 hours. There has been another case report of cervical epidural abscess that has been reported.[38]

Skeletal muscle myotoxicity has been demonstrated in experimental studies with the use of local anesthetic agents as they cause reversible myonecrosis. Histologic changes include hypercontracted myofibrils followed by lytic degeneration of striated muscle sarcoplasmic reticulum and myocyte edema and necrosis over 1 to 2 days. Muscle regeneration occurs within the next 3 to 4 weeks as myoblasts, basal laminae, and connective tissue elements remain intact. This effect has been seen in only a few case reports of myotoxic complications after local anesthetic administrations causing clinically relevant myopathy and myonecrosis after TPIs.[39] In experimental studies, procaine produces the least and bupivacaine causes the most severe muscle injury.

There has been one case report of severe hypokalemic paralysis after left iliopsoas muscle injection with ultrasound guidance that highlights the importance that high index of suspicion is warranted for prompt diagnosis and management.[40] It was postulated in this case that the cause of the hypokalemia was due to transcellular shifting due to epinephrine component of the TPI injectate.

Other complications that can occur include vasovagal syncope, allergic reaction, skin infection, and hematoma formation.[41] Proper preparation, taking adequate sterile precautions, and close monitoring of the patient during and after the procedure can minimize long-term effects.

TECHNIQUE FOR TPI (EXCLUDING PIRIFORMIS MUSCLE)
Technique for TPI

Preparation
TPIs should be performed by skilled professionals with adequate anticipation and preparation for complications such as vasovagal reaction and allergic reaction. After reviewing the contraindications as described earlier and after discussing the risks of the procedure including, but not limited to increased pain, infection, bleeding, allergic reaction, soft tissue injury, pneumothorax, cutaneous atrophy, bleaching of the skin (if steroid is administered), written informed consent is obtained.

Technique

The targeted areas are then identified and marked by the presence of discrete TrPs with localized tenderness, hypertonicity, and taut bands. Using the nondominant hand, the skin and underlying tissue is pinched between the index finger and thumb, and the needle attached to the syringe with the injectate is inserted using the dominant hand at a 30° angle until the taut band is reached. The needle is then advanced and retracted to various sites within the muscle until relaxation is achieved. At each site, after aspiration is performed to ensure negative return of blood or fluid, 0.2 to 0.5 mL of solution is injected. The needle is then withdrawn after all the injectate is administered in a fanlike distribution in the muscle and a sterile band-aid is applied.

EVIDENCE FOR THE USE OF IMAGE GUIDANCE FOR TPI (EXCLUDING PIRIFORMIS MUSCLE)

Traditionally, TPIs have been performed using blind technique without image guidance by palpating the TrPs and inserting the needle with or without injecting a solution. However, palpation of TrPs can be technically difficult in obese patients that can result in ineffective injection if placed in the soft tissues and can cause complications if inadvertently placed in other tissues. Several diagnostic methods including electromyography, magnetic resonance elastography, and ultrasonography have been studied to determine the location and characteristics of myofascial TrPs.[22,42,43] All these methods were shown to have limitations in proper identification. However, subsequent studies have supported the use of ultrasound, which is considered to be safe, portable, and inexpensive imaging modality for identification and evaluation of the effectiveness of therapeutic interventions in myofascial TrPs.[23,44]

The technique for using ultrasound guidance for TPIs was first described by Botwin and colleagues.[33] The authors described the muscle to have hyperechoic marbled appearance while adipose tissue had mixed echogenicity, using a 13-6 MHz 38 mm broadband linear array transducer. They demonstrated clear visualization of the injectate using a 25g 1.5-inch needle under direct ultrasound guidance that was further confirmed with color mode. A subsequent study also demonstrated ultrasound can differentiate myofascial tissue with and without active TrPs.[23] Several studies have shown that ultrasound-guided injections are extremely effective modality in various musculoskeletal locations and maximize injection accuracy and minimize potential complications.[45–48] Ultrasound may be considered by practitioners for guiding musculoskeletal injections to avoid complications from blind injections.

However, there are very limited number of studies on the effectiveness of ultrasound-guided injections for myofascial pain syndrome. Ultrasound-guided interfascial block with lidocaine between the rhomboids major and trapezius showed statistically significant improvement in pain and quality of life similar to pulsed radiofrequency treatment.[49] Ultrasound-guided deep injection using 12 to 18-MHz US transducer of the rhomboid major muscle was more effective than superficial injection of trapezius muscle for parameters of pain, disability, and quality of life in 61 patients with myofascial pain syndrome in a prospective randomized double-blinded study at 2 and 4 weeks post-treatment.[50] The author's findings corroborated with other studies that deep injections were superior to superficial injections and they concluded that ultrasound guidance can help to minimize the complications of blind injections such as pneumothorax, air embolism, inadvertent intrathecal injection, peripheral nerve injuries, and muscle injuries that are all rare reported complications, which is discussed in detail in the following section.[31]

Shear wave elastography using ultrasound has emerged as a quantitative method of measuring the mechanical properties of the soft tissue including skeletal muscle through external induction of the shear wave or with the use of the radiation force of the ultrasound.[51–53] A recent pilot feasibility study on 41 patients compared ultrasound-guided myofascial injections and blind injections with the use of shear wave elastography and showed statistically significant improvement in the pain (VAS) scores, neck disability scores (NDI), and shoulder pain disability score (SPADI) at baseline and at 4 weeks with significantly higher efficacy in the ultrasound group.[48]

Limitations of these studies comparing ultrasound-guided myofascial injections with blind injections are small sample size and lack of placebo intervention and short follow-up period.[50] Other efforts to characterize neuromuscular activation using surface electromyography signals using machine learning have been studied but have not been evaluated in clinical outcome studies.[54,55]

TECHNIQUE FOR PIRIFORMIS MUSCLE INJECTION AND EVIDENCE FOR THE USE OF IMAGE GUIDANCE

The use of imaging devices in the performance of piriformis injection procedures can help increase accuracy and reduce complications. It is important to select the appropriate image guidance to increase the success rate of procedures. Fluoroscopy and ultrasound are the most commonly used imaging techniques to perform piriformis injections. Ultrasound has been shown to provide higher accuracy in needle placement. In a study by Finnoff and colleagues, ultrasound-guided piriformis injections were found to be significantly more accurate than fluoroscopically guided contrast-controlled injections.[56] The authors concluded that despite the use of bony landmarks and contrast, most of the fluoroscopically attempted piriformis injections were placed superficially within the gluteus maximus.

The use of electromyography for localization of the piriformis muscle or other TrPs has been reported with mixed results. In a 2016 study, it was reported that there was no correlation between the location of a TrP and the position of peak EMG amplitude.[57] Fluoroscopic guidance relies on identification of bony target points that guide the practitioner to the piriformis muscle, whereas sonography can directly identify the piriformis muscles and provide a real-time image of surrounding soft tissues (nerves, muscles, vessels, etc.), an image of needle tip advancement relevant to surrounding structures, and visualization of injectate spread.[58] In addition, neither the patients nor clinicians are exposed to radiation during an ultrasound-guided procedure and therefore present as a much safer option long-term with the absence of cumulative doses of radiation associated with repeat procedures.[59]

For the fluoroscopically guided injection with EMG guidance, the patient is placed prone on a fluoroscopy table, and the inferior margin of the sacroiliac joint is imaged and marked. The needle insertion site is 1 to 2 cm caudal and 1 to 2 cm lateral to the inferior margin of the sacroiliac joint. After sterile preparation and infiltration of local anesthetic, a 7- to 10-cm insulated needle is inserted and advanced with the nerve stimulator turned on (1 mA, 2 Hz, 0.1 msec) until an evoked motor response of the sciatic nerve is achieved (dorsiflexion, plantar flexion, eversion, inversion) at 0.4 to 0.6 mA. The needle is then withdrawn until the sciatic stimulation disappears to avoid intraneural injection and 1 to 2 mL of contrast agent is injected. The contrast agent should outline the piriformis muscle belly with no sign of spillage (**Fig. 2**). After the characteristic spread of dye is achieved, a local anesthetic solution with steroid is administered.

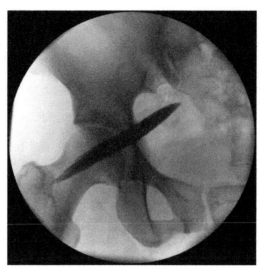

Fig. 2. Fluoroscopic-guided piriformis muscle injection.

For the ultrasonography-guided procedure, the piriformis is identified in long axis with the transducer in the oblique axial plane on the body just inferior to the sacroiliac joint and greater sciatic notch (**Fig. 3**). It is important to maintain visualization of the piriformis musculature, lateral edge of the sacrum, and sciatic nerve to avoid needle contact with the nerve itself.[60] Although the muscle is being visualized in the long axis, the nerve will be in the short axis and is typically seen deep to the piriformis when in the prone position. During this preprocedure scan, Doppler imaging should be used to locate vessels that will need to be avoided.[61] While maintaining visualization of the needle, the needle can then be inserted in plane with the transducer until it enters the piriformis muscle tissue at the targeted site. The needle trajectory can be adjusted as the needle is inserted to reach the desired location and to avoid the sciatic

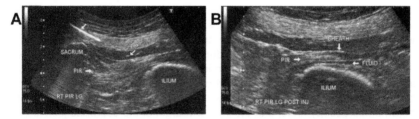

Fig. 3. (A) Longitudinal US view of the piriformis during needle placement using a medial-to-lateral approach parallel to the long axis of the transducer. The proximal end of the needle has been digitally enhanced to highlight the needle trajectory. (B) Postinjection tenogram at the level of the greater sciatic foramen. Anechoic injectate (FLUID) within the piriformis tendon sheath lies superficial and deep to the hyperechoic tendon. RT PIR LG, right side, piriformis, longitudinal view; TIP, needle tip. (Reproduced with permission from Archives of Physical Medicine and Rehabilitation, Authors Jay Smith, Mark-Friedrich Hurdle, Adam J. Locketz, Steven J. Wisniewski. December 2006. Copyright © 2006 American Congress of Rehabilitation Medicine and the American Academy of Physical Medicine and Rehabilitation. Published by Elsevier Inc. All rights reserved. (PERMISSIONS HAVE BEEN OBTAINED BY ALC).)

nerve. When the needle is in the correct position at the muscle, the medication can be injected and visualized entering the tissue.[62] Local anesthetic is visualized as anechoic, whereas corticosteroid may be hyperechoic with particulate steroids or anechoic in nonparticulate steroids.

Injectate Therapeutic Options

Saline, corticosteroids, a variety of local anesthetics including lidocaine and bupivacaine, botulinum toxin serotype A (BoNT-A), and dry needling have all been used and studied. Stimulation of the local twitch response in direct needling of the TrP is valuable in achieving immediate effect.[63] There is good evidence to suggest that there is no advantage of one injection therapy over another, or of any drug injectate over dry needling.[64] In a systemic review of 23 randomized controlled trials (RCTs), Cummings and White concluded that any effect derived from TPI is likely derived from the needle itself, rather than any specific substance injected, as there was no difference in therapeutic benefit of "wet" needling versus "dry" needling.[64] Their review also suggested that pain reduction with saline TPI is equal to pain reduction with local anesthetic TPI, both being significant.

Although adding corticosteroid preparation to local anesthetic is a common practice, it has not been reliably shown to reduce pain more than TPI with local anesthetic alone.[64,65] Botulinum toxin type A (BoNT-A) produces sustained and prolonged relaxation of muscles by inhibiting release of Ach at the motor endplate and is itself an analgesic inhibiting central sensitization.[66] Commercially prepared BoNT-A is expensive and should be used with care by a well-trained physician. Despite the widespread practice of TPI for myofascial pain, there is no consensus regarding the number of injection points, frequency of administration, and volume or type of injectate. Controlled studies are needed to evaluate the comparative efficacy of TPIs and their potential benefits in long-term pain reduction, if any.

OUTCOMES DATA AND DISCUSSION FOR TPIs WITH LOCAL ANESTHETIC ± STEROID

Over the years, few well-designed RCTs regarding TPIs have been performed with even fewer published in the last decade. Available literature investigated the efficacy of the injection for myofascial pain with diverse medications (**Table 1**). Initial studies evaluated the efficacy of TPI with various types of local anesthetics, concentrations of local anesthetics, and a variety of steroids.[65,67–70] The majority of these studies evaluated the injection techniques on the cervical neck, shoulder, masseter, abdominal/pelvic, and trapezius muscles. Regardless of medication used, the key component involved placing the needle into a taut band, which resulted in improved pain compared with baseline. Recent studies largely in the emergency medicine literature within the last 5 years have reaffirmed findings from earlier studies. In a study where patients presented to the emergency department with lumbar myofascial pain, patients were randomized to either intravenous (IV) nonsteroidal anti-inflammatory drugs (NSAIDs; 50 mg dexketoprofen) or TPI with 1.0% lidocaine. Of 54 patients enrolled in this RCT, TPIs were found to have superior analgesic effect compared with IV NSAIDs at all studied time points up to 60 minutes after intervention.[71] Though superior to pharmacologic, the type of injectate did not seem to make a substantial difference in most studies. Roldan and colleagues compared patients treated with either TPIs containing normal saline or lidocaine 1% with 40 mg triamcinolone who presented to the emergency department for management of lumbar myofascial pain. They found

Table 1
Outcomes data for trigger point injections with local anesthestic/steroid

Study Author	Study Type	Study Size	Metrics	Study Question	Outcomes
Hong CZ et al,[63] 1994	RCT	58	PS, Cervical ROM	Comparing 0.5% lidocaine TPI to dry needling in upper trapezius muscle MPS.	Lidocaine TPI resulted in more immediate soreness than dry needling. However, dry needling resulted in greater intensity and longer duration of soreness after procedure than lidocaine TPI
Tschopp KP et al,[67] 1996	RCT	107	PS	Comparing 0.25% bupivacaine to 1.0% lidocaine to saline TPI for MPS.	No difference in relief between groups so long as needle hits muscle belly.
Hameroff SR et al,[68] 1981	Crossover double-blind RCT	15	PS	Comparing bupivacaine to etidocaine to saline for TPI evaluating relief 7 days after injection for MPS.	Local preferred to saline alone.
Iwama H et al,[69] 2007	RCT	20	PS	Comparing 0.25% to 1.0% lidocaine for TPI for MPS.	0.25% lidocaine had less injection pain and better efficacy (14 d relief compared to 7 d)
Zaral idou AT et al,[70] 2009	RCT	68	PS	Comparing ropivacaine to levobupivacaine for TPI for MPS.	No significant differences were found between groups at 2 wk out.
Garvey TA et al,[65] 1989	Double-blind RCT	63	NRS	Comparing local anesthetic TPI, local anesthetic with steroid TPI, acupuncture, and cool spray with acupuncture for MPS.	No difference between types of procedural techniques was noted. Did not matter if medication was injected for procedure, both resulted in pain relief.

Study	Type	n	Outcome Measures	Comparison	Results
Kocak AO et al,[71] 2019	RCT	54	VAS	Comparing NSAID and TPI for low back MPS.	TPI was superior to NSAIDs when assessed with pain relief within the first hour of intervention.
Roldan CJ et al,[72] 2020	RCT	48	NRS	Comparing local anesthetic and steroid TPI to saline TPI in ED patients.	Resulted in similar change in pain relief in both groups.
Iwama H et al,[73] 2001	RCT	21	PS	Testing injection pain with dilute local anesthetic in volunteers as well as using dilute local anesthetic doses in patients with MPS.	Less pain with dilute local injections. Duration relief in MPS patients not affected by using dilute local at low enough doses.
Krishnan SK et al,[74] 2000	RCT	30	VAS	Comparing injection pain of bupivacaine, ropivacaine, bupivacaine with steroids, ropivacaine with steroids, and just needle insertion.	Ropivacaine was less painful (alone) compared to bupivacaine or either local anesthetic in combination with steroids.
Yoon SH et al,[75] 2007	RCT	77	VAS, NDI, SF-36	Comparing needle sizes on injection pain.	No difference was noted between sizes of needles used.
Ga H et al,[76] 2009	RCT	39	VAS, FACES, PPI, GDS-SF	Comparing TPI with 0.5% lidocaine with acupuncture for MPS.	No difference between groups.
Mitidieri AMS et al,[77] 2020	RCT	35	VAS, NCS, MPQ	Comparing acupuncture to TPI (local anesthetic) for pelvic pain from abdominal MPS.	No difference between outcomes when analyzed at 1 wk, 1 mo, 3 mo, and 6 mo out except for MPQ differences at 1 wk.

Abbreviations: FACES, Wong-Baker FACES Paine Scale; GDS-SF, Geriatric Depression Scale-Short Form; MPQ, McGill Pain Questionnaire; MPS, myofascial pain syndrome; NCS, Numeric Categorical Scale; NDI, Neck Disability Index; NPAD, Neck Pain and Disability Scale; NPQ, Neck Pain Questionnaire; NRS, numeric rating score; NSAID, nonsteroid anti-inflammatory drugs; PFDI-20, Pelvic Floor Distress Inventory - 20; PPI, Pressure Pain Intensity Scores; PS, pain score (internal system); RCT, randomized controlled trial; ROM, range of motion; SF-36, Medical Outcomes Study 36 Item Short Form Health Survey; TPI, trigger point injection; VAS, visual analog score.

that there was no statistically significant difference between the two groups immediately after injection or at 2 weeks follow-up.[72]

Aside from comparing efficacy of the injection for myofascial pain relief, studies have been performed evaluating if the concentrations of local anesthetic used affected the presence of pain on injection or its efficacy of relief.[69,73] Iwama and colleagues compared 0.25% lidocaine to 1.0% lidocaine TPI in patients with bilateral shoulder myofascial pain. It was found that injection pain was statistically significantly less with injection of 0.25% lidocaine compared with 1.0% with overall improved pain relief at 7 and 14 days postinjection.[69] A follow-up study performed by Iwama and colleagues compared water diluted 0.25% lidocaine TPI to water diluted 0.20% lidocaine TPI in patients with shoulder and cervical myofascial pain found that both patient cohorts reported statically significant pain relief for the same duration of time.[73] The same study evaluated diluted mepivacaine and bupivacaine along with diluted lidocaine to evaluate its effect on injection pain. The study found that diluted mepivacaine resulted in the least amount of pain with injection.

Other studies have also studied this phenomenon, finding that pain on injection varies among local anesthetics. Krishnan and colleagues studied intramuscular injection pain in healthy volunteers comparing the amount of injection pain when bupivacaine, ropivacaine, bupivacaine with steroids, and ropivacaine with steroids were used. In the study, bupivacaine injections were noted to be more painful than ropivacaine in intensity that was deemed not associated with the differences in the local anesthetic pH.[74] Needle size affecting the pain upon injection was investigated by Yoon and colleagues comparing 21-gauge to 23-gauge needles for TPIs in 77 patients with trapezius myofascial pain found no statistical difference in pain scores at the time of injection or visual analog scores at follow-up.[75] Injection pain aside, only one study in 1981 found indicate benefit of local anesthetic compared with normal saline for TPI 7 days after injection in a cohort of only 15 patients.[68] Ga and colleagues also found this similar trend when acupuncture was compared to TPI with 0.5% lidocaine in patients with myofascial pain. When both modalities were used resulting in a twitch response, there was no statistically significant difference in the amount of pain improvement in patients, up to 1 month out.[76] This was further validated by Mitideri and colleagues when Ashi acupuncture was compared to local anesthetic TPI in patients with pelvic pain from abdominal myofascial pain. When the taut band was intervened upon, they found equal efficacy in pain relief between both intervention groups.[77]

OUTCOMES DATA AND DISCUSSION FOR TPIs WITH BOTULINUM TOXIN

Similar to the studies evaluating local anesthetic and steroids for TPI, there is a paucity of well-designed RCTs evaluating the efficacy of botulinum toxin in the management of myofascial pain (**Table 2**). One of the earlier studies was performed by Wheeler and colleagues and was a double-blind RCT where 33 participants were randomized to receive either 50 or 100 units of BoNT-A or normal saline injection into symptomatic TrPs of the cervicothoracic area. Their findings showed significant improvement in pain scores, neck disability, and an increase in pressure pain threshold testing by algometer; however, there was no significant difference between BoNT-A groups and saline control groups.[78] Another study by Qerama and colleagues was a double-blind RCT in patients with chronic myofascial pain comparing TPI performed with 50 U BoNT-A to normal saline. This study found that there was no statistically significant difference in pain outcomes between the 2 groups at 28 days after injection.[79] Kwanchuay and colleagues compared the efficacy of BoNT-A TPI in patients for upper

Table 2
Outcomes data for trigger point injections with botulinum toxin

Study Author	Study Type	Study Size	Metrics	Study Question	Outcomes
Wheeler AH et al,[78] 1998	Double-blind RCT	33	NPAD, PS	Comparing 50 U BoNT-A, 100 U BoNT-A, and normal saline TPI for MPS.	All 3 groups improved pain. No statistically significant benefit between injection types.
Qerama E et al,[79] 2006	Double-blind RCT	30	NRS, PPDT, PPTT	Comparing BoNT-A TPI to saline TPI for MPS.	No difference in pain relief between groups at 28 d, but BoNT-A caused decreased EMG activity.
Kwanchuay P et al[80] 2015	Double-blind RCT	33	VAS, PPT	Comparing BoNT-A to saline TPI for MPS.	No difference between groups 6 wk out though BoNT-A TPI resulted statistically significant increase in pain threshold 6 wk out.
Dessie SG et al,[81] 2019	Double-blind RCT	59	VAS, PFDI-20	Comparing saline or BoNT-A TPI for abdominal MPS in pelvic pain for MPS.	No statistically significant difference between groups at 4 and 12 wk after injection.
Gobel H et al,[82] 2006	Double-blind RCT	145	PS	Comparing BoNT-A to saline TPI for MPS.	BoNT-A provided better relief between weeks 5 and 8.
Kamanli A et al,[83] 2005	Single-blind RCT	29	PPT, PS, VAS, NHP	Comparing BoNT-A TPI to dry needling to bupivacaine TPI for MPS.	TPI in general found to have better benefit than dry needling. Authors noted bupivacaine was best for TPI as it was fast acting meanwhile BoNT-A TPI should be used in medically refractory cases.
Ferrante FM et al,[84] 2005	Double-blind RCT	132	VAS, PPT	Comparing saline to 10, 25, or 50 U BoNT-A in up to 5 active TrPs for cervicothoracic MPS	No significant differences occurred between placebo and BoNT-A groups among all outcomes.
Harden RN et al,[85]	Double-blind RCT	23	PPT, Cervical ROM, MPQ, BDI, HSES, STAI, PDI, VAS	Comparing BoNT-A 25 U per trigger point (max 4 TrPs) to saline TPI for	Participants in the BoNT-A group reported greater reductions in

(continued on next page)

Table 2
(continued)

Study Author	Study Type	Study Size	Metrics	Study Question	Outcomes
				cervical MPS and chronic tension type headache	headache frequency compared with placebo.
Graboski et al,[86]	Double-blind RCT	18	VAS	Comparing BoNT-A 25 U per TrP to 0.5% bupivacaine for MPS	Both treatments were effective in reducing pain significantly but no difference between BoNT-A and bupivacaine groups.
Venancio et al[87] 2009	Double-blind RCT	45	VAS	Comparing dry needling, 0.25% lidocaine, and BoNT-A for MPS	All groups showed favorable reductions in pain; however, the BoNT-A group demonstrated less use of rescue medication, and less postinjection local sensitivity.
Nicol et al,[88] 2005	Double-blind RCT	114	NRS, SF-36, BPI, NDI	Comparing BoNT-A to saline TPI for cervical and shoulder girdle MPS	BoNT-A provided improved pain scores, headaches, and physical function parameters compared to saline TPI
Benecke et al,[89] 2011	Double-blind RCT	154	NRS	Comparing BoNT-A to saline TPI for cervical and shoulder MPS	BoNT-A provided improved pain relief compared to saline at 8 wk after TPI
Miller et al,[90] 2009	Double-blind RCT	47	VAS, MOPQ	Comparing BoNT-A to saline TPI for cervical and shoulder MPS	BoNT-A TPI led to improved pain intensity scores compared to saline TPI

BDI, Beck Depression Inventory; BoNT-A, botulinum toxin type A; HSES, Headache Specific Self-Efficacy Scale; MOPQ, Modified Oswestry Pain Questionnaire; MPQ, McGill Pain Questionnaire; MPS, myofascial pain syndrome; NDI, Neck Disability Index; NHP, Nottingham Health Profile; NRS, numeric rating score; PDI, Pain Disability Index; PPDT, pressure pain detection thresholds; PPT, pressure pain threshold; PPTT, pressure pain tolerance thresholds; PS, pain score (internal system); RCT, randomized controlled trial; ROM, range of motion; SF-36, Medical Outcomes Study 36 Item Short Form Health Survey; STAI, State-Trait Anxiety Inventory; TPI, trigger point injection; VAS, visual analog score.

trapezius myofascial pain to normal saline TPI. Their study found no difference in efficacy in VAS reduction; however, BoNT-A did increase the pressure pain threshold at 6 weeks after the injection in a statistically significant manner.[80] Dessie and colleagues also compared BoNT-A TPI to normal saline TPI in patients with pelvic myofascial pain syndrome where no statistically significant difference was found between the 2 groups at 4 and 12 weeks postprocedure.[81]

Other studies have found that BoNT-A may provide durable relief compared with other medications upon injection. In a double-blind RCT by Gobel and colleagues, patients with myofascial pain were randomized to receive either BoNT-A injections (10 sites, 40 U each) to saline TPI. The study found that BoNT-A did result in statistically significant pain control at 5 weeks with fewer days of pain between 5 and 12 weeks.[82] Kamanil and colleagues compared lidocaine TPI, BoNT-A TPI, and dry needling in patients with myofascial pain. At 1 month follow-up, patients receiving a TPI had statistically improved VAS compared with dry needling. However, all 3 modalities resulted in decreased VAS after treatment. Furthermore, in the study, it was argued by the authors that lidocaine TPI was less disruptive than dry needling and more cost-effective than BoNT-A TPI though BoNT-A may be useful for patients with MPS resistant to conventional treatment.[83]

Ferrante and colleagues found no statistically significant improvement compared to placebo with BoNT-A injection when injected directly into painful TrPs for cervico-thoracic MP.[84] They concluded that although it is intuitive for the clinician to consider therapeutic injection of BoNT-A as a treatment for MP (given its a priori similarity to TPI), peculiarities inherent to the use of toxin in lieu of dry needling or local anesthetic must be accounted for (ie, toxin spread through fascial planes), including the effects of dosing of toxin, volume of injectate, muscles chosen to inject, postural relations and abnormalities, and injection technique. Harden and colleagues were able to identify a short-term (12-week) reduction in MP of chronic tension-type headache with BoNT-A injection as compared with placebo.[85] Graboski and colleagues found no significant difference in BoNT-A versus 0.5% bupivacaine injected into TPs of patients with MPS, though both were effective in reducing pain below the baseline level.[86] Venancio and colleagues studied 45 MP patients who were assigned randomly to 1 of the following 3 groups: dry needling, 0.25% lidocaine TPI, and BoNT–A TPI, and assessed over a 12-week period.[87] Although all 3 groups showed favorable response to treatment, the BoNT-A group demonstrated less use of rescue medication, and less postinjection local sensitivity.[87] In another study, Nicol and colleagues reported that BoNT-A injected directly into painful muscle groups using a "follow the pain" and pattern injection technique in lieu of TrPs led to reduced average numerical pain scores, reduced number of headaches per week, and improvement in general activity and sleep quality of life measures.[88] Similar positive findings were seen in the studies by Benecke and colleagues[89] and Miller and colleagues[90] wherein patients with cervical myofascial pain received BoNT-A using a fixed-location injection technique.

OUTCOMES DATA AND DISCUSSION FOR PIRIFORMIS INJECTION WITH LOCAL ANESTHETICS ± STEROID

In patients who fail to respond to conservative treatment of piriformis syndrome that includes activity modification, rest, mobilizing soft tissue restrictions, medical management, physical therapy, and alternative therapies such as acupuncture or dry needling, invasive options have been suggested.[91,92] Injection interventions for piriformis TrPs with local anesthetics with or without steroids have been studied (**Table 3**). Early studies involving the analysis of 279 patients found that about 79% of the patients had at least 50% improvement when steroid (triamcinolone) injections to the piriformis were added to the physical therapy protocol suggesting the added benefit of injection treatment.[93] In a later study, 239 patients were injected with local anesthetic of bupivacaine and betamethasone demonstrated significant reduction of pain in 45% of patients for 2 to 4 months and 15% having 8 months or longer with significant improvement of pain.[94]

A subsequent study involving 162 patients, using MRI guidance and injection of local anesthetic provided complete relief without recurrence in 15% of patients and short-term relief up to 4 months with recurrence in 69% of patients.[94] Sixteen percent had no relief with injection. Another small study of 13 patients and 10 control subjects showed the potential benefit of CT-guided piriformis injection with local anesthetic and steroid with statistically significant improvement in VAS score at 5 to 7 days, 2,3,6, and 12 months.[95] A small case series showed 9 of 10 patients who received CT-guided piriformis injection had full and sustained recovery after piriformis injection.[96] In a study by Jeong and colleagues, 63 patients underwent ultrasound-guided piriformis injection of 40 mg triamcinolone, in which 40.5% of enrolled participants showed significant improvement with injection and 18.9% had partial improvement.[97]

As part of neural therapy to reduce pain and improve function, 51 patients with piriformis syndrome received 6 sessions of lidocaine injections that involved piriformis muscle injections, T11-S2 segmental injections and sacral canal injections along with stretching exercises.[98] Both the control group and the treatment group received stretching exercises as part of treatment and the study showed statistically significant improvement in pain and functional level in both groups with changes from baseline noticeably larger in the neural therapy group. This study showed that adding lidocaine injections can play a conjunctive role with other treatment options.

Steroid injections with local anesthetic have been studied in a recent cohort of 32 patients receiving injection therapy in the piriformis muscle using ultrasound guidance and showed statistically significant improvement in pain scale from baseline and at 1 month as well as 1 week to 1 month.[99] In another study of 49 patients with deep gluteal syndrome of which piriformis syndrome is one of the subtypes, ultrasound-guided injection of a mixture of 20 mLs of normal saline, 4 mLs of 2% lidocaine, and 1 mL of corticosteroid (40 mg of methyl-prednisone acetate) in the perisciatic region between the gluteus maximus and pelvic trochanteric muscles provided some level of pain relief in 73.7% with reduction in pain score from 8.3 preinjection to 2.8 postinjection. Recurrence of pain was reported in 50% of the patients and the effect lasted for 5.3 weeks.[100]

Although these previous studies have shown that piriformis injection with image guidance with local anesthetic and steroid had improvement in pain level at varying degrees, the effect of local anesthetic alone versus local anesthetic with a steroid was studied in a randomized controlled double-blinded study of 50 patients. This study failed to show a statistically significant difference in the pain level in 2 groups with and without steroid.[101] After a test injection and diagnosis of piriformis syndrome, one group (n = 22) received 5 mL of 2% lidocaine and other group (n = 25) received 4 mLs of 2% lidocaine and 1 mL of betamethasone. Both groups had a significant reduction in pain compared with baseline, there was no difference between the groups at rest, in motion, 1 month, or 3 months, suggesting that the addition of steroids may not have an added benefit over local anesthetic injections.

Another study has studied the effect of hydrodissection before injection of corticosteroid in piriformis syndrome and showed promising results. In this study, hydrodissection was performed by injecting fluid in the perineural tissue using ultrasound guidance to help reduce the adhesions and broaden the tissue space to deliver local

Table 3
Outcomes data for piriformis injection with local anesthestic ± steroid

Author/Year	Sample Size	Methods	Image guidance/ Additional Treatment	Injectate Used	Main findings/Outcome	Follow-up
Fishman LM et al,[93] 2002	279	Before-after trial of cohort of consecutive patients identified by operational definition	No image guidance/ received PT/serially reported pain and disability assessments	Lidocaine and triamcinolone	79% had >50% relief at 10 mo	48 mo
Filler AG et al[94] 2005	162	239 consecutive patients failed treatment of sciatica	MRI	Marcaine	15% complete relief, 16% no relief, recurrence in 69% at 4 mo	4 mo
Masala S et al,[95] 2012	23 (cases-13/ control-10)	Case-control study	CT	Methyl prednisone and lidocaine	Improvement in VAS at 5–7 d, 2,3,6, and 12 mo	12 mo
Ozisik PA et al,[96] 2014	10	Case series	CT	Depomedrol and marcaine	9/10 patients had full recovery, no pain or VAS score of 1–3	2 y
Nazlikul H et al,[98] 2018	102	Prospective randomized control study	No image guidance/ stretching exercises (n = 51), injections in neural therapy group (n = 51)	6 sessions of lidocaine injections with T11-S2 segmental injections and sacral canal injections	Improvement in VAS and ODI, more improvement in the neural therapy group	None
Terlemez et al,[99] 2019	30	Prospective cohort	Ultrasound	Lidocaine and betamethasone	Improvement in pain score from baseline at 1 wk and 1 mo	1 mo

(continued on next page)

Table 3
(continued)

Author/Year	Sample Size	Methods	Image guidance/ Additional Treatment	Injectate Used	Main findings/Outcome	Follow-up
Rosales J et al,[100] 2015	49	Prospective	Ultrasound	Lidocaine + saline + methyl-prednisone acetate	73.7% had some relief VAS-pre-8.3/post-2.8, relief lasted 5.3 wk	6 wk
Misirlioglu et al,[101] 2015	50	Prospective double-blinded, RCT	Ultrasound	Lidocaine only vs lidocaine and betamethasone	Pain reduction (NRS and LAS scale) from baseline but no difference between LA vs steroid group at 1 and 3 mo	3 mo
Burke CJ et al,[102] 2019	38	Consecutive patients	Ultrasound/ hydrodissection	LA and steroid (17-betamethasone, 21-triamcinolone)	84% immediate relief (pre-4.7/post-0.5), 47% continued relief at 33.6 d	1 mo

Table 4
Outcomes data for piriformis injection with botulinum toxin

Study (Year)	Intervention	Results
Porta,[103] 2000	BoNT-A (dose not reported), 0.5% bupivacaine, methylprednisolone	BoNT-A and steroid group had no significant differences in pain reduction at 1 mo; however, at 2 mo postinjection, there was a significant reduction in the BoNT-A group compared with the steroid group
Lang,[106] 2004	5000 u BoNT-B	Significant reduction in hip and buttock pain at 4, 12, and 16 wk
Fishman et al,[107] 2004	12,500 u BoNT-B	Combined with PT, 88.9% of patients injected had 50% improvement on the VAS
Yoon et al,[108] 2007	150 u BoNT-A vs 5 mg dexamethasone/1% lidocaine	Pain significantly lower in Dysport group at 4, 8, and 12 wk vs baseline $P < .0001$
Childers et al,[109] 2002	100 u BoNT-A	Significant improvement in pain, spasm, distress, and interference with activities
Fishman et al,[110] 2002	200 u BoNT-A vs 1.5 mL 2% lidocaine/20 mg triamcinolone, vs placebo	50% improvement at last 2 visits following 20 mg TL vs placebo injection: $P = .001$; BoNT-A vs TL: $P = .044$; BoNT-A vs placebo: $P = .001$
Fishman et al,[111] 2017	300 u BoNT-A vs saline	VAS score decreased significantly at 2,4,6,8,10, and 12 wk compared with placebo
Rodriguez-Pinero et al,[112] 2018	100 U BoNT-A	VAS scores and quality of life scores statistically significantly reduced at 1 and 6 mo after injection
Yan,[113] 2021	100 u BoNT-A/1% lidocaine/0.5% bupivacaine vs 1% lidocaine/0.5% bupivacaine/4 mg dexamethasone	Median pain-free days were 30 d for the BoNT-A group and 1 d for the non–BoNT-A group

Dr Chadwick has served as a consultant for Swing Therapeutics and receives research funding from the National Institutes of Health, National Institute of General Medical Sciences, Grant # K23GM123320.

anesthetic and steroid. Of the 38 patients studied, 17 received betamethasone and 21 received triamcinolone. Thirty-two patients (84%) received immediate pain relief with a reduction in pain score from 4.7/10 to 0.5/10. Of the 19 patients followed up at 33.6 days, 9 patients (47%) reported continuous pain relief.[102] Further large-scale studies are needed to compare the effect of hydrodissection before injection treatment.[91]

OUTCOMES DATA AND DISCUSSION FOR PIRIFORMIS INJECTION WITH BoNT

Piriformis muscle injection with BoNT-A is an increasingly common injection when the duration of effect from local anesthetic/corticosteroid injections is insufficient. A typical dose would be 100 units in a 2-mL volume.[103] Owing to its paralytic effect on the muscle, it causes atrophy and fatty degeneration of the muscle over time as evidenced by MRI.[104] This reduction in muscular volume would decrease pressure on the sciatic nerve and is the mechanism of analgesia[93,105–112] but is a more profoundly effective treatment when combined with physical therapy.[93,107,110] Several uncontrolled studies have evaluated the use of BoNT-A, often in combination with physical therapy, and reported high rates of success that lasted for months (**Table 4**).[103,106–111] A controlled study demonstrated superiority of BoNT-A over placebo injection for 10 weeks.[109] Other controlled studies have reported that the efficacy of botulinum toxin is superior to that of local anesthetic/steroid or normal saline injections for the treatment of piriformis syndrome.[110,113]

SUMMARY

Myofascial pain and myofascial pain syndromes are among some of the most common acute and chronic pain conditions. The pathophysiology of myofascial pain includes biomechanical and postural factors that likely interact with neurologic factors, psychological elements including depression and anxiety, and hormonal and nutritional imbalances. These factors (in total or in part) may create peripheral sensitization, autonomic dysregulation, and ultimately, central spinal cord sensitization, which can amplify the symptoms experienced by patients with myofascial pain. Many interventional procedures can be performed in both an acute and chronic pain setting to address myofascial pain syndromes. Injections can be achieved with or without imaging guidance such as fluoroscopy and ultrasound; however, the use of imaging in years past has been recommended to improve safety and accuracy of needle placement. Injections can be performed using no injectate (dry needling), or can involve the administration of local anesthetics, botulinum toxin, or corticosteroids, with the evidence suggesting that most injectates have minimal or no superiority over one another. A proper history and physical examination of the patient and imaging studies may prove to be helpful in identifying the correct myofascial pain syndrome and aiding in developing an appropriate treatment strategy for these very common conditions.

DISCLOSURE

Dr Chadwick receives research funding from the National Institutes of Health, National Institute of General Medical Sciences, grant # K23GM123320. Dr Chadwick has served as a consultant for Swing Therapeutics.

CLINICS CARE POINTS

- A trigger point is the hallmark of myofascial pain syndromes, which may be treated with physical therapy and trigger point injections.

- Common injectates used for trigger point injections include local anesthetics, corticosteroids, and botulinum toxins.

- The growing accessibility of ultrasound has improved available options for imaging guidance for trigger point injections and piriformis muscle injection.

- Ultrasound guidance may be used to improve safety and in the case of piriformis syndrome has been shown to improve accuracy of needle placement in the piriformis muscle.

- Outcomes data for trigger point injections have shown analgesic benefit with the use of local anesthetics, corticosteroids, and botulinum toxins for myofascial pain syndromes, with no evidence of superiority of any injectate.

- Outcomes data for piriformis muscle injections have shown that local anesthetic, steroid, and botulinum toxins are efficacious in reducing pain and improving symptoms. Botulinum toxins may provide superior analgesia and may be considered when local anesthetics/steroids are helpful but not providing long-term relief.

REFERENCES

1. Koukoulithras I, Plexousakis M, Kolokotsios S, et al. A Biopsychosocial Model-Based Clinical Approach in Myofascial Pain Syndrome: A Narrative Review. Cureus 2021;13(4):e14737.
2. Kuan TS. Current studies on myofascial pain syndrome. Curr Pain Headache Rep 2009;13(5):365–9.
3. Shah JP, Phillips TM, Danoff JV, et al. An in vivo microanalytical technique for measuring the local biochemical milieu of human skeletal muscle. J Appl Physiol (1985) 2005;99(5):1977–84.
4. Gerwin RD, Dommerholt J, Shah JP. An expansion of Simons' integrated hypothesis of trigger point formation. Curr Pain Headache Rep 2004;8(6):468–75.
5. Fernández-de-las-Peñas C, Cuadrado ML, Arendt-Nielsen L, et al. Myofascial trigger points and sensitization: an updated pain model for tension-type headache. Cephalalgia 2007;27(5):383–93.
6. Mendell LM, Wall PD. RESPONSES OF SINGLE DORSAL CORD CELLS TO PERIPHERAL CUTANEOUS UNMYELINATED FIBRES. Nature 1965;206:97–9.
7. Yoshihara T, Shigeta K, Hasegawa H, et al. Neuroendocrine responses to psychological stress in patients with myofascial pain. J Orofac Pain 2005;19(3): 202–8.
8. Russell IJ, Bieber CS. Myofascial pain and fibromyalgia syndrome. In: McMahon SB, Koltzenburg M, editors. Wall and Melzack's textbook of pain. 5th edition. Elsevier; 2006. p. 669–81.
9. Borg-Stein J, Stein J. Trigger points and tender points: one and the same? Does injection treatment help? Rheum Dis Clin North Am 1996;22(2):305–22.
10. Hua NK, Van der Does E. The occurrence and inter-rater reliability of myofascial trigger points in the quadratus lumborum and gluteus medius: a prospective study in non-specific low back pain patients and controls in general practice. Pain 1994;58(3):317–23.
11. Simons DGTJ, Simons LS. Myofasical pain and dysfunction: the trigger point manual. Wiliams & Wilkins; 1999.

12. Central SM. nervous system mechanisms of muscle pain: ascending pathways, central sensitization, and pain-modulating systems. In: Mense SGR, editor. Muscle pain: Understanding the mechanisms. Springer; 2010. p. 105–76.

13. Cummings M, Baldry P. Regional myofascial pain: diagnosis and management. Best Pract Res Clin Rheumatol 2007;21(2):367–87.

14. Ettlin T, Schuster C, Stoffel R, et al. A distinct pattern of myofascial findings in patients after whiplash injury. Arch Phys Med Rehabil 2008;89(7):1290–3.

15. Simons GD, Mense S. Understanding and measurement of muscle tone as related to clinical muscle pain. Pain 1998;75(1):1–17.

16. Rivner MH. The neurophysiology of myofascial pain syndrome. Curr Pain Headache Rep 2001;5(5):432–40.

17. Travell JG, Simons DG. Lower half of the body. Myofascial pain and dysfunction: the trigger point manual. Williams and Wilkins; 1999.

18. Gerwin RD, Shannon S, Hong CZ, et al. Interrater reliability in myofascial trigger point examination. Pain 1997;69(1–2):65–73.

19. Hsieh CY, Hong CZ, Adams AH, et al. Interexaminer reliability of the palpation of trigger points in the trunk and lower limb muscles. Arch Phys Med Rehabil 2000; 81(3):258–64.

20. Nice DA, Riddle DL, Lamb RL, et al. Intertester reliability of judgments of the presence of trigger points in patients with low back pain. Arch Phys Med Rehabil 1992;73(10):893–8.

21. Tantanatip A, Chang KV. Myofascial Pain Syndrome. StatPearls 2021.

22. Chen Q, Basford J, An KN. Ability of magnetic resonance elastography to assess taut bands. Clin Biomech (Bristol, Avon) 2008;23(5):623–9.

23. Sikdar S, Shah JP, Gebreab T, et al. Novel applications of ultrasound technology to visualize and characterize myofascial trigger points and surrounding soft tissue. Arch Phys Med Rehabil 2009;90(11):1829–38.

24. Benzon HT, Katz JA, Benzon HA, et al. Piriformis syndrome: anatomic considerations, a new injection technique, and a review of the literature. Anesthesiology 2003;98(6):1442–8.

25. Wun-Schen C. Bipartite piriformis muscle: an unusual cause of sciatic nerve entrapment. Pain 1994;58(2):269–72.

26. Probst D, Stout A, Hunt D. Piriformis Syndrome: A Narrative Review of the Anatomy, Diagnosis, and Treatment. PM R 2019;11(Suppl 1):S54–63.

27. Borg-Stein J, Simons DG. Focused review: myofascial pain. *Arch Phys Med Rehabil* Mar 2002;83(3 Suppl 1):S40–7, s48-S47.

28. Narouze S, Benzon HT, Provenzano D, et al. Interventional Spine and Pain Procedures in Patients on Antiplatelet and Anticoagulant Medications (Second Edition): Guidelines From the American Society of Regional Anesthesia and Pain Medicine, the European Society of Regional Anaesthesia and Pain Therapy, the American Academy of Pain Medicine, the International Neuromodulation Society, the North American Neuromodulation Society, and the World Institute of Pain. Reg Anesth Pain Med 2018;43(3):225–62.

29. Shafer N. Pneumothorax following "trigger point" injection. JAMA 1970;213(7): 1193.

30. Fitzgibbon DR, Posner KL, Domino KB, et al. Chronic pain management: American Society of Anesthesiologists Closed Claims Project. Anesthesiology 2004; 100(1):98–105.

31. Cheng J, Abdi S. Complications of Joint, Tendon, and Muscle Injections. Tech Reg Anesth Pain Manag 2007;11(3):141–7.

32. Zhao DY, Zhang GL. [Clinical analysis on 38 cases of pneumothorax induced by acupuncture or acupoint injection]. Zhongguo Zhen Jiu 2009;29(3):239–42.

33. Botwin KP, Sharma K, Saliba R, et al. Ultrasound-guided trigger point injections in the cervicothoracic musculature: a new and unreported technique. Pain Physician 2008;11(6):885–9.

34. Seol SJ, Cho H, Yoon DH, et al. Appropriate depth of needle insertion during rhomboid major trigger point block. Ann Rehabil Med 2014;38(1):72–6.

35. Alvarez DJ, Rockwell PG. Trigger points: diagnosis and management. Am Fam Physician 2002;65(4):653–60.

36. Park JS, Kim YH, Jeong SA, et al. Ultrasound-guided Aspiration of the Iatrogenic Pneumothorax Caused by Paravertebral Block -A Case Report. Korean J Pain 2012;25(1):33–7.

37. Nelson LS, Hoffman RS. Intrathecal injection: unusual complication of trigger-point injection therapy. Ann Emerg Med 1998;32(4):506–8.

38. Elias M. Cervical epidural abscess following trigger point injection. J Pain Symptom Manage 1994;9(2):71–2.

39. Zink W, Graf BM. Local anesthetic myotoxicity. Reg Anesth Pain Med 2004; 29(4):333–40.

40. Soriano PK, Bhattarai M, Vogler CN, et al. A Case of Trigger-Point Injection-Induced Hypokalemic Paralysis. Am J Case Rep 2017;18:454–7.

41. Hammi C, Schroeder JD, Yeung B. Trigger Point Injection. StatPearls 2021.

42. Ge HY, Fernandez-de-Las-Penas C, Yue SW. Myofascial trigger points: spontaneous electrical activity and its consequences for pain induction and propagation. Chin Med 2011;6:13.

43. Thomas K, Shankar H. Targeting myofascial taut bands by ultrasound. Curr Pain Headache Rep 2013;17(7):349.

44. Rha DW, Shin JC, Kim YK, et al. Detecting local twitch responses of myofascial trigger points in the lower-back muscles using ultrasonography. Arch Phys Med Rehabil 2011;92(10):1576–1580 e1.

45. Muir JJ, Curtiss HM, Hollman J, et al. The accuracy of ultrasound-guided and palpation-guided peroneal tendon sheath injections. Am J Phys Med Rehabil 2011;90(7):564–71.

46. Daniels EW, Cole D, Jacobs B, et al. Existing Evidence on Ultrasound-Guided Injections in Sports Medicine. Orthop J Sports Med 2018;6(2). 2325967118756576.

47. Koh SH, Lee SC, Lee WY, et al. Ultrasound-guided intra-articular injection of hyaluronic acid and ketorolac for osteoarthritis of the carpometacarpal joint of the thumb: A retrospective comparative study. Medicine (Baltimore) 2019;98(19): e15506.

48. Kang JJ, Kim J, Park S, et al. Feasibility of Ultrasound-Guided Trigger Point Injection in Patients with Myofascial Pain Syndrome. Healthcare (Basel) 2019;7(4). https://doi.org/10.3390/healthcare7040118.

49. Cho IT, Cho YW, Kwak SG, et al. Comparison between ultrasound-guided interfascial pulsed radiofrequency and ultrasound-guided interfascial block with local anesthetic in myofascial pain syndrome of trapezius muscle. Medicine (Baltimore) 2017;96(5):e6019. https://doi.org/10.1097/MD.0000000000006019.

50. Metin Okmen B, Okmen K, Altan L. Comparison of the Efficiency of Ultrasound-Guided Injections of the Rhomboid Major and Trapezius Muscles in Myofascial Pain Syndrome: A Prospective Randomized Controlled Double-blind Study. J Ultrasound Med 2018;37(5):1151–7.

51. Ballyns JJ, Turo D, Otto P, et al. Office-based elastographic technique for quantifying mechanical properties of skeletal muscle. J Ultrasound Med 2012;31(8): 1209–19.

52. Chen Q, Bensamoun S, Basford JR, et al. Identification and quantification of myofascial taut bands with magnetic resonance elastography. Arch Phys Med Rehabil 2007;88(12):1658–61.

53. Nightingale K, Soo MS, Nightingale R, et al. Acoustic radiation force impulse imaging: in vivo demonstration of clinical feasibility. Ultrasound Med Biol 2002; 28(2):227–35.

54. Lin YC, Yu NY, Jiang CF, et al. Characterizing the SEMG patterns with myofascial pain using a multi-scale wavelet model through machine learning approaches. J Electromyogr Kinesiol 2018;41:147–53.

55. Jiang CF, Lin YC, Yu NY. Multi-scale surface electromyography modeling to identify changes in neuromuscular activation with myofascial pain. IEEE Trans Neural Syst Rehabil Eng 2013;21(1):88–95.

56. Finnoff JT, Hurdle MF, Smith J. Accuracy of ultrasound-guided versus fluoroscopically guided contrast-controlled piriformis injections: a cadaveric study. J Ultrasound Med 2008;27(8):1157–63.

57. Barbero M, Falla D, Mafodda L, et al. The Location of Peak Upper Trapezius Muscle Activity During Submaximal Contractions is not Associated With the Location of Myofascial Trigger Points: New Insights Revealed by High-density Surface EMG. Clin J Pain 2016;32(12):1044–52.

58. Kim DH, Lee MS, Lee S, et al. A Prospective Randomized Comparison of the Efficacy of Ultrasound- vs Fluoroscopy-Guided Genicular Nerve Block for Chronic Knee Osteoarthritis. Pain Physician 2019;22(2):139–46.

59. Wagner LK, Eifel PJ, Geise RA. Potential biological effects following high X-ray dose interventional procedures. J Vasc Interv Radiol 1994;5(1):71–84.

60. Chang KV, Wu WT, Lew HL, et al. Ultrasound Imaging and Guided Injection for the Lateral and Posterior Hip. Am J Phys Med Rehabil 2018;97(4):285–91.

61. Jacobson J. Interventional techniques. Fundamentals of musculoskeletal ultrasound. 3rd ed. Elsevier; 2013. p. 357–8.

62. Bardowski EA, Byrd JWT. Piriformis Injection: An Ultrasound-Guided Technique. Arthrosc Tech 2019;8(12):e1457–61.

63. Hong CZ. Lidocaine injection versus dry needling to myofascial trigger point. The importance of the local twitch response. Am J Phys Med Rehabil 1994; 73(4):256–63.

64. Cummings TM, White AR. Needling therapies in the management of myofascial trigger point pain: a systematic review. Arch Phys Med Rehabil 2001;82(7): 986–92.

65. Garvey TA, Marks MR, Wiesel SW. A prospective, randomized, double-blind evaluation of trigger-point injection therapy for low-back pain. Spine (Phila Pa 1976) 1989;14(9):962–4.

66. Cui M, Khanijou S, Rubino J, et al. Subcutaneous administration of botulinum toxin A reduces formalin-induced pain. Pain 2004;107(1–2):125–33.

67. Tschopp KP, Gysin C. Local injection therapy in 107 patients with myofascial pain syndrome of the head and neck. ORL J Otorhinolaryngol Relat Spec 1996;58(6):306–10.

68. Hameroff SR, Crago BR, Blitt CD, et al. Comparison of bupivacaine, etidocaine, and saline for trigger-point therapy. Anesth Analg 1981;60(10):752–5.

69. Iwama H, Akama Y. The superiority of water-diluted 0.25% to neat 1% lidocaine for trigger-point injections in myofascial pain syndrome: a prospective, randomized, double-blinded trial. Anesth Analg 2000;91(2):408–9.

70. Zaralidou AT, Amaniti EN, Maidatsi PG, et al. Comparison between newer local anesthetics for myofascial pain syndrome management. Methods Find Exp Clin Pharmacol 2007;29(5):353–7.

71. Kocak AO, Ahiskalioglu A, Sengun E, et al. Comparison of intravenous NSAIDs and trigger point injection for low back pain in ED: A prospective randomized study. Am J Emerg Med 2019;37(10):1927–31.

72. Roldan CJ, Osuagwu U, Cardenas-Turanzas M, et al. Normal Saline Trigger Point Injections vs Conventional Active Drug Mix for Myofascial Pain Syndromes. Am J Emerg Med 2020;38(2):311–6.

73. Iwama H, Ohmori S, Kaneko T, et al. Water-diluted local anesthetic for trigger-point injection in chronic myofascial pain syndrome: evaluation of types of local anesthetic and concentrations in water. Reg Anesth Pain Med 2001;26(4):333–6.

74. Krishnan SK, Benzon HT, Siddiqui T, et al. Pain on intramuscular injection of bupivacaine, ropivacaine, with and without dexamethasone. Reg Anesth Pain Med 2000;25(6):615–9.

75. Yoon SH, Rah UW, Sheen SS, et al. Comparison of 3 needle sizes for trigger point injection in myofascial pain syndrome of upper- and middle-trapezius muscle: a randomized controlled trial. Arch Phys Med Rehabil 2009;90(8):1332–9.

76. Ga H, Choi JH, Park CH, et al. Acupuncture needling versus lidocaine injection of trigger points in myofascial pain syndrome in elderly patients–a randomised trial. Acupunct Med 2007;25(4):130–6.

77. Mitidieri AMS, Baltazar M, da Silva APM, et al. Ashi Acupuncture Versus Local Anesthetic Trigger Point Injections in the Treatment of Abdominal Myofascial Pain Syndrome: A Randomized Clinical Trial. Pain Physician 2020;23(5):507–18.

78. Wheeler AH, Goolkasian P, Gretz SS. A randomized, double-blind, prospective pilot study of botulinum toxin injection for refractory, unilateral, cervicothoracic, paraspinal, myofascial pain syndrome. Spine (Phila Pa 1976) 1998;23(15):1662–6 ; discussion 1667.

79. Qerama E, Fuglsang-Frederiksen A, Kasch H, et al. A double-blind, controlled study of botulinum toxin A in chronic myofascial pain. Neurology 2006;67(2):241–5.

80. Kwanchuay P, Petchnumsin T, Yiemsiri P, et al. Efficacy and Safety of Single Botulinum Toxin Type A (Botox(R)) Injection for Relief of Upper Trapezius Myofascial Trigger Point: A Randomized, Double-Blind, Placebo-Controlled Study. J Med Assoc Thai 2015;98(12):1231–6.

81. Dessie SG, Von Bargen E, Hacker MR, et al. A randomized, double-blind, placebo-controlled trial of onabotulinumtoxin A trigger point injections for myofascial pelvic pain. Am J Obstet Gynecol 2019;221(5):517 e1–9.

82. Gobel H, Heinze A, Reichel G, et al. Dysport myofascial pain study g. Efficacy and safety of a single botulinum type A toxin complex treatment (Dysport) for the relief of upper back myofascial pain syndrome: results from a randomized double-blind placebo-controlled multicentre study. Pain 2006;125(1–2):82–8.

83. Kamanli A, Kaya A, Ardicoglu O, et al. Comparison of lidocaine injection, botulinum toxin injection, and dry needling to trigger points in myofascial pain syndrome. Rheumatol Int 2005;25(8):604–11.

84. Ferrante FM, Bearn L, Rothrock R, et al. Evidence against trigger point injection technique for the treatment of cervicothoracic myofascial pain with botulinum toxin type A. Anesthesiology 2005;103(2):377–83.

85. Harden RN, Cottrill J, Gagnon CM, et al. Botulinum toxin a in the treatment of chronic tension-type headache with cervical myofascial trigger points: a randomized, double-blind, placebo-controlled pilot study. Headache 2009;49(5): 732–43.

86. Graboski CL, Gray DS, Burnham RS. Botulinum toxin A versus bupivacaine trigger point injections for the treatment of myofascial pain syndrome: a randomised double blind crossover study. Pain 2005;118(1–2):170–5.

87. Venancio Rde A, Alencar FG Jr, Zamperini C. Botulinum toxin, lidocaine, and dry-needling injections in patients with myofascial pain and headaches. Cranio 2009;27(1):46–53.

88. Nicol AL, Wu II, Ferrante FM. Botulinum toxin type a injections for cervical and shoulder girdle myofascial pain using an enriched protocol design. Anesth Analg 2014;118(6):1326–35.

89. Benecke R, Heinze A, Reichel G, et al. Botulinum type A toxin complex for the relief of upper back myofascial pain syndrome: how do fixed-location injections compare with trigger point-focused injections? Pain Med 2011;12(11):1607–14.

90. Miller D, Richardson D, Eisa M, et al. Botulinum neurotoxin-A for treatment of refractory neck pain: a randomized, double-blind study. Pain Med 2009;10(6): 1012–7.

91. Vij N, Kiernan H, Bisht R, et al. Surgical and Non-surgical Treatment Options for Piriformis Syndrome: A Literature Review. Anesth Pain Med 2021;11(1): e112825.

92. Michel F, Decavel P, Toussirot E, et al. Piriformis muscle syndrome: diagnostic criteria and treatment of a monocentric series of 250 patients. Ann Phys Rehabil Med 2013;56(5):371–83.

93. Fishman LM, Dombi GW, Michaelsen C, et al. Piriformis syndrome: diagnosis, treatment, and outcome–a 10-year study. Arch Phys Med Rehabil 2002;83(3): 295–301.

94. Filler AG, Haynes J, Jordan SE, et al. Sciatica of nondisc origin and piriformis syndrome: diagnosis by magnetic resonance neurography and interventional magnetic resonance imaging with outcome study of resulting treatment. J Neurosurg Spine 2005;2(2):99–115.

95. Masala S, Crusco S, Meschini A, et al. Piriformis syndrome: long-term follow-up in patients treated with percutaneous injection of anesthetic and corticosteroid under CT guidance. Cardiovasc Intervent Radiol 2012;35(2):375–82.

96. Ozisik PA, Toru M, Denk CC, et al. CT-guided piriformis muscle injection for the treatment of piriformis syndrome. Turk Neurosurg 2014;24(4):471–7.

97. Jeong HS, Lee GY, Lee EG, et al. Long-term assessment of clinical outcomes of ultrasound-guided steroid injections in patients with piriformis syndrome. Ultrasonography 2015;34(3):206–10.

98. Nazlikul H, Ural FG, Ozturk GT, et al. Evaluation of neural therapy effect in patients with piriformis syndrome. J Back Musculoskelet Rehabil 2018;31(6): 1105–10.

99. Terlemez R, Ercalik T. Effect of piriformis injection on neuropathic pain. Agri Nov 2019;31(4):178–82.

100. Rosales J, Garcia N, Rafols C, et al. Perisciatic Ultrasound-Guided Infiltration for Treatment of Deep Gluteal Syndrome: Description of Technique and Preliminary Results. J Ultrasound Med 2015;34(11):2093–7.

101. Misirlioglu TO, Akgun K, Palamar D, et al. Piriformis syndrome: comparison of the effectiveness of local anesthetic and corticosteroid injections: a double-blinded, randomized controlled study. Pain Physician 2015;18(2):163–71.
102. Burke CJ, Walter WR, Adler RS. Targeted Ultrasound-Guided Perineural Hydro-dissection of the Sciatic Nerve for the Treatment of Piriformis Syndrome. Ultra-sound Q 2019;35(2):125–9.
103. Porta M. A comparative trial of botulinum toxin type A and methylprednisolone for the treatment of myofascial pain syndrome and pain from chronic muscle spasm. Pain 2000;85(1–2):101–5.
104. Al-Al-Shaikh M, Michel F, Parratte B, et al. An MRI evaluation of changes in pir-iformis muscle morphology induced by botulinum toxin injections in the treat-ment of piriformis syndrome. Diagn Interv Imaging 2015;96(1):37–43.
105. Santamato A, Micello MF, Valeno G, et al. Ultrasound-Guided Injection of Botu-linum Toxin Type A for Piriformis Muscle Syndrome: A Case Report and Review of the Literature. Toxins (Basel). 2015;7(8):3045–56.
106. Lang AM. Botulinum toxin type B in piriformis syndrome. Am J Phys Med Reha-bil 2004;83(3):198–202.
107. Fishman LM, Konnoth C, Rozner B. Botulinum neurotoxin type B and physical therapy in the treatment of piriformis syndrome: a dose-finding study. Am J Phys Med Rehabil 2004;83(1):42–50, quiz 51-3.
108. Yoon SJ, Ho J, Kang HY, et al. Low-dose botulinum toxin type A for the treatment of refractory piriformis syndrome. Pharmacotherapy 2007;27(5):657–65.
109. Childers MK, Wilson DJ, Gnatz SM, et al. Botulinum toxin type A use in piriformis muscle syndrome: a pilot study. Am J Phys Med Rehabil 2002;81(10):751–9.
110. Fishman LM, Anderson C, Rosner B. BOTOX and physical therapy in the treat-ment of piriformis syndrome. Am J Phys Med Rehabil 2002;81(12):936–42.
111. Fishman LM, Wilkins AN, Rosner B. Electrophysiologically identified piriformis syndrome is successfully treated with incobotulinum toxin a and physical ther-apy. Muscle Nerve 2017;56(2):258–63.
112. Rodríguez-Piñero M, Vidal Vargas V, Jiménez Sarmiento AS. Long-Term Efficacy of Ultrasound-Guided Injection of IncobotulinumtoxinA in Piriformis Syndrome. Pain Med 2018;19(2):408–11.
113. Yan K, Xi Y, Hlis R, et al. Piriformis syndrome: pain response outcomes following CT-guided injection and incremental value of botulinum toxin injection. Diagn In-terv Radiol 2021;27(1):126–33.

Spinal Cord Stimulation
A Psychiatric Perspective

Mehul J. Desai, MD, MPH[a,b,*], Ryan Aschenbrener, MD[a],
Eduardo J. Carrera, MD[c], Nirguna Thalla, MD[d,e]

KEYWORDS

- Spinal cord stimulation • Neuromodulation • Paresthesia-free waveforms

KEY POINTS

- Over the past several decades, there has been a rapid evolution in spinal cord stimulation (SCS).
- Significant greater ability to customize therapy now exists.
- The development of a number of new and novel waveforms and programming methodologies has ushered in this ability to customize therapy.
- The potential to optimize therapy and expand indications is now being realized.

INTRODUCTION

Since its inception in 1967 by Shealy and colleagues,[1] the use of spinal cord stimulation (SCS) has increased dramatically. A tremendous evolution in technology over the past decade to a great extent spurred this growth. Technological advances, novel waveforms, imaging conditionality, and adaptation to recalcitrant pain syndromes formed the backbone of this development.[2] Furthermore, a greater understanding of the mechanisms behind SCS has been developed recently.

MECHANISMS

Over the first 5 to 6 decades of SCS use, its analgesic activity was hypothesized to occur as a result of Gate Control Theory as proposed by Wall and Melzack in 1965.[3] This theory postulates that the activation of cutaneous touch signals

[a] International Spine, Pain & Performance Center, 2021 K Street NW Suite 615, Washington, DC 20006, USA; [b] The George Washington University, School of Medicine and Health Sciences, 2300 I Street NW Washington, DC 20052, USA; [c] Department of Physical Medicine and Rehabilitation, University of Colorado, School of Medicine, 2631 East 17th Avenue, #1201, Auroro, CO 80045, USA; [d] Department of Rehabilitation Medicine, MedStar Georgetown University, Washington, DC, USA; [e] MedStar National Rehabilitation Hospital, Physical Medicine and Rehabilitation, 102 Irving Street NW Washington, DC 20010, USA
* Corresponding author.
E-mail address: drdesai@isppcenter.com

Phys Med Rehabil Clin N Am 33 (2022) 335–357
https://doi.org/10.1016/j.pmr.2022.01.003
1047-9651/22/© 2022 Elsevier Inc. All rights reserved.

transmitted via larger myelinated A-beta fibers may subdue afferent pain signals transmitted by smaller C fibers by gating output from the dorsal horn shared by these inputs. Fundamentally, SCS was conceived on this premise.[1] More recently, this premise has fallen under intense scrutiny as other potential mechanisms have emerged. Several alternate hypotheses have recently been proposed, including:

- Paresthesia-free waveforms. Jensen and Brownthorne suggested that SCS provides analgesia by stimulating the dendrites of GABAergic dorsal horn islet cells, which are oriented in the same rostro-causal direction as SCS electrodes.[4]
- Reducing dorsal horn glial cell activity. Glial cells contribute to neuropathic pain via modulation of neurotransmitters and cytokine concentrations.[5] SCS has been shown to decrease glial cell activity in rat models in conjunction with reducing hyperalgesia.[6] Stimulation of the dorsal horn also increases acetylcholine and GABA and decreases excitatory amino acids.[7,8]
- Cortical activity. SCS has been found to decrease sensory evoked potentials, although this reduction was not consistently correlated with pain relief in human subjects.[9]
- Endogenous opioid activation. In animal studies, rats given mu or delta opioid antagonists were found to experience a decrease in SCS analgesia effectiveness at certain stimulation frequencies.[10]

While significant disagreements persist regarding the ultimate mechanism of action of SCS, significant progress in this understanding has been made recently.

FEATURES

Physiatrists may tailor SCS therapy to their patient's pain complaints by adjusting a variety of device settings. These include but are not limited to:

- Basic parameters.
  - Amplitude.
  - Pulse width.
  - Frequency.
- Advanced parameters.
  - Contact configuration.
  - Contact location.
- Programs.
  - Tonic.
  - Burst.
  - High-frequency.
  - Ultra-low frequency.

Basic Parameters

The fundamentals of device programming include the modification of basic parameters including amplitude, pulse width, and frequency (**Fig. 1**).

Amplitude, measured in milliamperes (mA) or voltage (V), correlates with the power output from the internal or external pulse generator (IPG/EPG). Higher amplitude correlates with higher energy output. Currently, all commercially available SCS systems use a constant current (CC) setting. Patients seem to prefer CC systems over constant voltage (CV) systems,[11] likely because fluctuations in resistance can impact the amount of current being delivered, as per Ohm's Law (see **Fig. 1**).

$$C = I * R \ (C = \text{Current}, I = \text{Voltage and } R = \text{Resistance})$$

Fig. 1. Ohm's Law $C = I * R$ (C = Current, I = voltage and R = resistance).

Therefore, as resistance or impedance changes, CC systems adjust voltage such that the current experienced by the patient remains consistent.

Pulse width, measured in microseconds (μs), is the amount of time for which each pulse of energy is generated. Together, amplitude and pulse width determine the amount of charge-per-pulse generated (**Fig. 2**).[12] As the threshold for neuronal action potential generation is proportional to charge-per-pulse, wider pulse widths can compensate for lower amplitudes to increase energy density. Increasing pulse width may also increase the area of stimulation to broaden the region of spinal coverage. This, however, carries the risk of off-target stimulation.

Frequency is measured in Hertz (Hz). It is adjusted to impact neuronal depolarization frequency and overall strength of stimulation.[12] Although conventional frequencies range from 40 to 100 Hz,[13] newer devices have the capacity to operate at up to 10 kHz.

Advanced Parameters

Lead contact configuration is determined based on several factors. Lead contacts are programmed into anodes (positive charges) and cathodes (negative charges). As electrons flow away from a cathode ("active" contact), depolarization of nearby cells creates action potentials. The number of contacts used per lead, the intra-contact distance, and the lead-to-lead distance all impact the geometry of the electrical field created, and thereby the portion of the dorsal columns activated.[14]

Lead location is a key determinant of anatomic coverage in both paresthesia and paresthesia-free stimulation parameters. Prior work by Holsheimer and Barolat was key in determining placement as it correlated to analgesic effect.[15,16]

Programs

Over the past decade, a multitude of novel programs has emerged (see **Fig. 2**). Previously, tonic SCS waveforms and conventional range frequencies (40–100 Hz) were commonplace.[17] The first transformative development was the introduction of high-frequency stimulation coupled with subperceptive amplitudes.[17] This was found to achieve paresthesia-free analgesia, eliminating the need for intraoperative testing. High-frequency stimulation is thought to preferentially block large-diameter fibers

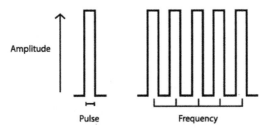

Fig. 2. Basic parameters for spinal cord stimulation when plotting current versus time. *(Modified from* Caylor, J., Reddy, R., Yin, S. et al. Spinal cord stimulation in chronic pain: evidence and theory for mechanisms of action. Bioelectron Med 5, 12 (2019). https://doi.org/10.1186/s42234-019-0023-1)

which convey vibratory sensation, while recruiting medium-diameter fibers to maintain the analgesic effect, although this hypothesis has not been proven further.[18]

Burst stimulation is an additional paresthesia-free modality. This program delivers five 1-μs spikes at 500 Hz in CC mode, repeated with an inter-burst frequency of 40 Hz.[19] Burst stimulation has been found to demonstrate an increase in electroencephalogram (EEG) activity of the dorsal anterior cingulate and dorsolateral prefrontal cortex.[20] Further, it has been noted to activate both medial and lateral spinothalamic pathways and wide dynamic range (WDR) neurons.[20] In BurstDR, a subtype of burst stimulation, wave amplitude increases over a five-spike train, followed by a passive charge balance.[21] The BurstDR waveform mimics physiologic discharges and may create longer lasting carryover benefits in between bursts.[21] BurstDR devices have been found to remain effective with intermittent doses, which may prolong battery life.[21,22] **(Fig. 3)** While this clear difference does exist between "burst stimulation" and "BurstDR stimulation," the rest of this article will refer to this programming paradigm as "burst stimulation" as an interchangeable term.

While work has recently been conducted in ultra-low frequency settings as low as 10 Hz, definitive data are still pending.[23]

Historically, SCS systems have been open-loop, requiring an external user to program a fixed amplitude that may vary based on patient position. This was despite significant evidence that patient position affects the cerebrospinal fluid thickness[24] and the distance between SCS leads and the spinal cord affects electrically evoked compound action potentials (ECAPs), as do postural changes.[25,26] Closed-loop systems, by contrast, tailor electrical output based on a patient's real-time ECAPs. This maintains a consistent amount of spinal cord activation, theoretically maximizing the therapeutic effect.[26] However, this technology remains in late-stage clinical trials with limited commercial availability in the United States.

PATIENT SELECTION CRITERIA

The National Institute for Health and Care Excellence guidelines from 2008 recommend SCS as a treatment option for adults with chronic neuropathic pain for at least 6 months despite treatment with conventional management.[27] Kumar in 2006 suggested that outcomes were optimal within the first 2 years of onset of chronic

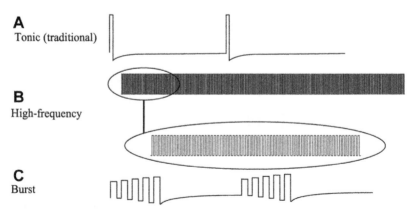

Fig. 3. Comparison of novel waveforms. (*Modified from* Caylor, J., Reddy, R., Yin, S. et al. Spinal cord stimulation in chronic pain: evidence and theory for mechanisms of action. Bioelectron Med 5, 12 (2019). https://doi.org/10.1186/s42234-019-0023-1)

pain.[28] Typically, selection of appropriate patients for SCS involves an in-depth discussion between multiple stakeholders, including the patient, patient's family, and physician. Physicians should focus on realistic expectations including those that pertain to pain relief, function, and quality of life (QoL). Medication issues should also be addressed, including expectations of tapering or weaning off opioid medications if they exist. Lifestyle modifications such as weight loss, tobacco use, and concomitant behavioral issues should be a central theme of discussions. Most commonly, various insurance providers now recommend a pre-SCS behavioral health consultation and clearance before proceeding with the next steps.[29] Care should also be taken to thoroughly review pre-SCS imaging studies, as there are cases whereby the epidural placement of leads is rendered impossible or inadvisable. When necessary, updated imaging to include entry levels and target levels should be ordered and reviewed.[29]

PROCEDURE

Following initial screening as above, an SCS trial is conducted. During the trial, temporary leads are placed into the epidural space and advanced to the target level. During the trial, particularly if the physician is planning to use tonic stimulation, intraoperative testing should be conducted to confirm appropriate placement with concordant paresthesia at the painful locations.[29] These temporary leads typically remain in place for 4 to 10 days and are secured to the patient's skin. At the conclusion of the trial, as the leads are removed, it may be advisable to consider an end-of-trial radiograph, particularly if coverage and pain relief changed substantially during the trial. This may provide further guidance regarding the optional surgical placement of the electrodes. NACC recommendations for proceeding with implantation include greater than 50% pain relief during the trial, with stable levels of activity and without an increase in pain medications.[30] A substantial improvement in activities of daily living (ADLs) or QoL may serve as alternates in lieu of achieving the 50% benchmark for pain relief.[30]

Assuming the above criteria are achieved, the patient may consider moving forward with device implantation. This may be accomplished either via surgical or percutaneous placement (**Figs. 4–8**). Surgical placement is performed by an orthopedic spine surgeon or a neurosurgeon, in which a flat unidirectional paddle electrode is placed via a laminotomy/laminectomy under direct visualization of the epidural space along with an IPG placement in the flank or buttock. Percutaneous placement is performed via small spinal and flank/buttock incisions under fluoroscopic guidance. This is a

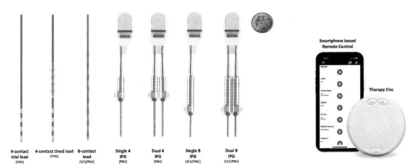

Fig. 4. Nalu leads, IPG, Therapy Disc.

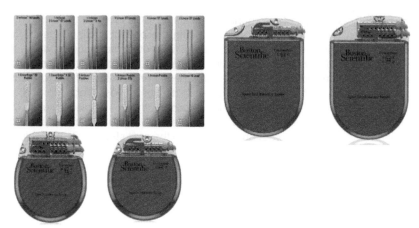

Fig. 5. Boston Scientific Leads and IPGs.

commonly used approach by interventional pain physicians. Patient factors should be paramount when determining the implanting physician.[29]

RISKS AND CONTRAINDICATIONS

Generally speaking, SCS is a safe and reversible procedure. Advances in technique and hardware have greatly improved and continue to improve the safety of this procedure. As with any interventional procedure, awareness of risks may help patients and providers make the most informed decisions and remain alert for complications. The overall reported complication rate stands between 30% and 40%.[31] Complications may be categorized as hardware-related or biologic. Hardware-related complications include: lead migration, fracture or malfunction; implant-related pain; IPG migration; and battery malfunction. Biologic complications include: infection, undesirable paresthesias, habituation, seroma, hematoma, spinal cord injury, and dural puncture. Most complications are hardware-related.[31] Common or major risks are discussed in **Table 1**.

Contraindications to SCS placement include: failure of trial stimulation, uncontrolled psychiatric conditions, inability to comply with therapy, persistent systemic or local infection, immunosuppression, use of diathermy, and anticoagulation or antiplatelet

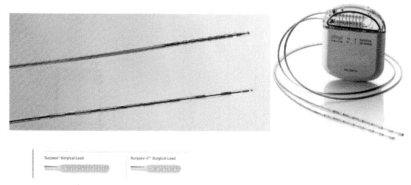

Fig. 6. Nevro Leads and IPG.

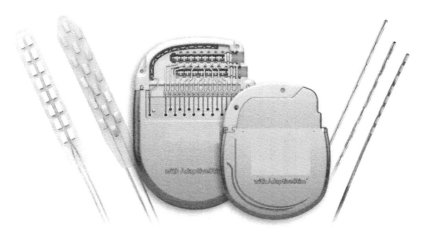

Fig. 7. Medtronic Leads and IPG.

therapy that cannot be suspended.[5,29,51] Relative contraindications include inconsistent history or examination and occupational risks such as climbing ladders, operating machinery, or vehicles.[51] Safety and effectiveness have not been established in pregnancy or pediatric use.[51]

OUTCOME DATA

Spinal cord stimulation has been well-studied in the treatment of chronic pain following FBSS, painful diabetic neuropathy (PDN), CRPS, angina, and painful peripheral vascular disease. Angina and painful peripheral vascular disease are common indications in Europe. While extensive retrospective and prospective noncontrolled studies on SCS exist for each indication, the discussion later in discussion is focused primarily on the seminal randomized controlled trials (RCTs) (**Table 2**).

Tonic (<100 Hz) Spinal Cord Stimulation for Failed Back Surgery Syndrome

Three major RCTs compared tonic SCS to conservative management or reoperation for the treatment of FBSS. North and colleagues[52] published the first major RCT in

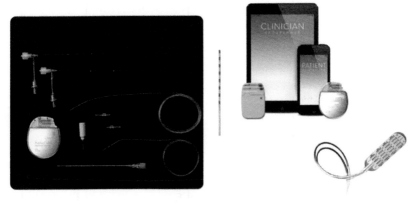

Fig. 8. Abbott Leads and IPG.

Table 1
Risks following SCS implant

Risk	Frequency	Details
Lead migration, fracture, or malfunction	Lead migration occurs at a mean reported rate of 15.49%.[31] Incidence of cylindrical lead migration requiring revision is 2%–9%, similar to rates reported for paddle leads.[32] The mean reported rate of lead fracture or malfunction is 6.37%.[31]	Rate of lead migration is twice as high in the cervical compared to the lumbar spine due to more motion in cervical spine.[28] Increased contacts per lead, improved suturing and anchoring systems and strain-relief loops have improved the rate of revision.[32]
Infection	General infection rate is 2.4%–3.1%.[33,34] Incidence of epidural infection is 0.1%.[34]	Methicillin-sensitive Staphylococcus aureus (MSSA) is the common infectious agent.[35] Infection rate is higher with longer trial duration and implant revisions.[36,37]
Implant-related pain	Mean reported rate of 6.15%.[31]	Most common reasons for pain include trauma to the IPG site, device migration or rotation, uncomfortable contact of the IPG with the ribs or clothing, and device malfunction.
Undesirable stimulation	In one retrospective review, 8% of all implanted patients and 26% of explants had paresthesias uncomfortable enough to pursue explantation.[38]	The intensity of stimulation from tonic SCS varies depending on lead location, stimulation parameters, and the thickness of the posterior CSF layer. The latter factor varies depending on location in the spinal cord and patient position. Technological advancements like closed-loop systems and alternative stimulation modalities can reduce or eliminate paresthesias.[27,39,40]
Loss of therapeutic effect	Retrospective studies suggest that loss of therapeutic effect occurs in 13.7% of patients and accounts for 39% of explants and 16.1% of revisions.[36]	Causes of loss of therapeutic effect include lead migration, malfunction, habituation, disease progression, epidural fibrosis, or alteration of the psychological status of the patient. Limited data exist on the use of "salvage therapy,"

Major Complications	The rate of spinal cord injury (SCI) varies between 0.1% and 2.13%. Catastrophic neurologic complications are rare following SCS.[42–44]	There does not appear to be significant differences in rates of SCI or epidural hematoma between the surgical paddle and percutaneous placement.[42] using an alternative stimulation or frequency pattern to regain therapeutic effect.[41]
Explantation	Rate of device explant 7.9% per year.[45] 30% of patients opted for explant in another study with a 14-y follow-up.[38]	The most common causes for explant include: • Loss of therapeutic effect (43.9%). • Complication (20.2%). • Need for magnetic resonance imaging (MRI) (19.2%). • Resolution of pain (6.1%). • Device malfunction (4.6%). • Other reasons (5.8%).[46] The risk of explantation increases with tobacco use, higher opioid use, pain medication polypharmacy, and cerebrovascular disease.[47]
Magnetic resonance imaging incompatibility	19.2% of explanted devices in one study were due to the need for MRI.[46]	Generally, SCS devices are either not suitable for MRI (MR Unsafe) or are suitable for MRI only under specific conditions (MR Conditional). These conditions could be limited to strictly head and neck MRI or full-body MRI under specific MRI machine parameters. Current devices for full-body imaging are limited to 1.5 T scanners. The need for MRI is meaningful and likely to increase with time.[48] Incorrect use of MRI scanners with SCS devices may damage the device or cause injury.[49,50]

Table 2
Summary of major SCS RCTs

Study	Population	Design	Follow-up	Outcome
North (2005)[51]	60 patients with FBSS with radicular predominant pain.	RCT Tonic SCS vs reoperation	2.9-y mean follow-up.	Greater pain relief and satisfaction in the tonic SCS group.
PROCESS Kumar (2007, 2008)[52,53]	100 patients with FBSS with radicular predominant pain.	RCT Tonic SCS + CMM vs CMM only	6 mo, then crossover allowed. 24-mo total follow-up.	Greater pain relief in tonic SCS + CMM group at 6 mo. After 2 y, tonic SCS + CMM group still had decreased leg pain but not back pain compared to baseline.
PROMISE Rigoard (2019)[53]	218 patients with FBSS with axial predominant pain.	RCT Tonic SCS + OMM vs OMM only.	6 mo, then crossover allowed. 24-mo total follow-up.	Greater pain relief in tonic SCS + OMM group at 6 mo. Within-group improvements in the tonic SCS + OMM group persisted at 12 and 24 mo.
SENZA Kapural (2015, 2016)[56,57]	198 patients with mixed axial and radicular. 77% with FBSS.	RCT 10-kHz SCS vs tonic SCS.	24-mo follow-up.	Greater back and leg pain relief in 10-kHz SCS group through 24-mo follow-up.
De Andres (2017)[58]	60 patients with FBSS with mixed axial and radicular pain.	RCT 10-kHz SCS vs tonic SCS.	12 mo	No difference in pain relief.
PROCO Thomson (2018)[58]	20 patients with axial predominant pain. 80% with FBSS.	Crossover RCT 1, 4, 7, and 10 kHz SCS in random order. Pulse	4 wk for each stimulation. 3 mo for preferred frequency.	No difference in pain relief between frequencies. 1 kHz used less charge.

Study	Patients	Study design	Duration	Results
			width and amplitude titrated.	
HALO Breel (2021)[60]	32 patients with FBSS. Unilateral leg pain predominant.	Crossover RCT 1 kHz SCS vs tonic SCS.	9 d, 5 washout, 9 d crossover.	No difference between 1 kHz SCS and 30 Hz SCS in crossover trial.
SUNBURST Deer (2018)[60]	100 patients with mixed axial and radicular pain. Heterogenous. 41.8% FBSS, 36.9% radiculopathy.	Crossover RCT Burst vs tonic SCS.	12 wk per stimulation setting. 6-mo follow-up with preferred setting.	Greater pain relief in burst setting vs tonic setting at 12 wk. More patients preferred burst at 1 y.
De Vos (2014)[66]	60 patients with PDN.	RCT Tonic SCS + CMM vs CMM only.	6 mo	Greater pain relief in tonic SCS + CMM group.
Slangen (2014)[67]	36 patients with PDN.	RCT Tonic SCS + BMT vs BMT only.	6 mo	Greater daytime and nighttime pain relief in tonic SCS + CMM group vs
SENZA-PDN Petersen (2021)[69]	216 patients with PDN.	RCT HF10 SCS + CMM vs CMM alone.	6 mo	Greater pain relief and neurologic improvement in HF10 SCS + CMM vs CMM only.
Kemler (2000, 2008)[71,72]	54 patients with CRPS type 1.	RCT Tonic SCS + PT vs PT only.	5 y	Greater pain relief in SCS + PT group for first 2 y. No difference in years 3–5.
Kriek (2017)[73]	29 patients with CRPS. Type 1 (93.1%), Type 2 (6.9%).	Crossover RCT Placebo, burst, 40 Hz, 500 Hz, 1200 Hz SCS in random order.	2 wk per phase, total of 10 wk.	All stimulation settings were superior to placebo. Most patients preferred 40 Hz stimulation.

2005, whereby 60 patients with FBSS were randomized to tonic SCS or repeat surgery. Candidates were patients with radicular pain equal to or greater than any axial low back pain and concordant with surgically remediable nerve root compression. Tonic SCS was superior to reoperation, with 47% of patients in the SCS group compared with 12% in the reoperation group meeting the composite primary outcome of ≥50% pain relief and patient satisfaction. SCS was also superior to reoperation in patients who crossed over to SCS after 6 months.

The PROCESS RCT, published in 2007, followed the landmark trial by North and colleagues One hundred patients with FBSS with predominant leg pain were randomized to tonic SCS and conservative medical management (CMM) or CMM alone. The tonic SCS and CMM group were superior to CMM alone, with 48% of patients in the former and 9% in the latter group meeting the primary outcome of ≥50% pain relief at 6 months.[53] Crossover was allowed after 6 months. On 2-year follow-up, patients in the tonic SCS and CMM group still had decreased leg pain but no difference in back pain compared with baseline.[54]

The study by North and colleagues and the PROCESS trial established level 1 evidence for the use of tonic SCS for the treatment of extremity-predominant pain in patients with FBSS compared with reoperation and CMM, respectively. However, the question remained whether tonic SCS could be effective for patients with low back-predominant pain and in a real-world application. The PROMISE trial, published in 2019, was a pragmatic RCT aimed to answer these questions by randomizing 218 patients with FBSS with predominant low back pain to tonic multicolumn SCS and optimal medical management (OMM) or OMM only.[55] Patients could cross over at 6 months. The tonic SCS and OMM group were superior to OMM only, with 13.6% of patients in the former and 4.6% in the latter group meeting the primary outcome of ≥50% reduction in low back pain at 6 months. In addition, the tonic SCS and OMM group showed significant improvement in Oswestry Disability Index (ODI) and SF-36 PCS scores compared with the OMM only group. Within-group improvements in the tonic SCS and OMM group persisted at 12 and 24 months. While the therapeutic effect on back pain was lower than expected, no prior RCT using tonic SCS had focused on the predominant low back pain population.

Subperception Spinal Cord Stimulation for Chronic Back and Leg Pain

Limitations from tonic SCS have included a limited effect of tonic SCS on back pain, undesirable paresthesia intensity, and increased procedure time required for paresthesia mapping.[56] Over the last decade, this has led to a shift in research from tonic SCS toward subperception (paresthesia-free) modalities such as high-frequency, burst, and high-density stimulation. These trials often enrolled heterogeneous populations, with the most common diagnoses being FBSS and radiculopathy.

The SENZA trial published in 2015 was the landmark trial providing level 1 evidence for the use of high-frequency 10-kHz SCS (HF10) for back and leg pain.[57] In this pragmatic RCT, 198 patients with mixed back and leg pain were randomized to HF10 or tonic SCS. Diagnostic criteria for FBSS were met by 77% of patients. Unlike prior studies, patients had similar back and leg pain at baseline. The composite primary outcome was ≥50% reduction in VAS without a neurologic deficit. There was a greater reduction in opioid use in the HF10 group (35.5%) compared with the conventional group (26.4%). At 3 months, patients in the HF10 group were more likely than patients in the tonic SCS group to be responders for back pain (84.5% vs 43.8%) and leg pain (83.1% vs 55.5%). Similarly, at 24-months follow-up patients on HF10 group were more likely than patients in the tonic SCS group to be responders for back pain (76.5% vs 49.3%) and leg pain (72.9% vs 49.3%).[58]

Several smaller RCTs demonstrate noninferiority but not the superiority of high-frequency stimulation to tonic SCS. De Andres and colleagues performed a randomized trial whereby 60 patients with FBSS with mixed axial and radicular pain were randomized to HF10 or tonic SCS. The study found no difference in VAS reduction or secondary outcomes between the 2 groups at 1 year.[59] Similarly, other smaller studies have shown no difference between 1 and 10 kHz as long as pulse width and amplitude were titrated,[60] as well as between 1 kHz and tonic SCS.[61]

The SUNBURST study published in 2018 was the primary landmark trial establishing the use of burst stimulation.[62] In this RCT, 100 patients were randomized to receive burst SCS or tonic SCS for 12 weeks, then the other stimulation mode for 12 weeks, after which patients could choose to continue with whichever waveform they preferred. The patient population was heterogeneous, with most patients diagnosed with FBSS (41.8%) or radiculopathy (36.9%). At 12 weeks, the study met the noninferiority and superiority criteria for VAS, with a difference of −5.1 mm. Responders were defined as patients with ≥30% reduction in VAS. 60% of patients in the burst SCS group were responders compared with 51% of patients in the tonic group. At 1 year of follow-up, 68.2% of patients preferred burst stimulation, whereas 23.9% preferred tonic stimulation. During the burst phase, 89% of patients experienced reduced or no paresthesias.[62] A meta-analysis of five studies including the SUNBURST in a predominant FBSS population yielded a mean VAS reduction of 1.64 cm for burst stimulation compared with tonic SCS.[63]

Taken in aggregate, subperception stimulation modalities such as burst and high-frequency stimulation seem to be at least noninferior to tonic stimulation for the treatment of chronic back and leg pain. There is also often greater patient preference for subperception modalities over tonic SCS.[64] Direct comparison between burst and high-frequency stimulation is lacking. The ongoing MULTIWAVE RCT will fill this gap by comparing conventional, burst, and high-frequency SCS in patients with FBSS.[65] Closed-loop systems have also been developed, which allow adjusting the stimulation intensity automatically based on the proximity of the lead to the dorsal columns, therefore, decreasing the chance of uncomfortable paresthesias due to overstimulation or lower therapeutic effect due to understimulation.[66] It remains to be seen how closed-loop tonic SCS systems compare to subperception modalities.

Painful Diabetic Neuropathy

De Vos and colleagues[67] published an open-label randomized parallel-group study in 2014 with 60 diabetic patients with PDN randomized 2:1 to medical therapy with tonic SCS or best medical therapy (BMT). The tonic SCS group was superior to BMT, with 60% of patients in the former and 5% in the latter group achieving ≥50% pain reduction at 6 months. The average VAS score decreased from 7.3 cm to 3.1 cm for the SCS group and remained at 6.7 cm for the BMT group at 6 months. There were also improvements in secondary outcomes for the SCS group, including QoL scores and use of analgesics.

Slangen and colleagues[68] published a randomized trial in 2014 comparing conventional SCS with BMT in 36 diabetic patients with PDN. The primary outcome was greater than 50% pain relief during daytime or nighttime or an improvement of ≥6 in pain and sleep on the Patient Global Impression of Change (PGIC) scale at 6 months. The tonic SCS group was superior to BMT, with 60% of patients meeting the primary outcome compared with 5% in the BMT group. 59% of patients in the SCS group compared with 7% of the BMT group met the primary outcome. In the SCS group, 41% of patients reported 50% or more pain relief during the day and 36% at night, compared with 0% during the day and 7% at night in the BMT group. Prospective follow-up data using patient data from the Slangen and colleagues study and a separate study demonstrated a decline over time of patients meeting the primary outcome from 86% of patients at 12 months to 55% of patients at 5-year follow-up.[68,69]

Most recently, the ZENSA-PDN trial was an open-label randomized trial published in 2021 comparing HF10 SCS with CMM to CMM alone in 216 patients with PDN.[70] The primary outcome of ≥50% pain relief on VAS was met by 79% of patients in the HF10 with CMM group compared with 5% in the CMM-only group. The mean VAS score was 7.6 cm at baseline and 1.7 cm at 6 months in the HF10 group, compared with 7.0 cm at baseline and 6.9 cm at 6 months for the CMM group. Interestingly, sensory, motor, and reflex improvements were noted in 62% of patients in the HF10 group compared with 3% in the CMM group. A 24-month follow-up study is ongoing.

The above trials demonstrate level 1 evidence for both tonic SCS and HF10 in the treatment of PDN. A gradual loss of therapeutic effect occurs over time with use of tonic SCS, similar to that seen in tonic SCS use in neuropathic pain conditions.[71] Long-term efficacy data for HF10 use in diabetic neuropathy still remain to be seen.

Complex Regional Pain Syndrome

While several retrospective and prospective cohort trials support the use of SCS for CRPS, 2 major randomized trials provide the highest quality evidence. Kemler and colleagues randomized 54 patients with CRPS to tonic SCS and physical therapy (PT) or PT-only.[72] There was a significant 3.6 cm improvement in the VAS scale for the SCS and PT group at 6 months compared with 0.2 cm worsening for the PT-only group.[72] The improvement in the SCS and PT group decreased over time, with differences persisting at the 2-year mark but missing cutoff for statistical significance between years 3 and 5.[73]

Kriek and colleagues[74] randomized 29 patients with CRPS through 2-week phases of placebo, burst, 40 Hz, 500 Hz, and 1200 Hz SCS. The 5 settings were programmed through random order for 2 weeks each without a washout period, for a total of 10 weeks. VAS scores were 39.89 mm (40 Hz), 40.13 mm (500 Hz), 42.89 mm (1200 Hz), 47.98 mm (burst), and 63.74 mm (placebo). All stimulation settings were significantly different compared with placebo. 48% of patients preferred the 40 Hz stimulation, whereas 52% preferred one of the other stimulation settings.

Nonsurgical Back Pain

Currently, no level 1 evidence exists for the use of SCS in the treatment of nonsurgical back pain. There is limited evidence from 2 uncontrolled prospective trials[75,76] and post hoc analysis of subgroups from 2 trials[77] supporting the efficacy of HF10 SCS for the treatment of nonsurgical back pain. At the time of writing of this article, there is an ongoing randomized control trial evaluating HF10 and CMM to CMM-alone for the treatment of nonsurgical back pain and an ongoing randomized trial comparing burst stimulation and CMM to CMM-alone for nonsurgical back pain.[78] The upcoming MODULATE-LBP trial will also compare HF10 to sham in patients with neuropathic low back pain who have not undergone surgery.[79]

DISCUSSION

This article highlights the common conditions that have been studied by clinical trials to date. An appraisal of the literature conducted by Harmsen and Colleagues assessed the literature of 212 studies on SCS since 1997. This analysis showed that the common indications of back/extremity pain, FBSS, SCI, neuropathy, and CRPS totaled a staggering 83.6% of all trials.[80] The best evidence continues to exist for these conditions. However, an increasing number of newly registered clinical trials continue to explore more novel indications, suggesting the growing nature of the field. These include neurologic disorders, cardiac disorders, gastrointestinal/genitourinary disorders, and neuropathic conditions outside of diabetic neuropathy.[80] The ability to blind studies with paresthesia-free stimulation allows us to explore true placebo-controlled randomizations for a wider array of disease processes. Improving the quality and the quantity of the available research and expanding the breadth of the field promises to show newer implementations for SCS.

Current Breadth of Evidence

On the basis of the various types of waveforms, the evidence continues to be variable. The different waveforms demonstrate varying degrees of evidence, with the more novel waveforms continuing to be carefully evaluated in ongoing studies. Traditional SCS has demonstrated excellent results in studies on efficacy for FBSS. CRPS also demonstrates positive results; however, longer term efficacy data remain inconclusive. Despite the inability to blind these studies, the studies conducted by North and colleagues and the PROCESS RCT conducted by Kumar and colleagues demonstrated pragmatic trial designs to show efficacy relative to reoperation and CMM, respectively, for the FBSS population.[52,54] These trial designs laid the groundwork for the wide use of SCS in this population cohort seen today. For CRPS, several important trials have solidified the strength of traditional SCS as a treatment modality. Kemler and colleagues' study of SCS and PT versus PT over the course of 2 years demonstrated a significant breakthrough in the measurement of long-term treatment outcomes for this population cohort.[71] Current evidence suggests that considerations should be made to implement SCS before last resort therapy for CRPS.[81] The International Association for the Study of Pain (IASP) has recommended that SCS be implemented in 12 to 16 weeks after the failure of conservative treatment measures.[81] With the development of newer waveforms, the focus of the studies has shifted to the comparison of waveforms as well as the study of new disease conditions.

For burst stimulation, the literature has been promising and has shown superiority to traditional SCS in a number of different studies.[71,82] With the ability to create double-blinded, placebo-controlled studies, the quality of evidence promises to be more robust. For example, Kriek and colleagues conducted a study in 2017 with 5 settings, including burst stimulation, versus placebo, for the treatment of CRPS. Burst, along with higher frequency settings, displayed promising results with 52% of the subjects preferring these nonstandard settings.[74] The evidence for burst SCS has expanded to other disease processes. Promising results have been published for PDN and nonsurgical back pain. The SUNBURST trial, a major prospective trial for burst stimulation, used a heterogenous population of trunk and lower back pain, of which a portion had not undergone previous surgery. The study was one of the first, larger scale studies to evaluate burst SCS. The study demonstrated that burst SCS is safe and effective. Burst stimulation was not only noninferior but also superior to tonic stimulation for the treatment of chronic pain.[61] De Ridder and colleagues conducted several smaller scale studies comparing traditional and burst stimulation (n = 15, n = 12) on limb and axial pain that showed a consensus preference for burst stimulation in all patients enrolled.[20] De Ridder and colleagues also conducted a larger scale (n = 102) multicenter, retrospective that demonstrated the ability of burst to be a promising modality in PDN but also demonstrating the potential as a "rescue" modality. 94.8% of responders to traditional SCS in the cohort of FBSS/PDN demonstrated improved pain relief with burst stimulation. An impressive 62% of nonresponders to Traditional SCS were salvaged with burst stimulation.[83] De Vos and colleagues conducted a similar study in a prospective manner on 48 patients for the FBSS/PDN cohort. The study participants were familiar with tonic SCS separating this study from previous prospective studies that test neuromodulation naive subjects. Again, burst stimulation displayed impressive results; 60% of patients experienced further pain reduction.[66]

Recent efficacy analyses of high-frequency SCS displaced stronger evidence. The SENZA trial introduced a larger scale, multicenter study that used a heterogeneous population with a cohort that was not limited to FBSS but expanded to a broader cohort of back and pain. Results of the study demonstrated the superiority of HF10 when compared with traditional SCS.[57,59] This major multicenter study set the stage for high-frequency SCS. However, given the contradictory studies that have followed, further evidence analysis is needed for more conclusive assessments and clinical recommendations.[59] One of the largest cohort multicenter studies conducted for PDN and neuromodulation also involves the use of HF10 SCS. The Zena-PDN study comparing HF10 with CMM versus CMM alone demonstrated positive results with the primary outcome of pain reduction on the VAS of 50%. 79% of those in the HF10 + CMM group met this endpoint versus just 5% in the CMM group.[66] These promising results demonstrate the viability of high-frequency SCS, although superiority studies are lacking. Given that PDN has been studied in previous waveforms, comparative studies will need to be conducted to assess for the superiority of the high-frequency stimulation.

Appraisal of Newer Studies

Several new studies highlight the current direction of neuromodulation. The newer studies can range from increasing our understanding of neuromodulation in previously poorly represented cohorts, gaining an understanding of superiority between waveforms, enhancing protocols and improving safety, and increasing our understanding of the mechanisms and newer technologies. Modulate LBP is a multicenter, randomized, double-blinded trial protocol that aims to assess patients undergoing HF SCS versus a sham treatment of chronic neuropathic low back pain in patients who have not had surgery.[78] The trial was developed to further our understanding of the non-FBSS cohort in addition to assessing high-frequency SCS. It also represents one of a few sham-controlled, double-blinded trials in neuromodulation. Increasing the quality of evidence will allow us to draw more sound conclusions. Similarly, Multiwave is a blinded, randomized trial protocol nearing completion that assesses the well-studied cohort of FBSS but aims to compare all 3 waveform stimulations in a randomized control crossover format.[65] This will be among the first study designs to assess all 3 modalities and the first to compare burst and high-frequency in a randomized, blinded format.

Several large-scale studies have scrutinized or have been scrutinized regarding safety protocols for SCS. The PROMISE RCT is a multinational RCT evaluating the effectiveness of surgical leads in SCS with CMM compared with CMM alone. An unplanned analysis for safety revealed higher infection rates in Belgium, whereby the trial durations averaged 21 days versus trial durations of the other countries, which averaged 6 days. A secondary analysis published in 2020 revealed a direct cause–effect relationship between infections and trial durations and concluded that prolonged durations should be avoided. Belgium adjusted the standard protocol to 10 days.[38] This is an example of the growing critical analysis of SCS studies that promise to create the framework for safer protocols in the future.

Cost-Effectiveness

Chronic low back and limb pain has been cited as the most common cause for disability and lost days of work in the industrialized world.[84] The utilization of health care resources in this population is tremendous. The goal of newer technologies and neuromodulation is to reduce the pain burden, minimize recurring treatments and improve the overall QoL for the patients. Achieving these results with a reasonable cost-benefit ratio is important, as it pertains to the practicality of a treatment option for the everyday individual. Kumar and colleagues conducted an assessment of cost-effectiveness of SCS in FBSS, CRPS, Peripheral Arterial Disease, and Refractory Angina Pectoris.[85] This study used a 20-year timeline and assessed 313 patients with a successful SCS implant and adjunctive CMM versus those with CMM alone. A Markov model was used to clearly define specific health states including optimal health, suboptimal health, and death. Health effects were measured using quality-adjusted life years. The costs considered for the SCS group included the preimplant costs, procedure costs, maintenance costs, adjunctive therapies costs, and pharmacotherapy costs. The costs considered for the control group included the cost of evaluations, imaging costs, costs of alternative therapies, pharmacotherapy costs, and intermittent hospitalization costs. Favorable results were seen in all 4 disease states for the SCS with adjunctive therapy cohort, demonstrating incremental net monetary benefit more than 20 years of greater than $100,000 USD each.[85] This study is one of the only available studies that have reviewed cost-effectiveness in a prospective manner. Hoelscher and colleagues published a comprehensive review analyzing 21 studies that have evaluated a cost utility component for SCS.[84] They noted a significant lack of higher level evidence analysis in this realm. Many of the existing studies are from small, retrospective, single-center institutions. Broad conclusions drawn from these studies are overwhelmingly in favor of long-term cost-effectiveness of SCS in chronic back, leg, and neuropathic conditions. Several of the studies analyzed note higher upfront and 1-year costs. One study by Kemler and colleagues noted the average first-year cost of SCS was $4000 more than traditional therapy, but the lifetime cost was $60,000 less.[86] Bell and colleagues observed savings at 5 years for all-comers with SCS and at 2.1 years with a very positive response to stimulation.[87] Higher quality data and prospective analyses are needed for the assessment of cost-effectiveness in SCS.

Despite the favorable results of these studies, the US health care system and insurance coverage for an SCS procedure continue to be challenging for many patients. Companies may argue against providing coverage for SCS given the market-style health care system. Many Americans link their health insurance to their employment. It has been estimated that the average American changes health insurance carriers every 3 years. Thus, third-party payers may not be incentivized to provide coverage for SCS systems if they believe the patient will likely switch insurance carriers in the near future.[84]

SUMMARY

The evolution of SCS has been remarkable over the past several decades. The expansion of waveforms and frequency alterations presents novel capabilities to alleviate pain signals. Patient selection and prudence to avoid peri-operative complications are imperative to achieving successful patient outcomes. Despite a growing body of evidence, indications for specific disease states remain limited. Furthermore, the overall quality and quantity of robust, non–industry-sponsored studies are also relatively minimal. It is imperative to note, however, that balanced clinician-industry collaboration remains key to the development of these therapies. The existing data in support of SCS provide good evidence for the studied disease states with the promise of further indication expansion. Exciting new modalities such as peripheral nerve stimulation and dorsal root ganglion stimulation have also emerged.

CLINICS CARE POINTS FOR PHYSIATRISTS

- SCS has evolved over the last 50 years. Development of paresthesia-free waveforms has revolutionized the industry, allowing for higher-quality analysis.
- SCS has played a significant role as a nonopioid alternative to refractory chronic pain conditions.
- Traditional SCS has robust evidence for FBSS, CRPS, PAD, and refractory angina pectoris.
- Burst stimulation has shown superiority in a number of studies and might be a potential "salvage" treatment of traditional SCS nonresponders.
- Burst stimulation has improved neuromodulation evidence for axial-predominant pain and PDN.
- High-frequency stimulation has shown noninferiority in a number of studies, but data are lacking regarding superiority to existing waveforms. Data tend to be more conflicting, but with the emergence of new trials comparing waveforms, high-frequency SCS has the potential to expand in the marketplace.
- Newer technologies, such as ECAP, have the potential to deliver more targeted treatment with real-time adjustments based on internal physiology. Robust studies are still needed for these technologies.
- The most significant complications of SCS continue to be minor infections and lead migration.
- Safety protocols continue to improve; overall complication rates have been decreasing with improved technologies.
- Cost-effectiveness in the first postoperative year tends to be higher for SCS, but overall lifetime costs have shown significant cost savings, especially for very positive responders.

DISCLOSURE

Dr M.J. Desai is a consultant for Abbott. His institution has received research support from Abbott, Nalu, and Nevro.

REFERENCES

1. Shealy CN, Taslitz N, Mortimer JT, et al. Electrical inhibition of pain: experimental evaluation. Anesth Analg 1967;46(3):299–305.
2. Chakravarthy K, Fishman MA, Zuidema X, et al. Mechanism of action in burst spinal cord stimulation: review and recent advances. Pain Med 2019;20(Suppl 1): S13–22.
3. Melzack R, Wall PD. Pain mechanisms: a new theory. Science 1965;150(3699): 971–9.
4. Jensen MP, Brownstone RM. Mechanisms of spinal cord stimulation for the treatment of pain: still in the dark after 50 years. Eur J Pain 2019;23:652–9.
5. Watkins LR, Milligan ED, Maier SF. Glial activation: a driving force for pathological pain. Trends Neurosci 2001;24(8):450–5.
6. Sato KL, Johanek LM, Sanada LS, et al. Spinal cord stimulation reduces mechanical hyperalgesia and glial cell activation in animals with neuropathic pain. Anesth Analg 2014;118(2):464–72.
7. Schechtmann G, Song Z, Ultenius C, et al. Cholinergic mechanisms involved in the pain relieving effect of spinal cord stimulation in a model of neuropathy. Pain 2008;139(1):136–45.

8. Cui JG, O'Connor WT, Ungerstedt U, et al. Spinal cord stimulation attenuates augmented dorsal horn release of excitatory amino acids in mononeuropathy via a GABAergic mechanism. Pain 1997;73(1):87–95.

9. Wolter T, Kieselbach K, Sircar R, et al. Spinal cord stimulation inhibits cortical somatosensory evoked potentials significantly stronger than transcutaneous electrical nerve stimulation. Pain Physician 2013;16(4):405–14.

10. Sato KL, King EW, Johanek LM, et al. Spinal cord stimulation reduces hypersensitivity through activation of opioid receptors in a frequency-dependent manner. Eur J Pain 2013;17(4):551–61.

11. Washburn S, Catlin R, Bethel K, et al. Patient-perceived differences between constant current and constant voltage spinal cord stimulation systems. Neuromodulation 2014;17(1):28–35 [discussion: 35-6].

12. Miller JP, Eldabe S, Buchser E, et al. Parameters of spinal cord stimulation and their role in electrical charge delivery: a review. Neuromodulation 2016;19(4): 373–84.

13. North RB, Kidd DH, Zahurak M, et al. Spinal cord stimulation for chronic, intractable pain: experience over two decades. Neurosurgery 1993;32(3):384–94 [discussion: 394-5].

14. Sankarasubramanian V, Buitenweg JR, Holsheimer J, et al. Triple leads programmed to perform as longitudinal guarded cathodes in spinal cord stimulation: a modeling study. Neuromodulation 2011;14(5):401–10 [discussion 411].

15. Holsheimer J, Barolat G, Struijk JJ, et al. Significance of the spinal cord position in spinal cord stimulation. Acta Neurochir Suppl 1995;64:119–24.

16. Chakravarthy K, Richter H, Christo PJ, et al. Spinal Cord stimulation for treating chronic pain: reviewing preclinical and clinical data on paresthesia-free high-frequency therapy. Neuromodulation 2018;21(1):10–8.

17. North JM, Hong KJ, Cho PY. Clinical outcomes of 1 kHz subperception spinal cord stimulation in implanted patients with failed paresthesia-based stimulation: results of a prospective randomized controlled trial. Neuromodulation 2016; 19(7):731–7.

18. Arle JE, Mei L, Carlson KW, et al. High-frequency stimulation of dorsal column axons: potential underlying mechanism of paresthesia-free neuropathic pain relief. Neuromodulation 2016;19(4):385–97.

19. De Ridder D, Vanneste S, Plazier M, et al. Burst spinal cord stimulation: toward paresthesia-free pain suppression. Neurosurgery 2010;66(5):986–90.

20. De Ridder D, Plazier M, Kamerling N, et al. Burst spinal cord stimulation for limb and back pain. World Neurosurg 2013;80(5):642–9.e1.

21. De Ridder D, Vancamp T, Falowski SM, et al. All bursts are equal, but some are more equal (to burst firing): burstDR stimulation versus Boston burst stimulation. Expert Rev Med Devices 2020;17(4):289–95.

22. Vesper J, Slotty P, Schu S, et al. Burst SCS microdosing is as efficacious as standard burst scs in treating chronic back and leg pain: results from a randomized controlled trial. Neuromodulation 2019;22(2):190–3.

23. Paz-Solís J, Thomson S, Jain R, et al. Exploration of high and low frequency options for subperception spinal cord stimulation using neural dosing parameter relationships: the HALO study. Neuromodulation 2021. https://doi.org/10.1111/ner. 13390.

24. Holsheimer J, den Boer JA, Struijk JJ, et al. MR assessment of the normal position of the spinal cord in the spinal canal. AJNR Am J Neuroradiol 1994;15(5):951–9.

25. Parker JL, Karantonis DM, Single PS, et al. Electrically evoked compound action potentials recorded from the sheep spinal cord. Neuromodulation 2013;16(4): 295–303 [discussion: 303].
26. Mekhail N, Levy RM, Deer TR, et al, Evoke Study Group. Long-term safety and efficacy of closed-loop spinal cord stimulation to treat chronic back and leg pain (Evoke): a double-blind, randomised, controlled trial. Lancet Neurol 2020; 19(2):123–34.
27. NICE. Technology. Appraisal Guidelines 159-spinal cord stimulation for chronic pain of neuropathic or ischaemic origin 2008. https://www.nice.org.uk/guidance/ta159.
28. Kumar K, Hunter G, Demeria D. Spinal cord stimulation in treatment of chronic benign pain: challenges in treatment planning and present status, a 22-year experience. Neurosurgery 2006;58(3):481–96 [discussion: 481-96].
29. Sheldon B, Staudt MD, Williams L, et al. Spinal cord stimulation programming: a crash course. Neurosurg Rev 2021;44(2):709–20.
30. Deer TR, Mekhail N, Provenzano D, et al, Neuromodulation Appropriateness Consensus Committee. The appropriate use of neurostimulation of the spinal cord and peripheral nervous system for the treatment of chronic pain and ischemic diseases: the Neuromodulation Appropriateness Consensus Committee. Neuromodulation 2014;17(6):515–50 [discussion 550].
31. Eldabe S, Buchser E, Duarte RV. Complications of spinal cord stimulation and peripheral nerve stimulation techniques: a review of the literature. Pain Med 2016; 17(2):325–36.
32. Gupta M, Abd-Elsayed A, Hughes M, et al. A retrospective review of lead migration rate in patients permanently implanted with percutaneous leads and a 10 kHz SCS device. Pain Res Management 2021;2021:e6639801.
33. Falowski SM, Provenzano DA, Xia Y, et al. Spinal cord stimulation infection rate and risk factors: results from a united states payer database. Neuromodulation 2019;22(2):179–89.
34. Hoelzer BC, Bendel MA, Deer TR, et al. Spinal cord stimulator implant infection rates and risk factors: a multicenter retrospective study. Neuromodulation 2017; 20(6):558–62.
35. Esquer Garrigos Z, Farid S, Bendel MA, et al. Spinal cord stimulator infection: approach to diagnosis, management, and prevention. Clin Infect Dis 2020; 70(12):2727–35.
36. Hayek SM, Veizi E, Hanes M. Treatment-limiting complications of percutaneous spinal cord stimulator implants: a review of eight years of experience from an academic center database. Neuromodulation 2015;18(7):603–8 [discussion: 608-609].
37. Simopoulos T, Aner M, Sharma S, et al. Explantation of percutaneous spinal cord stimulator devices: a retrospective descriptive analysis of a single-center 15-Year experience. Pain Med 2019;20(7):1355–61.
38. North R, Desai MJ, Vangeneugden J, et al. Postoperative infections associated with prolonged spinal cord stimulation trial duration (PROMISE RCT). Neuromodulation 2020;23(5):620–5.
39. Schultz DM, Webster L, Kosek P, et al. Sensor-driven position-adaptive spinal cord stimulation for chronic pain. Pain Physician 2012;15(1):1–12.
40. Malinowski MN, Kim CH, Deer TR. Complications of spinal cord stimulation. In: Krames ES, Peckham PH, Rezai AR, editors. Neuromodulation: Comprehensive Textbook of Principles, Technologies, and Therapies. 2nd edition. San Diego (CA): Academic Press; 2018. p. 660–2.

41. Reddy RD, Moheimani R, Yu GG, et al. A review of clinical data on salvage therapy in spinal cord stimulation. Neuromodulation 2020;23(5):562–71.
42. Petraglia FW, Farber SH, Gramer R, et al. The incidence of spinal cord injury in implantation of percutaneous and paddle electrodes for spinal cord stimulation. Neuromodulation 2016;19(1):85–90.
43. Labaran L, Jain N, Puvanesarajah V, et al. A retrospective database review of the indications, complications, and incidence of subsequent spine surgery in 12,297 spinal cord stimulator patients. Neuromodulation 2020;23(5):634–8.
44. Levy R, Henderson J, Slavin K, et al. Incidence and avoidance of neurologic complications with paddle type spinal cord stimulation leads. Neuromodulation 2011;14(5):412–22 [discussion: 422].
45. Van Buyten J-P, Wille F, Smet I, et al. Therapy-related explants after spinal cord stimulation: results of an international retrospective chart review study. Neuromodulation 2017;20(7):642–9.
46. Pope JE, Deer TR, Falowski S, et al. Multicenter retrospective study of neurostimulation with exit of therapy by explant. Neuromodulation 2017;20(6):543–52.
47. Sharan AD, Riley J, Falowski S, et al. Association of opioid usage with spinal cord stimulation outcomes. Pain Med 2018;19(4):699–707.
48. Desai MJ, Hargens LM, Breitenfeldt MD, et al. The rate of magnetic resonance imaging in patients with spinal cord stimulation. *Spine* (Phila Pa 1976 2015;40(9):E531–7.
49. Sayed D, Chakravarthy K, Amirdelfan K, et al. A Comprehensive practice guideline for magnetic resonance imaging compatibility in implanted neuromodulation devices. Neuromodulation 2020;23(7):893–911.
50. Atkinson L, Sundaraj SR, Brooker C, et al. Recommendations for patient selection in spinal cord stimulation. J Clin Neurosci 2011;18(10):1295–302.
51. North R, Shipley J, Prager J, et al. Practice parameters for the use of spinal cord stimulation in the treatment of chronic neuropathic pain. Pain Med 2007;8(Suppl 4):S200–75.
52. North RB, Kidd DH, Farrokhi F, et al. Spinal cord stimulation versus repeated lumbosacral spine surgery for chronic pain: a randomized, controlled trial. Neurosurgery 2005;56(1):98–106 [discussion: 106-107].
53. Kumar K, Taylor RS, Jacques L, et al. Spinal cord stimulation versus conventional medical management for neuropathic pain: a multicentre randomised controlled trial in patients with failed back surgery syndrome. Pain 2007;132(1–2):179–88. https://doi.org/10.1016/j.pain.2007.07.028.
54. Kumar K, Taylor RS, Jacques L, et al. The effects of spinal cord stimulation in neuropathic pain are sustained: a 24-month follow-up of the prospective randomized controlled multicenter trial of the effectiveness of spinal cord stimulation. Neurosurgery 2008;63(4):762–70 [discussion: 770].
55. Rigoard P, Basu S, Desai M, et al. Multicolumn spinal cord stimulation for predominant back pain in failed back surgery syndrome patients: a multicenter randomized controlled trial. Pain 2019;160(6):1410–20.
56. Head J, Mazza J, Sabourin V, et al. Waves of pain relief: a systematic review of clinical trials in spinal cord stimulation waveforms for the treatment of chronic neuropathic low back and leg pain. World Neurosurg 2019;131:264–74.e3.
57. Kapural L, Yu C, Doust MW, et al. Novel 10-kHz High-frequency therapy (HF10 Therapy) is superior to traditional low-frequency spinal cord stimulation for the treatment of chronic back and leg pain: the SENZA-RCT randomized controlled trial. Anesthesiology 2015;123(4):851–60.

58. Kapural L, Yu C, Doust MW, et al. Comparison of 10-kHz high-frequency and traditional low-frequency spinal cord stimulation for the treatment of chronic back and leg pain: 24-month results from a multicenter, randomized, controlled pivotal trial. Neurosurgery 2016;79(5):667–77.

59. De Andres J, Monsalve-Dolz V, Fabregat-Cid G, et al. Prospective, randomized blind effect-on-outcome study of conventional vs high-frequency spinal cord stimulation in patients with pain and disability due to failed back surgery syndrome. Pain Med 2017;18(12):2401–21.

60. Thomson SJ, Tavakkolizadeh M, Love-Jones S, et al. Effects of rate on analgesia in kilohertz frequency spinal cord stimulation: results of the PROCO randomized controlled trial. Neuromodulation 2018;21(1):67–76.

61. Breel J, Wille F, Wensing AGCL, et al. A comparison of 1000 Hz to 30 Hz spinal cord stimulation strategies in patients with unilateral neuropathic leg pain due to failed back surgery syndrome: a multicenter, randomized, double-blinded, cross-over clinical study (HALO). Pain Ther 2021;6:1189–202.

62. Deer T, Slavin KV, Amirdelfan K, et al. Success using neuromodulation With BURST (SUNBURST) study: results from a prospective, randomized controlled trial using a novel burst waveform. Neuromodulation 2018;21(1):56–66.

63. Karri J, Orhurhu V, Wahezi S, et al. Comparison of Spinal cord stimulation waveforms for treating chronic low back pain: systematic review and meta-analysis. Pain Physician 2020;23(5):451–60.

64. Peeters J-B, Raftopoulos C. Tonic, burst, high-density, and 10-kHz high-frequency spinal cord stimulation: efficiency and patients' preferences in a failed back surgery syndrome predominant population. review of literature. World Neurosurg 2020;144:e331–40.

65. Billot M, Naiditch N, Brandet C, et al. Comparison of conventional, burst and high-frequency spinal cord stimulation on pain relief in refractory failed back surgery syndrome patients: study protocol for a prospective randomized double-blinded cross-over trial (MULTIWAVE study). Trials 2020;21(1):696.

66. Mekhail N, Levy RM, Deer TR, et al. Long-term safety and efficacy of closed-loop spinal cord stimulation to treat chronic back and leg pain (Evoke): a double-blind, randomised, controlled trial. Lancet Neurol 2020;19(2):123–34.

67. De Vos CC, Meier K, Zaalberg PB, et al. Spinal cord stimulation in patients with painful diabetic neuropathy: a multicentre randomized clinical trial. Pain 2014; 155(11):2426–31.

68. Slangen R, Schaper NC, Faber CG, et al. Spinal cord stimulation and pain relief in painful diabetic peripheral neuropathy: a prospective two-center randomized controlled trial. Diabetes Care 2014;37(11):3016–24.

69. van Beek M, Geurts JW, Slangen R, et al. Severity of neuropathy is associated with long-term spinal cord stimulation outcome in painful diabetic peripheral neuropathy: five-year follow-up of a prospective two-center clinical trial. Diabetes Care 2018;41(1):32–8.

70. Petersen EA, Stauss TG, Scowcroft JA, et al. Effect of high-frequency (10-kHz) spinal cord stimulation in patients with painful diabetic neuropathy: a randomized clinical trial. JAMA Neurol 2021;78(6):687–98.

71. Duarte RV, Nevitt S, Maden M, et al. Spinal cord stimulation for the management of painful diabetic neuropathy: a systematic review and meta-analysis of individual patient and aggregate data. Pain 2021;9:2635–43.

72. Kemler MA, De Vet HCW, Barendse GAM, et al. The effect of spinal cord stimulation in patients with chronic reflex sympathetic dystrophy: Two years' follow-up of the randomized controlled trial. Ann Neurol 2004;55(1):13–8.

73. Kemler MA, de Vet HCW, Barendse GAM, et al. Effect of spinal cord stimulation for chronic complex regional pain syndrome Type I: five-year final follow-up of patients in a randomized controlled trial. J Neurosurg 2008;108(2):292–8.
74. Kriek N, Groeneweg JG, Stronks DL, et al. Preferred frequencies and waveforms for spinal cord stimulation in patients with complex regional pain syndrome: a multicentre, double-blind, randomized and placebo-controlled crossover trial. Eur J Pain 2017;21(3):507–19.
75. Baranidharan G, Feltbower R, Bretherton B, et al. One-Year results of prospective research study using 10 kHz spinal cord stimulation in persistent nonoperated low back pain of neuropathic origin: maiden back study. Neuromodulation 2021;24(3):479–87.
76. Al-Kaisy A, Palmisani S, Smith TE, et al. Long-term improvements in chronic axial low back pain patients without previous spinal surgery: a cohort analysis of 10-kHz high-frequency spinal cord stimulation over 36 months. Pain Med 2018; 19(6):1219–26.
77. Al-Kaisy A, Van Buyten JP, Kapural L, et al. 10 kHz spinal cord stimulation for the treatment of non-surgical refractory back pain: subanalysis of pooled data from two prospective studies. Anaesthesia 2020;75(6):775–84.
78. Patel N, Calodney A, Kapural L, et al. High-frequency spinal cord stimulation at 10 kHz for the treatment of nonsurgical refractory back pain: design of a pragmatic, multicenter, randomized controlled trial. Pain Pract 2021;21(2):171–83.
79. Al-Kaisy A, Royds J, Palmisani S, et al. Multicentre, double-blind, randomised, sham-controlled trial of 10 khz high-frequency spinal cord stimulation for chronic neuropathic low back pain (MODULATE-LBP): a trial protocol. Trials 2020; 21(1):111.
80. Harmsen IE, Hasanova D, Elias GJB, et al. Trends in clinical trials for spinal cord stimulation. Stereotactic Funct Neurosurg 2021;99:123–34.
81. Poree L, Krames E, Pope J, et al. Spinal cord stimulation as treatment for complex regional pain syndrome should be considered earlier than last resort therapy. Neuromodulation 2013;16(2):125–41.
82. Kirketeig T, Schultheis C, Zuidema X, et al. Burst spinal cord stimulation: a clinical review. Pain Med 2019;20(Suppl 1):S31–40.
83. Dirk De R, Lenders MWPM, De Vos CC, et al. A 2-center comparative study on tonic versus burst spinal cord stimulation: amount of responders and amount of pain suppression. Clin J Pain 2015;31(5):433–7.
84. Hoelscher C, Riley J, Wu C, et al. Cost-effectiveness data regarding spinal cord stimulation for low back pain. Spine 2017;42(Suppl 14):S72–9.
85. Kumar K, Rizvi S. Cost-Effectiveness of Spinal Cord Stimulation Therapy in Management of Chronic Pain. Pain Med 2013;14(11):1631–49. https://doi.org/10. 1111/pme.12146. Available from.
86. Kemler MA, Raphael JH, Bentley A, et al. The cost-effectiveness of spinal cord stimulation for complex regional pain syndrome. Value Health 2010;13(6):735–42.
87. Bell GK, Kidd D, North RB. Cost-effectiveness analysis of spinal cord stimulation in treatment of failed back surgery syndrome. J Pain Symptom Manage 1997; 13(5):286–95.

Dorsal Root Ganglion Stimulation

Steven T. Potter, DO, MS[a],*, Sean Welch, MD[a], Faye Tata, DO[a], Seth Probert, DO[a], Ameet Nagpal, MD, MS, MEd[b]

KEYWORDS

- Dorsal root ganglion stimulation • Neuromodulation • FDA approval

KEY POINTS

- Dorsal root ganglion stimulation was Food and Drug Administration approved in 2016 for placement at the levels of T10-S2.
- It is a novel targeted form of neuromodulation for the treatment of complex regional pain syndrome, causalgia, and chronic pelvic pain resistant to other treatments.
- Literature remains limited, but risk appears to be comparable to other forms of neuromodulation.
- The potential to optimize this targeted therapy and expand indications is promising.

INTRODUCTION

Neurostimulation is a well-established treatment option for people who suffer from chronic, refractory painful disorders.[1–7] Traditional spinal cord stimulation (SCS), where electrodes are implanted into the epidural space, has been an effective, generally safe and evidence-based treatment option for chronic pain syndromes that are refractory to conservative measures.[8,9] Despite ongoing efforts to improve localization by the advanced programming of current SCS techniques,[10] there continues to be poor patient satisfaction and high explantation rates in some patients.[11,12] SCS has shown effectiveness in many central neuropathic pain processes, but its effectiveness in the treatment of focal and peripheral lesions causing pain in the trunk, groin, knee and foot has been less reliable. Although SCS intervention has been most extensively used and has the most supportive literature, its limitations arise from the lack of specific dermatomal or peripheral targets. Furthermore, it is postulated that increased stimulation to the spinal cord may lead to increased tolerance and habituation to the therapy.[7] This has given rise to new neurostimulation techniques that provide

[a] Department of Rehabilitation Medicine, UT Health San Antonio, Mail Code 7798, 7703 Floyd Curl Drive, San Antonio, TX 78229-3900, USA; [b] Department of Anesthesiology, UT Health San Antonio, Mail Code 7798, 7703 Floyd Curl Drive, San Antonio, TX 78229-3900, USA
* Corresponding author.
E-mail address: potters@uthscsa.edu

Phys Med Rehabil Clin N Am 33 (2022) 359–378
https://doi.org/10.1016/j.pmr.2022.02.005
1047-9651/22/© 2022 Elsevier Inc. All rights reserved.

better localization of coverage, increased patient satisfaction, and fewer complications (**Fig. 1**).

Dorsal root ganglion stimulation (DRGS) has recently emerged as a newer neuromodulation modality for more localized treatment of neuropathic pain.[9] The dorsal root ganglia (DRG) are located at each segmental level of the spinal cord and lumbosacral spine (**Fig. 2**). They can be found in the intervertebral foramina as the nerve roots exit the spinal column. The DRG is the first cell body of the sensory pathway from the periphery to the central nervous system.[13] Because of its location within the epidural space, the DRG can be stimulated with more accurate lead positioning. This allows for greater lead excitability along with smaller contact size and spacing, all of which aid in providing greater pain relief.[14] Because of the proximity to the spinal cord, DRGS is often grouped along with SCS techniques.[9]

Increased excitability at the DRG is thought to contribute to chronic pain after injuries to the peripheral nerves, as is commonly seen in complex regional pain syndrome (CRPS) and other peripheral nerve injuries.[8,15] The DRG is thus an appropriate target for neurostimulation in these conditions. In 2016, the Food and Drug Administration (FDA) approved the use of DGRS for patients who suffer from CRPS I and II.[16] Furthermore, the Neuromodulation Appropriateness Consensus Committee (NACC) performed a literature review in 2018 and concluded that there is strong evidence for the use of DRG stimulation for patients with CRPS I and II and other chronic pain syndromes of the pelvic and lower extremity.[7] Although the current literature suggests DRGS may be superior to SCS, especially in the treatment of CRPS type I and II of the lower extremity,[9] there are many promising applications

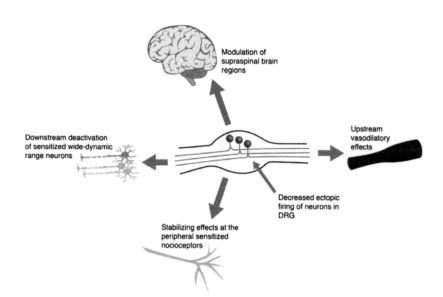

Modulation of supraspinal brain regions

Downstream deactivation of sensitized wide-dynamic range neurons

Upstream vasodilatory effects

Decreased ectopic firing of neurons in DRG

Stabilizing effects at the peripheral sensitized nocioceptors

Fig. 1. Effect of dysregulated DRG on peripheral nerve.[7] (*From* Deer, T. R., Pope, J. E., Lamer, T. J., Grider, J. S., Provenzano, D., Lubenow, T. R., FitzGerald, J. J., Hunter, C., Falowski, S., Sayed, D., Baranidharan, G., Patel, N. K., Davis, T., Green, A., Pajuelo, A., Epstein, L. J., Harned, M., Liem, L., Christo, P. J., Chakravarthy, K., ... Mekhail, N. (2019). The Neuromodulation Appropriateness Consensus Committee on Best Practices for Dorsal Root Ganglion Stimulation. Neuromodulation : journal of the International Neuromodulation Society, 22(1), 1–35.)

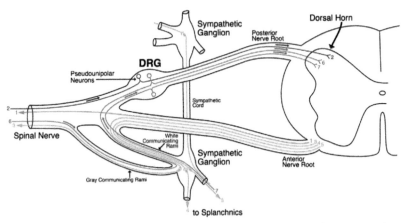

Fig. 2. Image of the DRG functions as a key check point in the pain pathway to block, propagate, or filter peripheral nerve action potentials. (1) Somatic efferent fibers; (2) somatic afferent fibers; (3–5) sympathetic efferent fibers; (6–7) sympathetic afferent fibers.[7] (*From Deer, T. R., Pope, J. E., Lamer, T. J., Grider, J. S., Provenzano, D., Lubenow, T. R., FitzGerald, J. J., Hunter, C., Falowski, S., Sayed, D., Baranidharan, G., Patel, N. K., Davis, T., Green, A., Pajuelo, A., Epstein, L. J., Harned, M., Liem, L., Christo, P. J., Chakravarthy, K., ... Mekhail, N. (2019). The Neuromodulation Appropriateness Consensus Committee on Best Practices for Dorsal Root Ganglion Stimulation. Neuromodulation : journal of the International Neuromodulation Society, 22(1), 1–35.*

yet to be more thoroughly researched. In this article, the authors discuss the patient selection criteria, risks/contraindications, and current outcome data for DRGS.

PATIENT SELECTION CRITERIA

Per the FDA, the only indication for DRGS is CRPS and/or peripheral causalgia in the groin and lower limb,[16] largely in part owing to the ACCURATE trial. In this well-known pragmatic randomized control trial, all patients met either Budapest criteria for CRPS type 1 or the authors' criteria for a diagnosis of causalgia: "a painful condition arising from damage to a nerve resulting in chronic pain, generally restricted to the innervation pattern of the damaged nerve or nerves, which may or may not have secondary symptoms."[9] In this population, the GRADE rating of evidence for the use of DRGS for the treatment of pain and improvement of function at 3-month and 12- month time points is low.[17–19] Still, there are many other studies that demonstrate notable pain reduction, as well as functional and mood improvements for patients with CRPS after DRGS.[9,20–22]

In addition, in 2018 the NACC announced that there is strong evidence for the use of DRGS for patients with CRPS I and II and other chronic pain syndromes of the pelvis and lower extremity with identified pathologic condition, despite its shard authorship with the ACCURATE trial. Recommendations for appropriate patient selection were also published and include considerations that mirror those pertinent to any neuromodulation, a notable point being that a potential recipient should be educated on the device, offered alternative options, and given the opportunity to ask questions.[7]

Stelter and colleagues,[23] together with the NACC recommendations, outline several other non-CRPS chronic pain syndromes that DRGS has been used for. Stelter and colleagues[23] recognize 4 common themes within pertinent publications: axial low back pain, pelvic and groin pain, other peripheral neuropathies (including diabetic neuropathy, phantom limb, and postsurgical pains), and multiple concomitant pain causes. GRADE rating of evidence for these indications is very low,[19] mainly because the data, apart from a single clinical trial, remain almost completely case studies and case series. These studies do, however, yield optimistic reductions in pain for these complicated patients.

As was the case in recent studies, DRGS should only be considered in non-CRPS diagnoses that are refractory to conventional treatments, including lifestyle modifications, and pharmacologic and interventional treatments alike. A definition of intractable or refractory pain has been suggested by Deer and colleagues[24]: "when 1) multiple evidence based biomedical therapies used in clinically appropriate and acceptable fashion have failed to reach treatment goals that may include adequate pain reduction and/or improvement in daily functioning or have resulted in intolerable adverse effects, and when 2) psychiatric disorders and psychosocial factors that could influence pain outcomes have been assessed and appropriately addressed."

RISKS AND CONTRAINDICATIONS

DRGS was approved by the FDA in 2016 for neuromodulation from the level of T10 and inferiorly,[7,25] but has been approved in Europe and Australia at any spinal level since 2011. Off-label use is performed by some providers in the United States superior to T10. Per NACC 2019 guidelines, experts think it is safe to use DRGS caudally to C6[7] and report that risks resemble neuromodulation implantation, such as SCS.[7,26] Overall, complication rates in SCS are approximately 30% to 40%.[27] DRGS safety literature is currently based on case reports/observational studies (**Table 1**). For more information from these tables please refer to the cited study.[19] 1 retrospective Manufacture and User Device Experience (MAUDE) database analysis (**Fig. 3**), and 1 industry-funded randomized clinical trial (RCT) (**Table 2**).[9,19,28] Discussed later are 3 key areas of complications in DRGS: (1) device related, (2) procedural, and (3) serious adverse events (SAE).[26]

Device-Related

Device-related complications were the most common cause of adverse event (AE) in DRGS, accounting for 47% and 69.2% when including implantable pulse generator (IPG) site pain and unwanted stimulation.[26] Lead migration was the primary device-related issue with more than 2 times that of lead damage. This is shown in **Fig. 3**, which is taken from a retrospective review of 979 unique complication episodes.[26] DRGS leads are thought to be more stable than SCS leads because of placement in the dural sheath and limited ability for signal to spread or be attenuated, as in SCS.[7] However, the ACCURATE trial showed no statistical difference in device-related and stimulation-related AE (see **Table 2**).[9] IPG site pain rates are likely to be like SCS given similar device and pocket design.[26] Other device considerations include MRI compatibility, allergic response, skin erosion, lead or extension changes, and component/battery failure.

Procedural

DRGS procedural complications accounted for the second most AE at 28% reported to the MAUDE database. In the ACCURATE trial, the most commonly reported AEs in the DRGS arm were at the incision sites (7.9%), IPG pocket pain (13.2%), and overstimulation (3.9%).[9] Per NACC 2017, the overall risk of AE resembles that of any other neuromodulation procedure regarding risks of infection, seroma, dural puncture, hematoma, or meningitis and encephalitis owing to lead placement proximity to the

Table 1
Adverse events and complications of case reports and observational studies from Nagpal and colleagues,[19] 2021

	AEs/Complications
Falowski,[16] 2019	None reported
Gravius,[17] 2019	Mild IPG pocket irritation (1), percutaneous placement restriction in a trial patient (1)
Hunter,[18] 2019	None reported
Huygen,[19] 2019	7 SAEs related to procedure: implant site infection (1), implanted neurostimulator pocket infection (4), transient motor deficit (1), dural puncture (1)
Morgalla,[20] 2019	None reported
Skaribas,[21] 2019	None reported
Eldabe,[22] 2018	2 AEs related to procedure: failure to capture primary pain area and dural puncture
Deer,[23] 2017	8 SAEs related to procedure; 2 infections required device explantation. Most frequent AEs reported were pain at incision site 17.9%), IPG pocket pain (13.2%), and overstimulation (3.9%)
Morgalla,[24] 2017	5 AEs related to procedure: lead breakage (2), infection (1), lead generator relocation (1), additional electrode (1)
Van Buyten,[25] 2017	3 AEs related to procedure: discomfort from stimulation, pain over IPG implant, intermittent calf cramping
Zuidema,[26] 2014	None reported
Liem,[27] 2013	70 events in 24 subjects included infection, cerebrospinal fluid hygroma, loss of paresthesia coverage, prolonged hospital stay, inflammation. temporary cessation of stimulation, and ataxia

From Nagpal A, Clements N, Duszynski B, Boies B. The Effectiveness of Dorsal Root Ganglion Neuro-stimulation for the Treatment of Chronic Pelvic Pain and Chronic Neuropathic Pain of the Lower Extremity: A Comprehensive Review of the Published Data. Pain Med. 2021 Feb 4;22(1):49-59. https://doi.org/10.1093/pm/pnaa369. PMID: 33260203, with permission.

epidural space.[7] Nonetheless, in the ACCURATE trial, DRGS procedural complications were significantly higher at 46.1% versus 23.1%, as seen in **Table 2**. This difference could be attributed to the increased number of lead implantation, up to 3 to 4 with DRGS, compared with 1 to 2 in SCS and lower provider expertise.[28]

Dural puncture is the greatest procedural risk, as shown in **Fig. 3**. Care should be taken when implanting at the L5-S1 level because of the thinner ligamentum flavum and tighter epidural space than other lumber levels.[7] Infection rate associated with DRG trials, implantation, and revision is suggested to be around 1.03%, 4.8%, and 3.85%, respectively.[28] One review of 217 pooled patients across 5 studies reported 13 infections (5.1%) with only 8 requiring explanation.[29] Hematoma formation was the least common AE related to DRG device implantation (see **Fig. 3**).[30] Regardless, care should be taken given the high morbidity associated with hematoma or infection near the spinal cord.

Serious Adverse Events

The ACCURATE trial data suggest that DRGS rates of SAE are comparable to those of SCS at 10.5% and 14.5%, respectively.[9] SAE were left undefined, but no deaths or unanticipated SAE events were reported in the study. In Sivanesan and colleagues,[26] SAE accounted for 2.4% of reported complication episodes (see **Fig. 3**). Liem and colleagues[31] reported 9 SAE out of 70 AE.

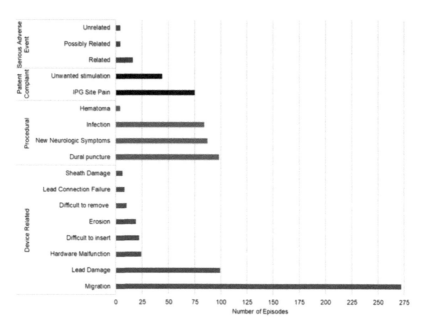

Fig. 3. Categorization of 979 unique reported complications into 16 specific types, from the 2019 MAUDE retrospective analysis.[26] (*From* Sivanesan E, Bicket MC, Cohen SP. Retrospective analysis of complications associated with dorsal root ganglion stimulation for pain relief in the FDA MAUDE database. Reg Anesth Pain Med. 2019;44(1):100-106. doi:10.1136/rapm-2018-000007)

Contraindications

Absolute and relative contraindications have been extrapolated from general neuro-modulation implantation guidelines and the FDA owing to limited independent safety studies.[7,9] Absolute contraindications for patients include (1) failure of DRGS trial, (2) anticoagulation therapy that cannot be suspended, (3) unstable psychiatric

Table 2
Related adverse events in the dorsal root ganglion stimulation arm compared with spinal cord stimulation from the ACCURATE trial[9]

	Rates of Related Adverse Events			
	DRG (N = 76 Subjects)		SCS (N = 76 Subjects)	
Adverse Event Characteristics	Events, n	Subjects, n/ N (%)	Events, n	Subjects, n/ N (%)
Relatedness to neurostimulator system or device	39	28/76 (36.8)	24	20/76 (26.3)
Relatedness to implant procedure	52	35/76 (46.1)	29	20/76 (26.3)
Relatedness to stimulation therapy	10	87/6 (10.5)	10	10/76 (13.2)

From Deer TR, Levy RM, Kramer J, Poree L, Amirdelfan K, Grigsby E, Staats P, Burton AW, Burgher AH, Obray J, Scowcroft J, Golovac S, Kapural L, Paicius R, Kim C, Pope J, Yearwood T, Samuel S, McRoberts WP, Cassim H, Netherton M, Miller N, Schaufele M, Tavel E, Davis T, Davis K, Johnson L, Mekhail N. Dorsal root ganglion stimulation yielded higher treatment success rate for complex regional pain syndrome and causalgia at 3 and 12 months: a randomized comparative trial. Pain. 2017 Apr;158(4):669-681. https://doi.org/10.1097/j.pain.0000000000000814. PMID: 28030470; PMCID: PMC5359787, with permission.

conditions, (4) poor surgical candidate, and (5) poor understanding of the procedure or device use.[7,25,27] Relative contraindications include hemoglobin A_{1C} greater than 8%, current smoker status, prior surgery at the level of implantation, foraminal stenosis, and epidural space stenosis.[7] Safety and efficacy have not been assessed in pregnant women or pediatric patients. To mitigate procedural complication, screening for poor surgical candidates is imperative. Recommendations for neuromodulation implantation anticoagulation management can be seen in **Table 3**.[1]

OUTCOME DATA

Currently, high-quality evidence for DRGS is limited to only 1 RCT, as well as prospective cohort studies, observational studies, case series, and case reports. The major indications for DRGS are for refractory cases of CRPS type I and causalgia, which correspond with most of the current literature. Unfortunately, most data for DRGS of alternative causes of pain, including but not limited to, axial back pain, pelvic pain, failed back surgery syndrome, and focal peripheral neuropathies, are limited to prospective cohort studies, observational studies, and case reports. The most common outcome measure used was the visual analog scale (VAS) with 50% or more reduction in pain being deemed a success. Follow-up intervals ranged from 1 week to 3 years (**Table 4**).[19] For more information from these tables please refer to the cited study. Other measures included function, mood, and medication usage.

Outcomes in Pain Intensity

Complex regional pain syndrome
The ACCURATE trial compared DRGS with more traditional SCS for the treatment of CRPS and causalgia. Outcome success data were defined as greater than 50% pain relief. For this study, 3-month treatment success was reported at 81.2% (95% confidence interval [CI]: 72% to 90.4%) in DRGS compared with SCS at 55.7% (95% CI: 44.1%–67.3%). **Tables 5** and **6** provide both continuous and categorical data from these studies.[19] For more information from these tables please refer to the cited study. Longer-term data, with follow-up at 12 months, demonstrated both noninferiority ($P<.0001$) and superiority ($P<.0004$) when compared with SCS. Success rates, again defined as greater than 50% pain relief, were reported at 74.2% (95% CI: 63.6%–84.8%) for DRGS and 53.0% (95% CI: 41%–65%) for SCS ($P = .01$). This study, however, is prone to bias given it was industry funded. In addition, the subject arms at this time point were decreased from n = 76 to 66 for unclear reasons.

Liem and colleagues in 2013[31] published the first prospective cohort study on DRGS. Thirty-two patients were enrolled with "intractable pain in the trunk, limbs and/or sacral region for a minimum of 6 months." Outcome data were measured at 3 and 6 months. The 3-month data collection demonstrated a decrease in pain of 50.8% (standard deviation [SD] ± 7.0%) with a VAS of 38.4 mm (SD ± 5.7; $P<.001$) compared with baseline. Again, at 6 months, the VAS continued to decrease with the average VAS down to 33.5 mm (SD 6 6.0; $P<.001$), a 56.3% reduction from baseline. A total of 41% (95% CI: 24%–58%) of subjects met the criteria for greater than 50% pain relief.

In 2019, Huygen and colleagues[20] conducted another prospective cohort study of 66 participants with a wider range of diagnoses than the ACCURATE trial. This included CRPS, failed back surgery syndrome, and peripheral nerve injury. Primary outcomes were measured at 6 months and 12 months. At 6 months, peripheral nerve injury/causalgia had an average reduction in VAS from 7.38 ± 1.97 to 4.03 ± 3.11. Subjects with CRPS type I had an average reduction in VAS from 8.44 ± 1.23 to 4.34 ± 3.11 at 6 months. At 12-months, 43% (95% CI: 30%–56%) achieved greater

Table 3
Antiplatelet and anticoagulation management recommendations for neuromodulation procedures, per the Neuromodulation Appropriateness Consensus Committee 2017[1]

Drug	Brain Neuromodulation	When to Stop Spinal Neuromodulation	Peripheral Neuromodulation	When to Restart[a]
Aspirin (ASA) and ASA combinations	• Primary prophylaxis: 6 d • Secondary prophylaxis: 6 d[b]	• Primary prophylaxis: 6 d • Secondary prophylaxis: shared assessment and risk-stratification	Shared assessment and risk-stratification	24 h
Nonaspirin NSAIDs	5 half-lives	5 half-lives	No	24 h
Diclofenac	1 d	1 d		
Ketorolac	1 d	1 d		
Ibuprofen	1 d	1 d		
Etodolac	2 d	2 d		
Indomethacin	2 d	2 d		
Naproxen	4 d	4 d		
Meloxicam	4 d	4 d		
Nabumetone	6 d	6 d		
Oxaprozin	10 d	10 d		
Piroxicam	10 d	10 d		
Phosphodiesterase inhibitors				
Cilostazol	2 d	2 d	No	24 h
Dipyridamole	2 d	2 d	No	
ASA combinations	Follow ASA recommendations	Follow ASA recommendations	Shared assessment and risk-stratification[a]	
Anticoagulants				
Coumadin	5 d, normal INR	5 d, normal INR	5 d, normal INR	24 h
Acenocoumarol	3 d, normal INR	3 d, normal INR	3 d, normal INR	24 h

IV heparin	4 h	4 h	4 h	24 h
Subcutaneous heparin, bid & tid[d]	8–10 h	8–10 h	8–10 h	24 h
LMWH: prophylactic	12 h	12 h	12 h	12–24 h
LMWH: therapeutic	24 h	24 h	24 h	12–24 h
Fibrinolytic agents	48 h	48 h	48 h	48 h
Fondaparinux	4 d	4 d	4 d	24 h
P2Y12 inhibitors				
Clopidogrel	7 d	7 d	7 d	12–24 h
Prasugrel	7–10 d	7–10 d	7–10 d	12–24 h
Ticagrelor	5 d	5 d	5 d	12–24 h
Cangrelor[c]	1–2 h	1–2 h	1–2 h	c
New anticoagulants				
Dabigatran	4–5 d 6 d (impaired renal function)	4–5 d 6 d (impaired renal function)	4–5 d 6 d (impaired renal function)	24 h
Rivaroxaban	3 d	3 d	3 d	24 h
Apixaban	3–5 d	3–5 d	3–5 d	24 h
Edoxaban	3 d (5–6 d in renal patients)	3 d (5–6 d in renal patients)	3 d (5–6 d in renal patients)	24 h
Glycoprotein IIb/IIIa inhibitors[d]				
Abciximab	2–5 d	2–5 d	2–5 d	8–12 h
Eptifibatide	8–24 h	8–24 h	8–24 h	8–12 h
Tirofiban	8–24 h	8–24 h	8–24 h	8–12 h

Abbreviations: INR, international normalized ratio; LMWH, low-molecular-weight heparin.

Deer TR, Narouze S, Provenzano DA, Pope JE, Falowski SM, Russo MA, Benzon H, Slavin K, Pilitsis JG, Alo K, Carlson JD, McRoberts P, Lad SP, Arle J, Levy RM, Simpson B, Mekhail N. The Neurostimulation Appropriateness Consensus Committee (NACC): Recommendations on Bleeding and Coagulation Management in Neurostimulation Devices. Neuromodulation. 2017 Jan;20(1):51-62. doi: 10.1111/ner.12542. Epub 2017 Jan 2. Erratum in: Neuromodulation. 2017 Jun;20(4):407. PMID: 28042905.

[a] When to restart after lead removal for trials (medications should be discontinued during the whole trial) or after permanent implant.

[b] In patients taking ASA for secondary prevention with high-risk factors for cardiovascular disease, and when discontinuing is not recommended, this should be considered a relative contraindication for brain neuromodulation.

[c] Cangrelor is a new intravenous P2Y12 inhibitor that was recently approved by the FDA. Neuromodulation procedures in patients on cangrelor are rarely encountered.

[d] It should be noted that neuromodulation procedures are mostly elective procedures, and these medications should be assessed case by case.

Table 4
Dorsal root ganglion stimulation studies from Nagpal and colleagues,[19] 2021

	DRGN	Design	Inclusion Criteria	Follow-Up Interval	Outcome Measures
Falowski,[16] 2019	8	Case series	Diagnosis of peripheral neuropathy; primarily lower-extremity pain; pain intractable to conventional treatment; successful DRG trial with >50% relief	6 wk postoperative	VAS, opioid consumption
Gravius,[17] 2019	12	Prospective cohort study	Chronic neuropathic pain	3 mo	NRS, BDI, PSQI
Hunter,[19] 2019	4	Case series	Severe chronic pelvic pain; successful DRGS trial with L1 and S2 DRGs	Variables	VAS, function, opioid consumption, satisfaction
Huygen,[19] 2019	56	Prospective observational cohort	Adults; psychologically appropriate for implantation; lower body pain; chronic pain of 6-mo duration; intractable pain; VAS >60 mm	1 wk and 1, 3, 6, and 12 mo	VAS, quality of life, EQ-5D, mood disturbance
Morgalla,[20] 2019	12	Prospective cohort study	Age >18 y; chronic NP unilaterally affecting groin or lower limb; probably NP pain based on NP grading scale; refractory pain control with conservative measures	1 and 6 mo	NRS, SF-36 (function)
Skaribas,[21] 2019	5	Case series	Age >18 y; chronic foot pain	1, 3, and 6 mo	NRS, opioid consumption
Eldabe,[22] 2018	7	Case series	Implantation of DRG neurostimulator for phantom limb or residual limb pain	6 and 12 mo	VAS

Study	DRGN	Study type	Inclusion criteria	Follow-up	Outcome measures
Deer,[23] 2017	76	Prospective RCT	Chronic intractable neuropathic pain with diagnosis of CRPS or causalgia; naive to neurostimulation; tried and failed 2 pharmacologic measures; free from psychological contraindications	3 and 12 mo	VAS, BPI, satisfaction, POMS, total mood disturbance
Morgalla,[24] 2017	30	Case series	Age >18 y; chronic neuropathic pain of the groin as a result of nerve injury; failure of conservative treatment; no indication for further surgical intervention	3 mo and 1, 2, and 3 y	VAS, PDI, BPI, opioid usage, PCS
Van Buyten,[25] 2017	8	Case series	Age >18 y; met Budapest criteria for the diagnosis of CRPS	1 wk, 1 mo, 5 wk, and 2, 3, and 6 mo	VAS, BPI, EQ-5D3L, POMS
Zuidema,[26] 2014	3	Case series	Refractory groin pain patient who underwent DRG stimulatory placement	3 mo	VAS
Liem,[27] 2013	32	Case series	Age >18 y; chronic intractable pain in the trunk, limbs, or sacral region for ≥6 mo; baseline VAS of ≥60 mm; stable pain medication dosage	1 wk and 1, 2, 3, and 6 mo	VAS

Abbreviations: DRGN, number of patients receiving DRG stimulation; NP, neuropathic pain; PSQI, Pittsburgh Sleep Quality Index; SF-36, Short Form 36 Questionnaire

From Nagpal A, Clements N, Duszynski B, Boies B. The Effectiveness of Dorsal Root Ganglion Neurostimulation for the Treatment of Chronic Pelvic Pain and Chronic Neuropathic Pain of the Lower Extremity: A Comprehensive Review of the Published Data. Pain Med. 2021 Feb 4;22(1):49-59. https://doi.org/10.1093/pm/pnaa369. PMID: 33260203, with permission.

Table 5			
Continuous data from Nagpal and colleagues, 2021			
	DRGN	Follow-Up Interval	% Mean Improvement Remaining Subjects at each Time Point
Falowski,[16] 2019	8	6 wk	80
Gravius,[17] 2019	12	3 mo	61
Huygen,[19] 2019	56	3 mo	62
		6 mo	52
		12 mo	49
Morgalla,[20] 2019	12	6 mo	69
Eldabe,[22] 2018	7	6 mo	66
		12 mo	64
Deer,[23] 2017	76	3 mo	81
		6 mo	75
		9 mo	77
		12 mo	69
Morgalla,[24] 2017	30	3 mo	63
		1 y	56
		2 y	50
		3 y	44
Van Buyten,[25] 2017	8	3 mo	68
		6 mo	63
		12 mo	62
Liem,[26] 2013	32	2 mo	51
		3 mo	51
		6 mo	56

From Nagpal A, Clements N, Duszynski B, Boies B. The Effectiveness of Dorsal Root Ganglion Neurostimulation for the Treatment of Chronic Pelvic Pain and Chronic Neuropathic Pain of the Lower Extremity: A Comprehensive Review of the Published Data. Pain Med. 2021 Feb 4;22(1):49-59. https://doi.org/10.1093/pm/pnaa369. PMID: 33260203, with permission.

than 50% reduction in VAS. Further breakdown by cause demonstrates greater reduction in pain in peripheral nerve injury/causalgia over CRPS type I with 60% (6/10) versus 33.3% (3/9) of subjects who report greater than 50% relief.

Pelvic and groin pain
Morgalla and colleagues[32] included 30 subjects in their study for neuropathic groin pain with follow-up for 3 years. VAS scores decreased from a baseline median score of 8.0 to 4.5, for a total of 63.5% ($\pm$10%, $P = .005$) improvement. Greater than 50% pain relief was achieved by 72.7% of subjects who completed follow-up. However, if lost to follow-up, subjects were accounted for as treatment failures, and the greater than 50% relief drops to 27% (95% CI: 11%–42%) of subjects at the 3-year mark.

In addition, 5 case reports using DRGS showed a promising response with a greater than 70% reduction in pain at last follow-up,[33–37] whereas 2 others demonstrated 69.7% and 43%, respectively.[38,39]

Table 6
Categorical data from Nagpal and colleagues, 2021[19]

	DRGN	Follow-Up Interval	>50% Improvement (95% CI)	>75% Improvement (95% CI)	100% Improvement (95% CI)
Falowski,[16] 2019	8	5 wk	88% (65%–100%)	50% (15%–85%)	25% (0%–55%)
Gravius,[17] 2019,	12	3 mo	58% (30%–86%)		
Hunter,[18] 2019	4	>3 mo	100%	75% (33%–100%)	25% (0%–67%)
Huygen,[19] 2019	56	12 mo	43% (30%–56%)		
Skaribas,[21] 2019	5	6 mo	100%	60% (17%–100%)	0%
Eldabe,[22] 2018	7	3 mo	43% (6%–80%)	29% (0%–62%)	14% (0%–40%)
		6 mo	43% (6%–80%)	29% (0%–62%)	14% (0%–40%)
		12 mo	29% (0%–62%)	29% (0%–62%)	14% (0%–40%)
Deer,[23] 2017	76	3 mo	81% (72%–90%)		
		12 mo	74% (64%–84%)		
Morgalla,[24] 2017	30	3 mo	83% (70%–97%)		
		3 y	27% (11%–42%)		
Van Buyten,[25] 2017	8	12 mo	63% (29%–96%)		
Zuidema,[26] 2014	3	2 mo	100%	100%	33% (0%–87%)
Liem,[27] 2013	32	2 mo	41% (24%–58%)		
		3 mo	47% (30%–64%)		
		6 mo	41% (24%–58%)		

From Nagpal A, Clements N, Duszynski B, Boies B. The Effectiveness of Dorsal Root Ganglion Neurostimulation for the Treatment of Chronic Pelvic Pain and Chronic Neuropathic Pain of the Lower Extremity: A Comprehensive Review of the Published Data. Pain Med. 2021 Feb 4;22(1):49-59. https://doi.org/10.1093/pm/pnaa369. PMID: 33260203, with permission.

Axial low back pain

Most literature on axial back pain management with DRGS is limited to observation studies, case series, and case reports (**Table 7**).[23] However, many of the studies seem promising by demonstrating greater than 50% pain reduction from baseline at the time of last follow-up.[40–42]

Outcomes in Function

Six studies used a function questionnaire, including Back Pain Inventory (BPI), Pain Disability Index (PDI), and the SF-36 Physical Functioning Scale.[9,21,31,32,35,43] The ACCURATE trial demonstrated improvements in SF-36 scores at 3 and 6 months in both the DRGS and the SCS groups ($P<.05$). However, by 12 months, the DRGS group had statistically greater improvement on 3 subscales of the SF-36 compared with the SCS group.

Morgalla and colleagues[32] found significant improvement in SF-36 domains related to physical functioning, energy/fatigue, and pain compared with baseline at 1 month and kept these improvements up to 12 months.

Outcomes in Mood

Six studies reported significant outcomes in mood following DRGS using multiple scales, including Profile of Mood States (POMS), Becks Depression Index (BDI), Total Mood Disturbance, and the Pain Catastrophizing Scale (PCS).[9,20,21,31,43,44]

Table 7
Studies reviewed in Stelter and colleagues,[23] 2021

Author/y Published	Study Type	Population Size	Patient Age (y)	Pain Syndrome	Lead Location and Number of Leads Used	Pain Outcome Measure	Pre-DRGS Pain	Post-DRGS Pain	Follow-up	Complications
Huygen et al,[20] 2017	Case series	N = 12	42–52	FBSS; low back pain with radicular pain	1–4 leads placed L1-L4, S1; Total 29 leads placed; L1 = 3.4%; L2 = 56.6%; L3 = 31%; L4 = 3.4%; S1 = 3.4%	VAS	77.6 ± 2 mm	49.2 ± 9.6 mm (38.2%); 44.6 ± 9.5 mm (44.2%)	6 mo, n = 12; 12 mo, n = 11	None reported
Kallewaard et al, 2018	Case series	N = 13	26–70	FBSS	1–3 leads placed L2, L3, L4, L5; 20 leads total	NPRS	8.64 ± 0.92	2.40 ± 2.38 (72.05%)	12 mo, n = 9	None reported
Weiner et al,[41] 2016	Case series	N = 11	37–78	FBSS; low back pain	1 lead per site; 11 leads total; L1 = 4; L2 = 1; L3 = 4; L4 = 2	VAS, % reduced	L1/2 = 5.9; L2/3 = 7.3; L3/4 = 6.5; L4/5 = 8.0	L1/2 = 3.0; L2/3 = 2.0; L3/4 = 2.3; L4/5 = 3.2 (63% pain reduction)	6 wk	Lead migration = 2
Kufakwaro et al, 2014	CA prospective randomized comparative study vs PRF	N = 21; 10 = PRF; 11 = DRGS	Not reported	Chronic low back pain and neuropathic leg pain	None reported	VAS	9	3 mo = 60% pain reduced; 6 mo = 55% pain reduced	3 mo; 6 mo	Not reported

Study	Design	N	Age	Indication	Outcome measure	Lead placement		Results	Follow-up	Complications
Chapman et al,[42] 2020	Case series	N = 17	34–71	Chronic low back pain and neuropathic leg pain	VAS	Avg number of leads per patient = 3.2 Bilateral T12 (17) At least 1 lead at L1 (3) At least 1 lead at S1 (10)	92.5 ± 8.0	22.3 ± 16.6 29.4 ± 15.4 20.6 ± 12.8 19.3 ± 16.4 (77.8% reduction from baseline at 12 mo)	1 mo, n = 15 3 mo, n = 16 6 mo, n = 16 12, n = 7	(4/17) Lead migrations requiring surgery = 2 Pocket pain = 1
Chapman et al,[42] 2020	Case series	N = 4	56–70	FBSS	VAS	4 leads placed T12, S1 4 leads placed T12, S1, L3, L4 3 leads placed T12, S1 2 leads placed T12, S1	Not reported	All patients had >60% pain reduction	26 mo	None reported

Abbreviations: CA, conference abstract; FBSS, failed back surgery syndrome; NPRS, numeric pain rating scale; PRF, pulsed radiofrequency ablation.

Stelter B, Karri J, Marathe A, Abd-Elsayed A. Dorsal Root Ganglion Stimulation for the Treatment of Non-Complex Regional Pain Syndrome Related Chronic Pain Syndromes: A Systematic Review. Neuromodulation. 2021 Jun;24(4):622-633. https://doi.org/10.1111/ner.13361. Epub 2021 Jan 26. PMID: 33501749.

The ACCURATE trial found that both SCS and DRGS groups showed improvement in POMS from baseline to 3 months. These changes were statistically greater in the DRGS group.[9]

Outcomes in Medication Consumption

Four studies reported a decrease in opioid consumption after a DRGS trial or permanent implantation.[35,43,45,46] Morgalla and colleagues,[43] during a case series (n = 30), reported 4 subjects (13.3%) no longer required their previous medication regimen following DRGS. Fourteen subjects (46.7%) were able to reduce their pain medication by 50%. Four subjects (13.3%) reduced their pain medication by 25% overall during their study, and 73.3% of the patients reduced their pain medication after DRGS.[43] Falowski and colleagues[45] looked at medication use following DRGS at 6 weeks and found 7/8 patients (87.5%) were able to reduce or eliminate pain medications. Hunter and Yang[35] reported a decreased use in opioids and neuropathic agents after DRGS. Skaribas and colleagues[46] reported a decrease in oral pain medications, but it was unclear whether opioid or nonopioid.

DISCUSSION

DRGS has demonstrated efficacy in the treatment of a variety of painful conditions. The best evidence for its use is for the treatment of the pain and dysfunction associated with CRPS. Other diagnoses, such as chronic pelvic pain, neuropathy, and axial low back pain, can be treated with DRGS, but the level of evidence is not as favorable at this time.

Although the evidence supports the use of DRGS as first-line treatment for CRPS, some caveats are warranted. First, the FDA has only approved DRGS for use at levels T10-S2, and this limits its utility to the lower extremity. Second, the single RCT demonstrating the value of DRGS used a different diagnosis for "causalgia" as that which is ordinarily accepted.[9] The International Association for the Study of Pain defines causalgia as "[a] syndrome of sustained burning pain, allodynia, and hyperpathia after a traumatic nerve lesion, often combined with vasomotor and sudomotor dysfunction and later trophic changes," which is analogous to CRPS type II.[47] The definition used by the investigators of the ACCURATE study is more vague, and therefore, likely includes a broader range of diagnoses. It is therefore reasonable to conclude that many lower-extremity neuropathies, refractory to conservative treatment, would be treated effectively with DRGS.

The body region with the most burgeoning evidence for the use of DRGS is the pelvis. Chronic pelvic pain is a ubiquitous condition, affecting 5.7% to 26.6% of women.[48] Two separate prospective case series have demonstrated benefit in pain and function for patients with chronic pelvic pain treated with DRGS.[35,36]

Ultimately, further RCTs are necessary to demonstrate the true effectiveness of DRGS for other neuropathic pain conditions. Because DRGS is largely a paresthesia-free form of stimulation, crossover design studies are possible, which would be valuable in assessing the explanatory benefits of DRGS.[49] Consideration must be given to each individual patient's unique disease state and medical history as well as the physician's comfort level with performing this procedure before pursuing DRGS.

SUMMARY

DRGS is a relatively new form of neuromodulation that is first-line therapy for the treatment of lower-extremity CRPS. Burgeoning evidence suggests that DRGS may be beneficial in the treatment of neuropathic pain/neuropathy, chronic pelvic pain, and axial LBP. Further RCTs are needed to understand the true effectiveness of this treatment option in refractory chronic pain syndromes.

CLINICS CARE POINTS

- Dorsal root ganglion stimulation is a form of neuromodulation that is first-line therapy for the treatment of complex regional pain syndrome of the lower extremities.
- Dorsal root ganglion stimulation should be considered in the treatment algorithm for patients with refractory neuropathic pain/neuropathy of the lower extremities, chronic pelvic pain, and/or axial low back pain.
- Dorsal root ganglion stimulation is only Food and Drug Administration approved for use from the levels of T10-S2.
- Dorsal root ganglion stimulation is technically more difficult to perform for the physician than traditional dorsal column stimulation, and technique improves with continued use of the device.
- Risks of performing dorsal root ganglion stimulation are similar to the risks of traditional dorsal column stimulation.
- Every patient who is a candidate for this procedure should have preprocedure imaging (ideally MRI) to review the foramen in question to ascertain whether there is sufficient room for the lead to be placed, as dorsal root ganglion injury can occur in the stenotic foramina.

DISCLOSURE

Nothing to disclosure.

REFERENCES

1. Deer TR, Narouze S, Provenzano DA, et al. The Neurostimulation Appropriateness Consensus Committee (NACC): recommendations on bleeding and coagulation management in neurostimulation devices. Neuromodulation 2017;20(1):51–62.
2. Deer TR, Provenzano DA, Hanes M, et al. The Neurostimulation Appropriateness Consensus Committee (NACC) recommendations for infection prevention and management. Neuromodulation 2017;20(1):31–50.
3. Deer TR, Lamer TJ, Pope JE, et al. The Neurostimulation Appropriateness Consensus Committee (NACC) safety guidelines for the reduction of severe neurological injury. Neuromodulation 2017;20(1):15–30.
4. Deer TR, Mekhail N, Provenzano D, et al. The appropriate use of neurostimulation of the spinal cord and peripheral nervous system for the treatment of chronic pain and ischemic diseases: the Neuromodulation Appropriateness Consensus Committee. Neuromodulation 2014;17(6):515–50.
5. Deer TR, Mekhail N, Petersen E, et al. The appropriate use of neurostimulation: stimulation of the intracranial and extracranial space and head for chronic pain. Neuromodulation 2014;17(6):551–70.
6. Deer TR, Mekhail N, Provenzano D, et al. The appropriate use of neurostimulation: avoidance and treatment of complications of neurostimulation therapies for the treatment of chronic pain. Neuromodulation 2014;17(6):571–98.

7. Deer TR, Pope JE, Lamer TJ, et al. The Neuromodulation Appropriateness Consensus Committee on best practices for dorsal root ganglion stimulation. Neuromodulation 2019;22(1):1–35.

8. Djouhri L. L5 spinal nerve axotomy induces sensitization of cutaneous L4 Aβ-nociceptive dorsal root ganglion neurons in the rat in vivo. Neurosci Lett 2016; 624:72–7.

9. Deer TR, Levy RM, Kramer J, et al. Dorsal root ganglion stimulation yielded higher treatment success rate for complex regional pain syndrome and causalgia at 3 and 12 months: a randomized comparative trial. Pain 2017;158(4):669–81.

10. Liem L, Russo M, Huygen FJPM, et al. One-year outcomes of spinal cord stimulation of the dorsal root ganglion in the treatment of chronic neuropathic pain. Neuromodulation 2015;18(1):41–9.

11. Thomson SJ, Tavakkolizadeh M, Love-Jones S, et al. Effects of rate on analgesia in kilohertz frequency spinal cord stimulation: results of the PROCO randomized controlled trial. Neuromodulation 2018;21(1):67–76.

12. Van Buyten JP, Wille F, Smet I, et al. Therapy-related explants after spinal cord stimulation: results of an International Retrospective Chart Review Study. Neuromodulation 2017;20(7):642–9.

13. Vancamp T, Levy RM, Peña I, et al. Relevant anatomy, morphology, and implantation techniques of the dorsal root ganglia at the lumbar levels. Neuromodulation 2017;20(7):690–702.

14. Vuka I, Marciuš T, Došenović S, et al. Neuromodulation with electrical field stimulation of dorsal root ganglion in various pain syndromes: a systematic review with focus on participant selection. J Pain Res 2019;12:803–30.

15. Koopmeiners AS, Mueller S, Kramer J, et al. Effect of electrical field stimulation on dorsal root ganglion neuronal function. Neuromodulation 2013;16(4):304–11.

16. Deer TR, Pope JE. Dorsal root ganglion stimulation approval by the Food and Drug Administration: advice on evolving the process. Expert Rev Neurother 2016;16(10):1123–5.

17. Guyatt G, Oxman AD, Akl EA, et al. GRADE guidelines: 1. Introduction - GRADE evidence profiles and summary of findings tables. J Clin Epidemiol 2011;64(4): 383–94.

18. Guyatt GH, Oxman AD, Vist GE, et al. GRADE: an emerging consensus on rating quality of evidence and strength of recommendations. BMJ 2008;336(7650): 924–6.

19. Nagpal A, Clements N, Duszynski B, et al. The effectiveness of dorsal root ganglion neurostimulation for the treatment of chronic pelvic pain and chronic neuropathic pain of the lower extremity: a comprehensive review of the published data. Pain Med 2021;22(1):49–59.

20. Huygen FJPM, Liem L, Nijhuis H, et al. Evaluating dorsal root ganglion stimulation in a prospective Dutch cohort. Neuromodulation 2019;22(1):80–6.

21. Van Buyten JP, Smet I, Liem L, et al. Stimulation of dorsal root ganglia for the management of complex regional pain syndrome: a prospective case series. Pain Pract 2015;15(3):208–16.

22. Zuidema X, Breel J, Wille F. Paresthesia mapping: a practical workup for successful implantation of the dorsal root ganglion stimulator in refractory groin pain. Neuromodulation 2014;17(7):665–9.

23. Stelter B, Karri J, Marathe A, et al. Dorsal root ganglion stimulation for the treatment of non-complex regional pain syndrome related chronic pain syndromes: a systematic review. Neuromodulation 2021;24(4):622–33.

24. Deer TR, Caraway DL, Wallace MS. A definition of refractory pain to help determine suitability for device implantation. Neuromodulation 2014;17(8):711–5.
25. *PMA P150004: FDA Summary of Safety and Effectiveness Data SUMMARY OF SAFETY AND EFFECTIVENESS DATA (SSED).* US Food and Drug Administration Website. https://www.accessdata.fda.gov/scripts/cdrh/cfdocs/cfpma/pma.cfm?id=P150004. Updated January 19, 2022. Accessed January 19, 2022.
26. Sivanesan E, Bicket MC, Cohen SP. Retrospective analysis of complications associated with dorsal root ganglion stimulation for pain relief in the FDA MAUDE database. Reg Anesth Pain Med 2019;44(1):100–6.
27. Eldabe S, Buchser E, Duarte R v. NEUROMODULATION SECTION Complications of Spinal Cord Stimulation and Peripheral Nerve Stimulation Techniques: A Review of the Literature. Pain Medicine 2016;17(2):325–36. https://doi.org/10.1093/pm/pnv025.
28. Moman RN, Peterson AA, Maher DP, et al. Infectious complications of dorsal root ganglion stimulation: a systematic review and pooled analysis of incidence. Neuromodulation 2021. https://doi.org/10.1111/ner.13473.
29. Huygen FJPM, Kallewaard JW, Nijhuis H, et al. Effectiveness and safety of dorsal root ganglion stimulation for the treatment of chronic pain: a pooled analysis. Neuromodulation 2020;23(2):213–21.
30. Petraglia FW, Farber SH, Gramer R, et al. The incidence of spinal cord injury in implantation of percutaneous and paddle electrodes for spinal cord stimulation. Neuromodulation 2016;19(1):85–9.
31. Liem L, Russo M, Huygen FJPM, et al. A multicenter, prospective trial to assess the safety and performance of the spinal modulation dorsal root ganglion neurostimulator system in the treatment of chronic pain. Neuromodulation 2013;16(5):471–82.
32. Morgalla MH, de Barros Filho MF, Chander BS, et al. Neurophysiological effects of dorsal root ganglion stimulation (DRGS) in pain processing at the cortical level. Neuromodulation 2019;22(1):36–43.
33. Schu S, Gulve A, Eldabe S, et al. Spinal cord stimulation of the dorsal root ganglion for groin pain-a retrospective review. Pain Pract 2015;15(4):293–9.
34. Patel KVM. Dorsal root ganglion stimulation for chronic pelvic pain. Obstet Gynecol 2019;133:223.
35. Hunter CW, Yang A. Dorsal root ganglion stimulation for chronic pelvic pain: a case series and technical report on a novel lead configuration. Neuromodulation 2019;22(1):87–95.
36. Giordano NL, van Helmond N, Chapman KB. Coccydynia treated with dorsal root ganglion stimulation. Case Rep Anesthesiol 2018;2018:1–4.
37. Hassanain M, Murphy P. Dorsal root ganglion stimulation for the treatment of bilateral intractable chronic testicular pain. Neuromodulation 2019;22(1):115–6.
38. Rowland DCL, Wright D, Moir L, et al. Successful treatment of pelvic girdle pain with dorsal root ganglion stimulation. Br J Neurosurg 2016;30(6):685–6.
39. Donaldson A. LKMP; (1) CPI and WFBMCKN (2) CPI and C for CRW-SN. Dorsal root ganglia (DRG) electrical stimulation for intractable pudendal neuralgia. AAPM 2018 Annual Meet Abstracts 2018;19(4):819–905. https://doi.org/10.1093/pm/pny044.
40. Huygen F, Liem L, Cusack W, et al. Stimulation of the L2–L3 dorsal root ganglia induces effective pain relief in the low back. Pain Pract 2018;18(2):205–13.
41. Weiner RL, Yeung A, Garcia CM, et al. Treatment of FBSS low back pain with a novel percutaneous DRG wireless stimulator: pilot and feasibility study. Pain Med (United States) 2016;17(10):1911–6.

42. Chapman KB, Nagrani S, Patel KV, et al. Lumbar dorsal root ganglion stimulation lead placement using an outside-in technique in 4 patients with failed back surgery syndrome: a case series. A A Pract 2020;14(10):e01300.

43. Morgalla MH, Bolat A, Fortunato M, et al. Dorsal root ganglion stimulation used for the treatment of chronic neuropathic pain in the groin: a single-center study with long-term prospective results in 34 cases. Neuromodulation 2017;20(8):753–60.

44. Gravius N, Chaudhry SR, Muhammad S, et al. Selective L4 dorsal root ganglion stimulation evokes pain relief and changes of inflammatory markers: part I profiling of saliva and serum molecular patterns. Neuromodulation 2019;22(1): 44–52.

45. Falowski S, Pope JE, Raza A. Early US experience with stimulation of the dorsal root ganglia for the treatment of peripheral neuropathy in the lower extremities: a multicenter retrospective case series. Neuromodulation 2019;22(1):96–100.

46. Skaribas IM, Peccora C, Skaribas E. Single S1 dorsal root ganglia stimulation for intractable complex regional pain syndrome foot pain after lumbar spine surgery: a case series. Neuromodulation 2019;22(1):101–7.

47. Terminology | International Association for the Study of Pain. Available at: https://www.iasp-pain.org/resources/terminology/#causalgia. Accessed January 27, 2022.

48. Ahangari A. Prevalence of chronic pelvic pain among women: an updated review. Pain Physician 2014;17(2):141–8.

49. Verrills P, Mitchell B, Vivian D, et al. Dorsal root ganglion stimulation is paresthesia-independent: a retrospective study. Neuromodulation 2019;22(8): 937–42.

Peripheral Nerve Stimulation for Chronic Pain and Migraine: A Review

Samantha C. Erosa, MD[a,b,*], Roya S. Moheimani, MD[a,b],
Jessica C. Oswald, MD, MPH[a,b,c], Joel P. Castellanos, MD[a,b],
Mickey E. Abraham, MD[b,d], Nathaniel M. Schuster, MD[a,b]

KEYWORDS

- Peripheral nerve stimulation • Neuromodulation • Chronic pain
- Interventional pain management

KEY POINTS

- Peripheral nerve stimulation (PNS) is an interventional option to consider for chronic pain conditions when conservative measures fail.
- Proper patient selection is essential and should include psychological screening.
- Recent advancements include novel systems specifically created for PNS.

INTRODUCTION

Peripheral nerve stimulation (PNS) is an emerging chronic pain treatment. PNS is achieved by modulating afferent pain pathways by providing a stimulus to a peripheral nerve. Over the last few years there have been new clinical trials studying PNS for indications including peripheral neuropathy, postamputation pain, back pain, hemiplegic shoulder pain (HSP) and nonhemiplegic shoulder pain, and chronic pelvic pain (CPP).[1–5] Here we review and analyze this growing evidence.

History

First described in 1967 for the treatment of focal mononeuropathy,[6,7] early PNS required surgical cut down and implantation of multicontact electrodes near or adjacent to the nerve. PNS was fret with complications to include iatrogenic nerve injury and an 85% revision rate.[8,9] In 1999, Weiner and Reed[10] described percutaneously

[a] Department of Anesthesiology, Division of Pain Medicine, University of California, San Diego, CA, USA; [b] Koman Family Outpatient Pavilion, Center for Pain Medicine, 9400 Campus Point Drive, MC 7328, La Jolla, CA 92037, USA; [c] Department of Emergency Medicine, University of California, San Diego, San Diego, CA, USA; [d] Department of Neurosurgery, University of California, San Diego, San Diego, CA, USA
* Corresponding author.
E-mail address: serosa@health.ucsd.edu

Phys Med Rehabil Clin N Am 33 (2022) 379–407
https://doi.org/10.1016/j.pmr.2022.01.007
1047-9651/22/© 2022 Elsevier Inc. All rights reserved.

implanted PNS to treat occipital neuralgia using spinal cord stimulator (SCS) leads and an implantable pulse generator (IPG) off-label. However, PNS using SCS systems had high rates of migration, lead fracture, and reoperation.[11] In recent years, new systems, most of which were developed specifically for PNS, have received Food and Drug Administration (FDA) clearance, including StimRouter, StimQ PNS, NALU (Nalu Medical, Inc, Carlsbad, CA), and SPRINT PNS (SPR Therapeutis, Inc; Cleveland, OH).

PNS has had growing popularity in recent years with the results of new clinical trials and FDA clearance of novel, dedicated PNS systems. PNS is less invasive and a more targeted therapy when compared with traditional SCS.[11,12] With some new PNS systems, an external pulse generator (EPG) is applied with skin adhesives and eliminates IPG-related discomfort and complications.[13]

Although tonic stimulation had been used historically, subperception programs including high-frequency and burst programming initially developed for SCS have been incorporated into PNS systems.[4,14]

Mechanism of Action

There are several theories for PNS's mechanism of action. The original and most widely studied is the gate control theory of pain, in which presynaptic stimulation and depolarization blocks and modulates the afferent firing of pain sensory fibers.[6,7] PNS is postulated to activate Aδ fiber groups and subsequently inhibit spinothalamic tract afferent pain signals.[15] It is also theorized that central or cortical reorganization may occur with repetitive nerve stimulation.[16,17]

Mechanistically, the applied electric current creates a magnetic field that inhibits the painful afferent signal[18]; it was originally tested within the range of 0.5 to 20 Hz with higher frequencies providing more robust inhibition of painful stimuli. The efficacy of the electrically induced magnetic field is highly dependent on the relative distance of the electrode to the target, along with the target nerve fiber diameter. In addition, repetitive stimuli are noted to be more potent than a stronger single stimulus.[18] **Fig. 1** provides an example of PNS at the right knee used to treat painful distal extremity neuropathy.

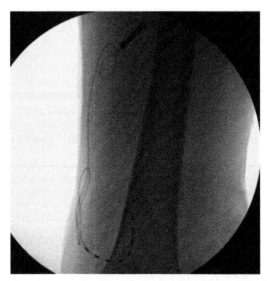

Fig. 1. A NALU peripheral nerve stimulator device implanted to treat painful right superficial peroneal neuropathy. The system was placed just distal to the sciatic bifurcation.

PATIENT SELECTION CRITERIA

Studies evaluating PNS often select patients with at least 3 to 6 months of focal chronic pain that is refractory to conservative treatment.[3,19,20] Some indications include but are not limited to peripheral neuropathy, postamputation pain (PAP), and chronic mechanical low back, shoulder, and pelvic pain.[1–5] It is recommended that patients remain on a stable pain medication.[21]

Risks and Contraindications

The International Neuromodulation Society created the Neurostimulation Appropriateness Consensus Committee (NACC) to review currently available literature and provide treatment guidelines.[22] NACC recommends avoiding PNS in patients who are unsafe to come off of anticoagulation or antiplatelet therapy for the duration of the trial and implantation procedures.[21] Cognitive decline is a relative contraindication because patients may be unable to participate in the aftercare, with an exception if caregivers are able to assist in the patient's maintenance of the device.[21] Psychology evaluations are strongly recommended for permanent implanted devices including PNS.[21] Psychiatric conditions and active substance use disorders are poor prognostic factors for neuromodulation success and should be addressed before pursuing PNS.[21]

PNS devices should not be placed in close proximity to hardware such as cardiac pacemakers and defibrillators. Leads must be placed 6 in or more from any metallic hardware.

After review of the evidence for PNS, NACC's strong consensus was that PNS has not been associated with direct neurologic trauma (level 2–3 evidence) and image guidance as well as intermittent nerve stimulation should be used for percutaneous lead placement (level 2).[22] Finally, there was level 3 evidence and strong consensus that specialized equipment designed for PNS will improve efficacy and reduce adverse events (AEs).

To reduce AEs, NACC suggests adopting practices used to reduce AEs in SCS which also apply to PNS placement. Sedation, if used, should be managed to allow patients the ability to report paresthesia when percutaneous lead placement is near the nerve.[23]

Mechanical or hardware complications of PNS include lead failure, fracture, and/or migration.[24] Biologic complications include infection, bleeding, skin irritation, and/or neurologic damage. Hardware complications are more common than biologic complications, and, overall, the rate of serious complications is low. Infections with PNS, which were estimated to be less than 0.0001%, seem to be affected by the lead design, with lower rates with the noncoil design.[13] The NACC recommends optimization of immunosuppression and consideration of patient pathology that may predispose to infection and hamper wound healing,[21] and this includes timing PNS procedures with the assistance of oncology to avoid poor wound healing or increased risk of wound infection.

Evaluation for recent skin or systemic infection, preprocedural antibiotics, hair removal, and chlorhexidine gluconate for antiseptic technique are recommended to reduce the risk of surgical site infections (SSIs).[21,25] Proper care should be taken in the preprocedural period to monitor for development of SSIs. Infection rate was estimated to be less than 0.0001%, with lower rates with noncoiled versus coiled design.[13]

As with other neuromodulation devices, there is potential for eventual habituation and loss of efficacy after implantation.[14]

CURRENT EVIDENCE AND OUTCOME DATA

PNS is used for a variety of chronic pain conditions. A review of the current literature and pertinent outcomes by pain subtype is provided in **Tables 1–5**. For categorical data of interest, the authors of this review calculated the 95% confidence intervals (CIs) about means; when the 95% CIs were overlapping, the finding was not significant, whereas when the 95% CIs were not overlapping, the finding was significant. These data are presented together with *P* values reported in the original article by the investigators. For studies of interest where the investigators reported per-protocol (PP) analyses, the authors of this review calculated intention-to-treat (ITT) analyses with considering dropouts as nonresponders.

Neuropathic Pain

Deer and colleagues[19] performed a randomized controlled trial (RCT) evaluating the safety and efficacy of the StimRouter PNS (Stimrouter, Bioness, Inc, Valencia, CA) system with an EPG to treat pain of neuropathic origin. The investigators randomized 94 individuals to receive electrical stimulation placed with fluoroscopic or ultrasound guidance (treatment group) or no therapeutic stimulation (control group) and the option to crossover after the 90-day treatment period. The study included patients with neuropathic pain of the upper extremity, lower extremity, or trunk; neither targeted nerves nor pain cause was reported in the article. The primary outcome was response rate, defined as at least 30% reduction in numerical rating scale (NRS) without increase in pain medications, at 3 months. Patients receiving active stimulation achieved a significantly higher response rate (38%, 95% CI, 23.6%–51.9%) versus control (10%, 95% CI, 1.7%–18.7%, *P* = .0048). At 3 months there was also a significantly greater mean percentage pain reduction in the treatment (27.2%) versus control group (2.3%, *P* < .0001). Although these differences are statistically significant between groups, readers should consider that this reduction in NRS was modest. No serious device-related AEs occurred, but 51 device-related events were reported with 80.4% described as mild such as skin rash, redness, or soreness at the surgical site.[19]

In a retrospective case series of 26 consecutive patients with chronic neuropathic pain of the upper extremity secondary to complex regional pain syndrome type 1 or 2 or other peripheral nerve injury, cylindrical quadripolar electrode (Medtronic, Minneapolis, MN, USA) SCS leads were implanted percutaneously under ultrasound guidance to the suprascapular nerve or cervical nerve roots with a surgically placed IPG.[3] The stimulation voltage was set below the threshold of inducing paresthesias or muscle contractions. Twenty (76.9%) patients had a mean follow-up of 27.5 months with a reported mean pain relief of 67.1%; 50% responder rates were 17 of 26 (65.4%, 95% CI, 47.1%–83.7%), and 70% responder rates were 12 of 26 (46.2%, 95% CI, 27.0%–65.3%). Of 26 patients 7 (26.9%) reported complications of lead fractures (n = 2), lead migration (n = 1), superficial infection (n = 1), and unpleasant shocklike sensations resulting in termination of therapy (n = 3).[3] **Table 1** provides a summary of the aforementioned studies.

Postamputation Pain

Chronic PAP includes residual limb pain (RLP) and phantom limb pain (PLP). In a survey of 914 amputees, 79.9% and 67.7% reported experiencing PLP and RLP symptoms, respectively.[26] **Table 2** summarizes the below-mentioned studies.

A double-blind, placebo-controlled trial by Gilmore and colleagues[27] (NCT01996254) randomized 28 traumatic lower extremity amputees to receive either 8 weeks of the SPRINT temporary PNS system with EPG to the sciatic and femoral

Table 1
Characteristics of included studies that evaluated peripheral nerve stimulation for neuropathic pain

Reference (Year)	Type of Study	Patient Population	Study Duration	N	Device	Treatment	Comparator	Scale	Mean/Median Pain Score	Outcome and Results
Deer et al,[19] 2016	Prospective, multicenter, randomized, double-blind, partial crossover study	Adults >22 year old with chronic pain of peripheral nerve origin with posttraumatic or postsurgical neuralgia	90 d	94	StimRouter System	Electrical stimulation from the StimRouter System and stable dosing of pain medication for 90 d	No therapeutic stimulation and a stable dose of pain medications for 90 d	BPI	8.1 ± 1.1 (baseline for treatment) 8.0 ± 1.1 (baseline for control) 6.7 ± 2.3 (3 mo follow-up treatment) 7.6 ± 2.0 (3 mo follow-up control)	Statistically significant improvement between randomized groups The treatment group achieved a mean pain reduction of 27.2% from baseline to month 3 compared with a 2.3% reduction in the control group (P < .0001)
Bouche et al,[3] 2016	Retrospective cohort study	Chronic refractory neuropathic pain of the upper limb	Mean 27.5 mo	26	PiscesQuad, Medtronic	PNS of BP cervical nerve roots	PNS of SSN	% of pain relief	Mean pain relief of 67.1%	Treating the SSN or BP roots, PNS provided an effective option to reduce upper limb neuropathic pain.

(continued on next page)

Table 1
(continued)

Reference (Year)	Type of Study	Patient Population	Study Duration	N	Device	Treatment	Comparator	Scale	Mean/Median Pain Score	Outcome and Results
										50% responder rates were 17/26 (65.4%, 95% CI 47.1%–83.7%) and 70% responder rates were 12/26 (46.2%, 95% CI 27.0%–65.3%)

Abbreviations: BP, brachial plexus; BPI, Brief Pain Inventory; CI, confidence interval; PNS, peripheral nerve stimulation; SSN, suprascapular nerve.

Table 2
Characteristics of included studies that evaluated peripheral nerve stimulation for postamputation pain

Reference	Type of Study	Patient Population	Study Duration	N	Device	Treatment	Comparator	Scale	Mean/Median Pain Score	Outcome and Results
Gilmore et al,[27] 2019	Multicenter, double-blinded, randomized, placebo-controlled study	Chronic neuropathic postamputation pain	8 wk	28	SPRINT	US-guided implantation of percutaneous PNS leads and received PNS for 8 wk	Placebo for 4 wk, then n = 10 crossed over and received PNS for 4 weeks	NRS for RLP & PLP	Average reductions in RLP and PLP in the PNS therapy group were 36% and 56%, respectively, compared with 27% and 33% in the placebo group	Significantly greater proportion of subjects in the PNS group demonstrated ≥50% reduction in average postamputation pain at 8 wk (8/12, 67%) compared with those who received placebo (2/14, 14%)
Gilmore et al,[1] 2020	Open-label extension phase of a randomized, double-blind, placebo-controlled trial[26]	Chronic neuropathic postamputation pain	12 mo	28 (15 followed up through 12 mo)	SPRINT	US-guided implantation of percutaneous PNS leads and received PNS for 8 wk	Placebo for 4 wk, then n = 10 crossed over and received PNS for 4 weeks	NRS for RLP & PLP	6.4 ± 1 (RLP treatment baseline) 6.4 ± 1.3 (RLP control baseline) 2.3 ± 1.2 RLP treatment 12 mo	Significantly more individuals in the PNS group reported ≥50% reduction in average

(continued on next page)

Table 2
(continued)

Reference	Type of Study	Patient Population	Study Duration	N	Device	Treatment	Comparator	Scale	Mean/Median Pain Score	Outcome and Results
									3.2 ± 2.5 RLP control 12 mo 6.9 ± 1.7 PLP treatment baseline 6.8 ± 1.7 PLP control baseline 3.8 ± 3.8 PLP treatment 12 mo 3.5 ± 2.6 PLP control 12 mo	weekly pain scores at 12 mo (6/9, 67%) compared with 0% of participants in the placebo group
Rauck et al,[20] 2013	Prospective case series	Moderate-to-severe postamputation pain in the lower extremity	8 wk	16	Rehabilicare	US-guided PNS to sciatic and/or femoral nerves for 2 wk	N/A	BPI5	Average pain reduction in second week of stimulation: RLP: (72% ± 28%, N = 7) PLP: (81% ± 28%, N = 7)	At 4-week follow-up after the end of stimulation, reductions in RLP and PLP were 42% ± 27% (N = 7) and 47% ± 48%, (N = 7), respectively

Abbreviations: BPI3, Brief Pain Inventory Question 5; N/A; PLP, phantom limb pain; PNS, peripheral nerve stimulation; RCT, randomized controlled trial; RLP, residual limb pain; US, ultrasound.

Table 3
Characteristics of included studies that evaluated peripheral nerve stimulation for musculoskeletal pain

Reference (Year)	Type of Study	Patient Population	Study Duration	N	Device	Treatment	Comparator	Scale	Mean/Median Pain Score	Outcome and Results
Wilson et al,[28] 2014	Single-site, pilot, RCT	Chronic HSP	16 wk	25	Rehabilicare	PNS to middle and posterior deltoid muscles	8 h of outpatient PT over a 4-week period in addition to prescribed daily home exercises	BPI-SF question 3	PNS group: Pre: 7.5 ± 0.7 Post: 3.0 ± 0.7 Control group: Pre: 7.6 ± 0.7 Post: 6.1 ± 0.8	At the end of the 4-wk treatment period, both groups demonstrated improvement in pain but only the stimulation group maintained 60% pain reduction compared with 20% reduction in the PT group at 12 wk
Wilson et al,[29] 2018	Prospective multisite case series	Chronic HSP	12 mo	28	Rehabilicare or SPRINT	Axillary nerve PNS	N/A	BPI-SF question 3	Individuals implanted (n = 5): Baseline: 8.2 Postoperative: 0.8 ± 0.7	Of the 28 participants who underwent the trial stage, 5 individuals progressed into the implant stage.

(continued on next page)

Table 3
(continued)

Reference (Year)	Type of Study	Patient Population	Study Duration	N	Device	Treatment	Comparator	Scale	Mean/Median Pain Score	Outcome and Results
										All 5 experienced ≥50% pain reduction at 6 and 12 mo
Mansfield et al,[30] 2019	Retrospective case series	Chronic shoulder pain	44–733 d (mean 445 d)	8	Bioness StimRouter	Permanent axillary PNS	N/A	NPRS	8.14 (average NPRS preimplant) 2.71 (average NPRS postimplant)	88% of participants achieved at least 50% reduction in pain and 100% reported decreased opioid use after PNS placement with an average reduction of 88%
Gilmore et al,[2] 2020	Prospective case series	Chronic low back pain	12 mo	9	SPRINT	Percutaneous leads placed bilaterally to target the medial branches of the dorsal rami nerves under image guidance	N/A	BPI-SF	Baseline: 6.5 Post 1 mo treatment: 1.25	At the 12-mo follow-up 66.7% (6/9) of individuals reported sustained pain relief with an average reduction of 63%.

Gilmore et al,[31] 2021	Prospective, multi-site case study	Chronic low back pain	12 mo	74	SPRINT	Percutaneous leads placed bilaterally to target the medial branches of the dorsal rami nerves under image guidance	N/A	BPI-5	Baseline: 6.1 Post 2-mo treatment: 3.3	At the end of the 2-mo treatment period, 73% of participants (54/74) reported ≥30% reduction of pain with an average 58% reduction in pain intensity. Study is ongoing.

Abbreviations: BPI-5, Brief Pain Inventory-Question 5; BPI-SF, Brief Pain Inventory-Short Form; CI, confidence interval; HSP, hemiplegic shoulder pain; N/A; NPRS, numerical pain rating scale; PNS, peripheral nerve stimulation; PT, physical therapy; RCT, randomized controlled trial; UC, usual care.

Table 4
Characteristics of included studies that evaluated peripheral nerve stimulation for chronic migraine

Reference	Type of Study	Patient Population	Study Duration	N	Device	Treatment	Comparator	Scale	Mean/Median Pain Score	Outcome and Results
Saper et al,[33] 2010	Multicenter, randomized, blinded, controlled feasibility study	Chronic migraine	36 mo	110	Medtronic model 7427 Synergy and model 7427 V Synergy Versitrel	ONS randomized to AS or PS	MM	Overall pain intensity (0–10 scale)	Reduction in overall pain intensity: AS: 1.5 ± 1.6, PS: 0.5 ± 1.3, MM: 0.6 ± 1.0	At 3 mo, 39% of patients in the AS group achieved at least a 50% reduction in number of headache days per month or at least a 3-point reduction in overall pain intensity compared with baseline as opposed to 6% in the PS group and 0% in the MM group

Study	Study design	Condition	Duration	N	Device	Target	Control	Outcome measure	Results	Conclusions
Lipton et al,[34] 2010	Multicenter, double-blind, randomized, sham controlled study	Chronic migraine	12 wk	132	Boston Scientific Precision	ONS	Sham stimulation	Migraine days per month	A reduction of 5.5 migraine days in the active stimulation group compared with 3.9 d in sham stimulation group ($P = .29$)	This study demonstrated no statistically significant difference between groups when comparing the reduction of migraine days per month
Silberstein et al,[35] 2012	Randomized, multicenter, double-blinded, controlled study	Chronic migraine	12 wk	157	Genesis, St. Jude Medical Neuromodulation	PNS of the occipital nerve	Sham device	VAS (mm)	PNS group: Baseline: 59.9 ± 16.8 Control: Baseline: 56 ± 17 Primary outcome ≥50% reduction in VAS: 17.1% in PNS group compared with 13.5% in control ($P = .55$)	Although the study did not meet its primary outcome, there was a significant difference in participants reporting at least a 30% reduction in pain scores ($P = .01$), reduction in number of headache days ($P = .008$), and reduction in migraine-related disability ($P = .001$)

(continued on next page)

Table 4
(continued)

Reference	Type of Study	Patient Population	Study Duration	N	Device	Treatment	Comparator	Scale	Mean/Median Pain Score	Outcome and Results
Serra et al,[36] 2012	Randomized cross-over study	Chronic migraine	12 mo	34	Medtronic Synergy Versitrel™	ONS	Stimulation Off	MIDAS	Stimulation On: baseline: MIDAS A = 70 MIDAS B = 8 1-y follow-MIDAS A = 14 MIDAS B = 5	At 1-y follow-up participants were noted to have reductions in the Migraine Disability assessment ($P < .001$), improvements in quality of life ($P < .05$), and overall reduction in triptan and nonsteroidal anti-inflammatory use ($P < .001$)
Slotty et al,[5] 2015	Randomized, crossover study	Patients with existing ONS for chronic migraine	3 mo	8	St. Jude Medical Octrode	ONS (effective stimulation and subthreshold stimulation)	No stimulation	VAS	Mean baseline: 8.20 ± 1.22 Posttreatment: ES: 1.98 ± 1.56 SS: 5.65 ± 2.11 NS: 8.45 ± 0.99	This study suggests that suprathreshold stimulation is more effective than subthreshold stimulation or no stimulation

Abbreviations: AS, adjustable stimulation; CM, chronic migraine; ES, effective stimulation; MIDAS, migraine disability assessment; MM, medical management; NS, no stimulation; ONS, occipital nerve stimulation; PS, preset stimulation; SS, subthreshold stimulation; VAS, visual analog scale.

Table 5
Characteristics of included studies that evaluated peripheral nerve stimulation for pelvic pain

Reference (Year)	Type of Study	Patient Population	Study Duration	N	Device	Treatment	Comparator	Scale	Mean/Median Pain Score	Outcome and Results
Kabay et al,[38] 2009	Randomized controlled trial	Therapy-resistant pelvic pain	12 wk	89	Medtronic	Percutaneous PTNS	Sham treatment	NIH-CPSI	PTNS group: Baseline: 23.6 ± 6.3 Post: 10.2 ± 3.6 Sham: Baseline: 22.8 ± 5.4 Post: 21.4 ± 4.6	Significant reductions in VAS pain scores and the NIH-CPSI were demonstrated in the treatment group with no significant changes noted in the sham group ($P < .001$)
Istek et al,[39] 2014	Randomized controlled trial	CPP	6 mo	33	CystoMedix	Percutaneous PTNS	No stimulation	PPI-VAS	PTNS group: Baseline: 8.4 ± 1.1 6-mo: 4.5 ± 3.7 Control: 6.5 ± 1.1 6-mo: 5.9 ± 2.2	Significant improvement noted in all domains of the SF-MPQ and SF-36 in the PTNS group was maintained at 6-mo follow-up

(continued on next page)

Table 5
(continued)

Reference (Year)	Type of Study	Patient Population	Study Duration	N	Device	Treatment	Comparator	Scale	Mean/Median Pain Score	Outcome and Results
Gokyildiz et al,[40] 2012	Randomized clinical trial	Females with CPP	12 wk	24	Percutaneous PTNS	Percutaneous PTNS	No PTNS	VAS	PTNS group: Baseline: 8.08 ± 1.72 Post: 2.62 ± 2.70 Control: Baseline: 7.95 ± 1.03 Post: 7.87 ± 0.88	This study sought to determine the effects of PTNS on quality of life and sexual function of patients with CPP. Participants reported reduction in pain frequency & intensity, improved quality of life (SF-36), and decreased pain during sexual intercourse (FSFI) after receiving PTNS

Study	Design	Condition	Duration	N		Intervention		Outcome	Results	Conclusions
Van Balken et al,[41] 2003	Prospective, single-arm, open label study	CPP	12 wk	33	CystoMedix	Percutaneous PTNS	N/A	VAS	Baseline: 6.5 (5.3–7.7) Post: 5.4 (4.2–6.8)	Only 21% of the participants were found to have a VAS decrease of ≥50% but all individuals had significant improvements in quality of life assessed by the SF-36 questionnaire
Kim et al,[44] 2007	Prospective, single-arm, open-label study	CPP	12 wk	15	Percutaneous PTNS	Percutaneous PTNS	N/A	VAS	Baseline: 8.1 ± 0.2 Post: 4.1 ± 0.6	The study reported 60% of individuals to have at least a 50% reduction in VAS pain score followed by 30% of participants with a 25%–50% reduction in pain scores
Congregado Ruiz et al,[45] 2004	Clinical trial	Lower urinary tract irritative symptoms	21 mo (range 6–36)	51	Percutaneous PTNS	Percutaneous PTNS	N/A	Presence of hypogastric pain	Baseline: 21 patients Post: 7 patients	This study found statistically significant improvements in frequency/ urgency and quality of life ($P < .001$).

(continued on next page)

Table 5
(continued)

Reference (Year)	Type of Study	Patient Population	Study Duration	N	Device	Treatment	Comparator	Scale	Mean/Median Pain Score	Outcome and Results
										Of the individuals with hypogastric pain, 33.3% reported pain relief after treatment ($P < .001$)
Ragab et al,[46] 2015	Prospective cohort study	Refractory IC/BPS	12 wk	20	Urgent PC	Percutaneous PTNS	N/A	VAS	Baseline: 5.6 ± 1.1 Post: 5.2 ± 1.5	There were no significant changes in frequency, voiding volume, VAS pain score, or patient satisfaction after a successive 12-wk PTNS treatment course

| Zhao et al,[47] 2008 | Prospective open study | Percutaneous PTNS | 5 wk | 18 | Percutaneous PTNS | Percutaneous PTNS | N/A | ICPI | Baseline 12.5 ± 1.5 Post: 10.22 ± 1.7 | There were no significant changes in VAS pain sores but significant changes were noted in nighttime bladder volume, ICPI, and the ICSI |

Abbreviations: BPS, bladder pain syndrome; CPP, chronic pelvic pain; FSFI, female sexual function index; IC, interstitial cystitis; ICPI, Interstitial Cystitis Problem Index; ICSI, O'Leary/Sant Interstitial Cystitis Symptoms Index; NIH-CPSI, National Institutes of Health Chronic Prostatitis Symptom Index; PPI-VAS, present pain intensity-visual analog scale; PTNS, posterior tibial nerve stimulation; SF-36, 36-Item Short Form Survey; SF-MPQ, Short-Form McGill Pain Questionnaire; VAS, visual analog scale.

nerves or 4 weeks of sham stimulation (no stimulation delivered), followed by crossover to 4 weeks of active PNS (control group). Using ITT analysis, a greater proportion of patients receiving active PNS during weeks 1 to 4 experienced 50% or more reduction in pain (7 of 12, 57.3%, 95% CI, 30.4%–86.2%) versus control (2 of 14, 14%, 95% CI, -4.0% to 32.6%, P = .037). During weeks 5 to 8, with both groups now receiving active stimulation, the percentage of patients in the control group with 50% pain reduction remained 14% (2 of 14). A possible explanation for this (and a limitation of this study) is that when the leads were placed in the control group stimulation feedback was not used to maintain blinding; this possibly resulted in suboptimal lead placement and, therefore, suboptimal stimulation in the control group during the crossover period. At least a 50% reduction in pain interference—the degree to which pain interferes with cognitive, physical, social, and recreational activities—was significantly greater in treatment group in the PP analysis (8 of 10, 80%, 95% CI, 55.2%–1.05%) compared with the control group (2 of 13, 15.4%, 95% CI, -4.2% to 35.0%, P = .003). Using ITT analysis, responder rate was 8 of 12 (66.7%, 95% CI, 40.0%–93.3%) in the treatment group versus 2 of 14 in the control group (14.3%, 95% CI, -4.0% to 32.6%).

Gilmore and colleagues[1] published a prospective 12-month follow-up study of the aforementioned RCT. Of 12 patients randomized to the treatment group (true stimulation weeks 1–8), 9 had 12-month follow-up data. Six of 9 (67%, 95% CI, 35.9%–97.5%) reported greater than or equal to 50% reduction in average weekly pain at 12 months, with ITT responder rate of 6 of 12 (50%, 95% CI, 21.7%–78.3%). In comparison, the 50% responder rate at 12 months in the control group was 1 of 6 (16.7, 95% CI, -13.2 to 46.5%). These control patients received true stimulation during weeks 5 to 8, albeit as mentioned earlier with leads placed without stimulation feedback.

Rauck and colleagues[20] conducted an earlier feasibility study of PNS in patients with moderate to severe PAP in the lower extremity by using a fine-wire lead (Rehabilicare, St Paul, MN, USA) placed percutaneously under ultrasound guidance. Nine patients completed the 2-week treatment period and reported an 81% reduction in PLP and a 72% mean reduction in RLP determined by the Brief Pain Inventory-Short Form with reductions maintained after the 4-week follow-up period. Patients also experienced a 43% mean reduction in depression measured by the Beck Depression Inventory II and 70% mean reduction in disability as measured by the Pain Disability Index. Limitations of this study include its short duration and lack of a sham comparator.

Of these PNS studies for lower extremity PAP, none reported any serious AEs.[1,20,27] A limitation of these studies is the small sample sizes.

Musculoskeletal Pain

Hemiplegic shoulder pain

Wilson and colleagues[28] performed a single-site, pilot RCT to compare 3 weeks of PNS using a fine-wire percutaneous lead and an external stimulator ((Rehabilicare, Inc, New Brighton, MN)) with standard physical therapy (PT) for the treatment of HSP in patients at least 3 months after stroke. Twenty-five patients were randomized to receive 6 hours per day of percutaneous stimulation to the middle and posterior deltoid muscles for 3 weeks or 8 hours of outpatient PT over a 4-week period coupled with home exercises. Thirteen patients were randomized to PNS and 12 to PT. At the end of the 4-week treatment period, both groups demonstrated improvement in pain, but the stimulation group maintained 60% pain reduction, whereas the PT group maintained approximately a 20% pain reduction at 12 weeks. Limitations include lack of patient blinding and missing data regarding analgesic use during the study. AEs included pain after implantation (15.4%), pruritus (46.2%), electrode dislodgement requiring reimplantation (7.7%), and retained electrode fragment during explantation (21.4%).[28]

Wilson and colleagues[29] later conducted a prospective multisite case series using a fully implantable single-lead PNS system (Micropulse Inc, Columbia City, IN, USA) for axillary nerve PNS for the treatment of chronic HSP. The study used a 2-phase design beginning with a 3-week trial phase using 2 external stimulators (Rehabilicare or SPRINT). Of the 28 patients who underwent the trial phase, 5 received the IPG and all reported at least a 50% reduction in pain at 6 and 12 months and improvement in pain interference. Twelve serious AEs were reported: 11 were unrelated to the device or procedure and 1 participant was hospitalized for chest pain of uncertain origin.[29] Forty AEs were reported, including lead fracture (n = 7) and erythema or pruritus at the lead exit site, electrodes, or bandages.

Nonhemiplegic shoulder pain
In a retrospective case series by Mansfield and Desai[30], 8 adult patients with chronic nonhemiplegic shoulder pain underwent permanent axillary nerve PNS. Causes of chronic shoulder pain included subacromial impingement syndrome, rotator cuff pathology, glenohumeral joint arthritis, acromioclavicular joint arthritis, adhesive capsulitis, and biceps tendinopathy; 88% of participants achieved at least 50% reduction in pain and 100% reported decreased opioid use after PNS placement with an average reduction of 88%. No AEs were reported.

Axial low back pain
In a prospective case series, Gilmore and colleagues[2] investigated the efficacy of percutaneous SPRINT PNS for the treatment of chronic axial low back pain. Nine participants received percutaneous leads targeting the medial branches of the dorsal rami under ultrasound guidance implanted at the segmental level of their pain as identified by manual palpation; specific levels were not reported. After the 1-month treatment period leads were removed and 66.7% (6 of 9) of individuals reported at least a 50% reduction in average pain intensity. At the 12-month follow-up 66.7% (6 of 9) of individuals reported sustained pain relief with an average reduction of 63%. Skin irritation was reported (n = 2), but no serious AEs occurred.

Following this case series, Gilmore and colleagues[31] designed a larger prospective study to evaluate the efficacy of SPRINT PNS for the treatment of chronic axial low back pain in a population of 74 individuals. Percutaneous leads were placed under ultrasound and/or fluoroscopic guidance to target the vertebral level central to the region of pain. Stimulation was provided for 6 to 12 hours per day for up to 60 days and then was removed. The primary end point was defined as the proportion of participants experiencing at least a 30% reduction in average pain intensity at the end of the 2-month treatment; 73% of participants (54 of 74) were responders for the primary end point with an average 58% in average back pain intensity. The study is conducting follow-up through 12 months following the 2-month treatment period and is ongoing. A total of 89 AEs have been reported to date, and the majority include skin irritation (n = 34), pruritus (n = 21), granuloma/discoloration/urticaria (n = 8), new pain (n = 8), worsening pain (n = 5), and infection (n = 2).

An additional study (NCT04538430) was terminated early due to coronavirus disease 2019 and other factors after enrolling 7 patients.

Chronic knee pain
A registered clinical trial evaluating the efficacy of PNS to treat chronic knee pain (NCT04580732) is planned.

A limitation of these studies is the small sample sizes. **Table 3** provides a summary of the aforementioned studies.

Migraine

According to a recent global burden of disease study, headache disorders are the second leading cause of disability worldwide.[32] PNS is an option for chronic headaches refractory to conservative treatments. **Table 4** summarizes the following studies.

The ONSTIM feasibility study by Saper and colleagues[33] was a sham-controlled RCT investigating the preliminary safety and efficacy of occipital nerve stimulation (ONS) using the Medtronic Synergy IPG and quadripolar leads in individuals with chronic migraine (NCT00200109). A total of 75 individuals who responded to an occipital nerve block were randomized to be in the treatment group receiving adjustable stimulation (AS) or to one of 2 control groups: a sham group receiving 1 min/d of preset stimulation (PS) or a medical management (MM) group. At 3 months, 39% (11 of 28, 95% CI, 21.2%–57.4%) of patients in the AS group achieved at least a 50% reduction in the number of headache days per month or at least a 3-point reduction in overall pain intensity compared with baseline as opposed to 6% (1 of 16, 95% CI, -5.6 to 18.1%) in the PS group and 0% (0 of 17) in the MM group. There was no significant improvement over baseline when comparing headache days, pain, and duration in the AS group with those in the control groups, PS and MM. A total of 56 AEs occurred: 3 individuals required hospitalizations due to implant site infection, lead migration, or postoperative nausea. The most frequent AE reported in 24% of subjects (12 of 51) was lead migration.

Two other double-blind RCTs assessing the effectiveness of ONS for chronic migraine did not show significant benefits in primary outcomes when compared with sham stimulation.[34,35] The Precision Implantable Stimulator for Migraine (PRISM) study, published as an abstract only, randomized 132 participants to receive either bilateral active or sham stimulation (Precision, Boston Scientific Precision, Marlborough, MA) for 12 weeks (NCT00286078).[34] There was no significant between-group difference in reduction of migraine days per month: a reduction of 5.5 migraine days in the active stimulation group compared with 3.9 days in sham stimulation group ($P = .29$). The most common device-related AEs were sensory symptoms, pain at implant site, and infection. Silberstein and colleagues[35] published an RCT (NCT00615342) using the Genesis System (St. Jude Medical, Inc), which resulted in no significant difference in the primary outcome, defined as participants with at least a 50% reduction in mean daily visual analog scores, between the active (18 of 105 [17%, 95% CI, 9.9%–24.4%]) and control groups (7 of 52 [13.5%, 95% CI, 4.2%–22.7%]). However, there was a significant difference in participants reporting at least a 30% reduction in pain scores ($P = .01$), reduction in number of headache days ($P = .008$), and reduction in migraine-related disability ($P = .001$). The most common AEs included persistent pain at lead site (21.5%), lead migration (18.7%), and unintended stimulation events (6.5%).

Serra and Marchioretto[36] conducted a randomized crossover study to determine safety and efficacy of ONS (Medtronic) for chronic migraine and medication overuse headache. Thirty patients were randomized to "stimulation on" or "stimulation off" with crossover at 4 weeks. However, due to worsening symptoms in the "stimulation off" group, crossover occurred at a mean of 4.9 ± 3.9 days that allowed transition into the "stimulation on" group. Headache intensity and frequency were significantly lower in the "on" arm group ($P < .05$). Using pooled data from both treatment groups, reductions in the Migraine Disability assessment ($P < .001$), improvements in quality of life ($P < .05$), and overall reduction in triptan and nonsteroidal anti-inflammatory use

(P < .001) were noted among participants who completed the 1-year follow-up. Five AEs were reported: 2 severe implantation site infections and 3 lead migrations, none of which resulted in long-term complications or nerve damage. Limitations to this study include the earlier crossover and unblinded design.

A smaller RCT trial by Slotty and colleagues[5] using the Octrode system (St. Jude Medical Inc) sought to determine the "significance of paresthesia and possible placebo effects" in patients with ONS for the treatment of chronic migraine. The study recruited individuals with occipital nerve stimulators and at least 30% stable pain relief for 3 months. Eight participants were included and randomized to 3 treatment groups: effective stimulation, subthreshold stimulation, and no stimulation. A significant improvement in pain was found between suprathreshold stimulation compared with subthreshold stimulation (visual analog scale [VAS] 1.98 ± 1.56 vs 5.65 ± 2.11, $P = .0003$) and between subthreshold stimulation compared with no stimulation (VAS 5.65 ± 2.11 vs 8.45 ± 0.99, $P = .0031$), suggesting that suprathreshold stimulation is most effective. No AEs or complications were reported.

Pelvic and Urogenital Pain

PNS has been studied for various pelvic and urogenital pain syndromes including CPP, chronic prostatitis (CP), bladder pain syndrome (BPS), groin/ilioinguinal pain, and genital pain.[37] **Table 5** summarizes the following studies.

Percutaneous posterior tibial nerve stimulation for chronic pelvic pain

Three RCTs evaluated the effects of temporarily placed posterior tibial nerve stimulation (PTNS) for the treatment of CPP.[38–40] PTNS was developed for the treatment of lower urinary tract dysfunction, urge incontinence, and urgency/frequency symptoms.[41–43] The mechanism of action of PTNS is thought secondary to its delivery of electrical stimulation to the sacral micturition center via the sacral plexus with subsequent modulation of the C-fiber and $A\delta$-afferent fibers from the bladder.[37]

In the double-blind, sham-controlled study by Kabay and colleagues,[38] 89 males diagnosed with CP and CPP were randomized to receive Medtronic PTNS using landmarks (5 cm superior to medial malleolus and posterior edge of tibia) and stimulation to confirm placement or sham treatment for 12 weekly 30-minute treatment sessions. The investigators found that 66.7% (30 of 45, 95% CI, 52.9%–80.4%) of participants in the treatment group reported at least a 50% decrease in pain scores compared with 40.9% (18 of 44, 95% CI, 26.4%–55.4%) in the sham group. Overall, significant reductions in VAS pain scores and the National Institutes of Health Chronic Prostatitis Symptom Index were demonstrated in the treatment group with no significant changes noted in the sham group (P < .001).

The second RCT, an open-label study by Istek and colleagues,[39] randomized 33 women with CPP to receive either 12 weekly 30-minute PTNS treatment sessions with the Cystomedix neuromodulation system (Cogentix Medical Inc, Minnetonka, MN, USA) using landmarks and stimulation to confirm placement (treatment group) or oral analgesics (control group). The primary outcome of the study was patient-reported improvement in symptoms; 56.3% (9 of 16, 95% CI, 31.9%–80.6%) in the PTNS group reported being cured or much improved following treatment compared with 11.8% (2 of 17, 95% CI, -3.6% to 27.1%) in the control group. Additionally, significant improvement noted in all domains of the Short-Form McGill Pain Questionnaire and 36-Item Short Form Survey (SF-36) in the PTNS group were maintained at 6-month follow-up. A limitation of this study was the lack of sham stimulation in the control group.

In a study by Gokyildiz and colleagues,[40] 24 women with CPP were randomized to receive either 30 minute sessions of PTNS once a week for 12 weeks or conventional management. Pain intensity significantly decreased in the experimental group, 8.08 ± 1.72 on average at baseline to 2.62 ± 2.70 on average after treatment ($P = .00$). There was no significant change in the control group with 7.95 ± 1.03 average pain intensity at baseline compared with an average 7.87 ± 0.88 at the end of 12 weeks. In addition, the treatment group reported improved quality of life measured by SF-36 and decreased pain during sexual intercourse measured by the female sexual function index after receiving PTNS. One patient had a hematoma, and 4 patients had slight pain with sessions. No other AEs were reported.

Two small, prospective, single-arm, open-label studies investigated the benefits of PTNS in patients with CPP.[41,44] Each study used anatomic landmarks and stimulation to confirm placement of the percutaneous needle at the tibial nerve target. In each of the studies, 12 weekly sessions each lasting 30 minutes were administered in the outpatient setting; time end point was at the completion of the 12 weekly sessions. Van Balken and colleagues[41] reported only 21% of the participants to have a VAS decrease of at least 50% but all individuals (n = 33) had significant improvements in quality of life assessed by the SF-36 questionnaire. In a population of 15 patients, Kim and colleagues[44] reported 60% of individuals to have at least a 50% reduction in VAS pain score followed by 30% of participants with a 25% to 50% reduction in pain scores.

Percutaneous posterior tibial nerve stimulation for bladder pain syndrome and interstitial cystitis

Three prospective cohort studies investigated the effect of PTNS on lower urinary tract irritative symptoms in women including those related to BPS and interstitial cystitis.[45–47] Congregado Ruiz and colleagues[45] administered weekly stimulations of 30 minutes for 10 consecutive weeks in 51 patients and found statistically significant improvements in frequency/urgency and quality of life ($P < .001$). In addition, of the individuals with hypogastric pain, 33.3% reported pain relief after treatment ($P < .001$). The remaining 2 studies did not show a significant benefit for individuals with interstitial cystitis and BPS after treatment with PTNS.[46,47] In a population of 20 patients, Ragab and colleagues[46] did not find significant changes in frequency, voiding volume, VAS pain score, or patient satisfaction after a successive 12-week PTNS treatment course. Zhao and colleagues[47] also found no significant change in VAS pain indexes after 18 participants received 10 sessions of biweekly PTNS treatments but did note significant changes in nighttime bladder volume, Interstitial Cystitis Problem Index (ICPI), and the O'Leary/Sant Interstitial Cystitis Symptoms Index (ICSI).

DISCUSSION

Recent advances in PNS have included new systems specifically developed for PNS and results of new clinical trials.

Evidence supporting PNS for neuropathic pain includes both an RCT and multiple case series.[3,4,19] The randomized, sham-controlled trial by Deer and colleagues[19] showed modest but significant improvement of pain at 3 months with true versus sham PNS. A limitation of this study is that it included numerous neuropathic pain etiologies without subgroup reporting by diagnosis. With 38% of patients reporting a 30% response rate and a mean 27.2% pain reduction with true PNS in the study by Deer and colleagues,[19] further research delineating which subpopulations may benefit most from PNS are warranted, as are comparative effectiveness studies comparing PNS with spinal cord stimulation and dorsal root ganglion stimulation for distal extremity neuropathic pain.

For PAP there are multiple studies including an RCT.[1,20,27] In the RCT, patients received temporary PNS stimulation with SPRINT PNS for 60 days. There was a clinically significant reduction in pain and improvement in quality of life in the treatment arm when compared with sham. In an open-label extension of this RCT, sustained benefit was seen at 12 months. Of note, the sample size for this study was small (N = 28), and with only 12 patients randomized to receive PNS, the results have large 95% CIs.

There is a small, unblinded RCT evaluating PNS efficacy for HSP.[28] Future studies should include larger, blinded RCTs comparing PNS versus sham stimulation and should study quality of life and functional outcomes. There is sparse published evidence on PNS for nonstroke shoulder pain, with only one retrospective case series of 8 patients with promising results.[30] The evidence for axial low back pain is only supported by a prospective case series of 9 patients with promising results. A clinical trial is planned studying PNS for chronic knee pain. Additional larger studies are needed to establish the role of PNS for musculoskeletal pain.

The largest number of sham-controlled RCTs for PNS has been conducted studying ONS for chronic migraine.[33-36] These were conducted with SCS systems, which likely contributed to their high rate of lead migration. Choice of primary outcome in these studies was selected based on the information that the investigators had at the time; since then ensuing research and International Headache Society guidelines have provided investigators with standardized outcomes to use in chronic migraine prevention research.[48] Future studies may find better efficacy and lower complication rates with dedicated PNS systems, novel and/or multiple waveforms, and combined treatment of supraorbital nerve stimulation and ONS.[49,50]

Pelvic pain includes CPP, CP, BPS, groin/ilioinguinal pain, and genital pain. The RCTs and prospective studies to date have studied 30-minute weekly sessions of temporarily placed PTNS. There are 3 RCTs evaluating PTNS for CPP: 1 in males comparing PTNS to sham stimulation and 2 in females comparing PTNS to medical management.[38-40] There have been case reports and small retrospective case series of other PNS treatments for ilioinguinal neuralgia, genitofemoral neuralgia, and testicular pain; prospective studies and RCTs are needed to evaluate these treatments.[51-53] Studies of implantable PNS systems providing more frequent and longer treatment than 30-minute weekly sessions are also warranted.

SUMMARY

Overall, PNS has been studied for many chronic pain conditions including neuropathic pain, PAP, musculoskeletal pain, migraine, and pelvic pain. Additional and larger, sham-controlled RCTs incorporating advancements in PNS devices and waveforms would strengthen the evidence supporting PNS for its many possible indications.

CLINICS CARE POINTS

- Before discussing PNS with a patient, providers should be familiar with the literature supporting PNS for the given indication, with attention given to the magnitude of benefit seen in clinical trials as well as the number of patients studied.

- The PNS landscape now includes numerous novel dedicated PNS, which have decreased lead migration and fracture rates. Differences between these systems include temporary (60-day) versus permanent implantation and whether or not a trial is performed before permanent implantation.

• When considering PNS, proper patient selection is essential and should include psychological screening.

DISCLOSURE

S.C. Erosa, MD, R.S. Moheimani, MD, and M.E. Abraham, MD, have nothing to disclose. J.C. Oswald, MD, receives honorarium from Averitas Pharma. J.P. Castellanos, MD, is a scientific advisor for Tryp Therapeutics. N.M. Schuster, MD, receives research funding from Migraine Research Foundation; personal fees from Eli Lilly & Company, Lundbeck, Averitas, and UMEHEAL; and is on the editorial boards of *Pain Medicine*, *Interventional Pain Medicine*, and *Annals of Headache Medicine*.

REFERENCES

1. Gilmore CA, Ilfeld BM, Rosenow JM, et al. Percutaneous 60-day peripheral nerve stimulation implant provides sustained relief of chronic pain following amputation: 12-month follow-up of a randomized, double-blind, placebo-controlled trial. Reg Anesth Pain Med 2020;45(1):44–51.
2. Gilmore CA, Kapural L, McGee MJ, et al. Percutaneous peripheral nerve stimulation for chronic low back pain: prospective case series with 1 year of sustained relief following short-term implant. Pain Pract 2020;20(3):310–20.
3. Bouche B, Manfiotto M, Rigoard P, et al. Peripheral nerve stimulation of brachial plexus nerve roots and supra-scapular nerve for chronic refractory neuropathic pain of the upper limb. Neuromodulation 2017;20(7):684–9.
4. Manning A, Ortega RG, Moir L, et al. Burst or conventional peripheral nerve field stimulation for treatment of neuropathic facial pain. Neuromodulation 2019;22(5): 645–52.
5. Slotty PJ, Bara G, Kowatz L, et al. Occipital nerve stimulation for chronic migraine: a randomized trial on subthreshold stimulation. Cephalalgia 2015;35(1):73–8.
6. Wall PD, Sweet WH. Temporary Abolition of Pain in Man. Science 1967;155(3758): 108–9.
7. Campbell JN, Long DM. Peripheral nerve stimulation in the treatment of intractable pain. J Neurosurg 1976;45(6):692–9.
8. Nielson KD, Watts C, Clark WK. Peripheral nerve injury from implantation of chronic stimulating electrodes for pain control. Surg Neurol 1976;5(1):51–3.
9. Nashold BS, Goldner JL, Mullen JB, et al. Long-term pain control by direct peripheral-nerve stimulation. J Bone Joint Surg Am 1982;64(1):1–10.
10. Weiner RL, Reed KL. Peripheral neurostimulation for control of intractable occipital neuralgia. Neuromodulation 1999;2(3):217–21.
11. Chakravarthy KV, Xing F, Bruno K, et al. A review of spinal and peripheral neuromodulation and neuroinflammation: lessons learned thus far and future prospects of biotype development. Neuromodulation Technol Neural Interf 2018;22(3): 235–43.
12. Chakravarthy K, Nava A, Christo PJ, et al. Review of recent advances in peripheral nerve stimulation (PNS). Curr Pain Headache Rep 2016;20(11):60.
13. Ilfeld BM, Gabriel RA, Saulino MF, et al. Infection rates of electrical leads used for percutaneous neurostimulation of the peripheral nervous system. Pain Pract 2017;17(6):753–62.
14. Reddy RD, Moheimani R, Yu GG, et al. A review of clinical data on salvage therapy in spinal cord stimulation. Neuromodulation 2020;23(5):562–71.

15. Chung JM, Lee KH, Hori Y, et al. Factors influencing peripheral nerve stimulation produced inhibition of primate spinothalamic tract cells. Pain 1984;19(3):277–93.
16. Ridding MC, Brouwer B, Miles TS, et al. Changes in muscle responses to stimulation of the motor cortex induced by peripheral nerve stimulation in human subjects. Exp Brain Res 2000;131(1):135–43.
17. Chen R, Corwell B, Hallett M. Modulation of motor cortex excitability by median nerve and digit stimulation. Exp Brain Res 1999;129(1):77–86.
18. Reilly JP. Peripheral nerve stimulation by induced electric currents: Exposure to time-varying magnetic fields. Med Biol Eng Comput 1989;27(2):101.
19. Deer T, Pope J, Benyamin R, et al. Prospective, multicenter, randomized, double-blinded, partial crossover study to assess the safety and efficacy of the novel neuromodulation system in the treatment of patients with chronic pain of peripheral nerve origin. Neuromodulation 2016;19(1):91–100.
20. Rauck RL, Cohen SP, Gilmore CA, et al. Treatment of post-amputation pain with peripheral nerve stimulation. Neuromodulation 2014;17(2):188–97.
21. Deer TR, Pope JE, Lamer TJ, et al. The neuromodulation appropriateness consensus committee on best practices for dorsal root ganglion stimulation. Neuromodulation Technol Neural Interf 2018;22(1):35.
22. Deer TR, Lamer TJ, Pope JE, et al. The Neurostimulation Appropriateness Consensus Committee (NACC) safety guidelines for the reduction of severe neurological injury. Neuromodulation 2017;20(1):15–30.
23. Deer TR, Mekhail N, Provenzano D, et al. The appropriate use of neurostimulation: Avoidance and treatment of complications of neurostimulation therapies for the treatment of chronic pain. Neuromodulation 2014;17(6):571–97.
24. Eldabe S, Buchser E, Duarte RV. Complications of spinal cord stimulation and peripheral nerve stimulation techniques: a review of the literature. Pain Med 2015; 17(2):325–36.
25. Provenzano DA, Deer T, Luginbuhl Phelps A, et al. An international survey to understand infection control practices for spinal cord stimulation. Neuromodulation 2016;19(1):71–84.
26. Ephraim PL, Wegener ST, MacKenzie EJ, et al. Phantom pain, residual limb pain, and back pain in amputees: results of a national survey. Arch Phys Med Rehabil 2005;86(10):1910–9.
27. Gilmore C, Ilfeld B, Rosenow J, et al. Percutaneous peripheral nerve stimulation for the treatment of chronic neuropathic postamputation pain: a multicenter, randomized, placebo-controlled trial. Reg Anesth Pain Med 2019;44(6):637–45.
28. Wilson RD, Gunzler DD, Bennett ME, et al. Peripheral nerve stimulation compared with usual care for pain relief of hemiplegic shoulder pain: a randomized controlled trial. Am J Phys Med Rehabil 2014;93(1):17–28.
29. Wilson RD, Bennett ME, Nguyen VQC, et al. Fully Implantable Peripheral Nerve Stimulation for Hemiplegic Shoulder Pain: A Multi-Site Case Series With Two-Year Follow-Up. Neuromodulation 2018;21(3):290–5.
30. Mansfield JT, Desai MJ. Axillary peripheral nerve stimulation for chronic shoulder pain: a retrospective case series. Neuromodulation 2020;23(6):812–8.
31. Gilmore CA, Desai MJ, Hopkins TJ, et al. Treatment of chronic axial back pain with 60-day percutaneous medial branch PNS: Primary end point results from a prospective, multicenter study. Pain Pract 2021;21(8):877–89.
32. James SL, Abate D, Abate KH, et al. Global, regional, and national incidence, prevalence, and years lived with disability for 354 Diseases and Injuries for 195 countries and territories, 1990-2017: a systematic analysis for the Global Burden of Disease Study 2017. Lancet 2018;392(10159):1789–858.

33. Saper JR, Dodick DW, Silberstein SD, et al. Occipital nerve stimulation for the treatment of intractable chronic migraine headache: ONSTIM feasibility study. Cephalalgia 2011;31(3):271–85.
34. Schwedt TJ, Silberstein SD. 14th International headache congress: Clinical highlights. Headache 2010;50(3):509–19.
35. Silberstein SD, Dodick DW, Saper J, et al. Safety and efficacy of peripheral nerve stimulation of the occipital nerves for the management of chronic migraine: results from a randomized, multicenter, double-blinded, controlled study. Cephalalgia 2012;32(16):1165–79.
36. Serra G, Marchioretto F. Occipital nerve stimulation for chronic migraine: A randomized trial. Pain Physician 2012;15(3):245–53.
37. Roy H, Offiah I, Dua A. Neuromodulation for pelvic and urogenital pain. Brain Sci 2018;8(10):180.
38. Kabay S, Kabay SC, Yucel M, et al. Efficiency of posterior tibial nerve stimulation in category IIIB chronic prostatitis/chronic pelvic pain: a sham-controlled comparative study. Urol Int 2009;83(1):33–8.
39. Istek A, Gungor Ugurlucan F, Yasa C, et al. Randomized trial of long-term effects of percutaneous tibial nerve stimulation on chronic pelvic pain. Arch Gynecol Obstet 2014;290(2):291–8.
40. Gokyildiz S, Kizilkaya Beji N, Yalcin O, et al. Effects of percutaneous tibial nerve stimulation therapy on chronic pelvic pain. Gynecol Obstet Invest 2012;73(2):99–105.
41. Van Balken MR, Vandoninck V, Messelink BJ, et al. Percutaneous Tibial Nerve Stimulation as neuromodulative treatment of chronic pelvic pain. Eur Urol 2003;43(2):158–63.
42. Vandoninck V, Van Balken MR, Agrò EF, et al. Posterior tibial nerve stimulation in the treatment of urge incontinence. Neurourol Urodyn 2003;22(1):17–23.
43. Van Der Pal F, Van Balken MR, Heesakkers JPFA, et al. Correlation between quality of life and voiding variables in patients treated with percutaneous tibial nerve stimulation. BJU Int 2006;97(1):113–6.
44. Kim SW, Paick JS, Ku JH. Percutaneous posterior tibial nerve stimulation in patients with chronic pelvic pain: a preliminary study. Urol Int 2007;78(1):58–62.
45. Congregado Ruiz B, Pena Outeiriño XM, Campoy Martínez P, et al. Peripheral afferent nerve stimulation for treatment of lower urinary tract irritative symptoms. Eur Urol 2004;45(1):65–9.
46. Ragab MM, Tawfik AM, Abo El-Enen M, et al. Evaluation of percutaneous tibial nerve stimulation for treatment of refractory painful bladder syndrome. Urology 2015;86(4):707–11.
47. Zhao J, Bai J, Zhou Y, et al. Posterior tibial nerve stimulation twice a week in patients with interstitial cystitis. Urology 2008;71(6):1080–4.
48. Tassorelli C, Diener HC, Dodick DW, et al. Guidelines of the International Headache Society for controlled trials of preventive treatment of chronic migraine in adults. Cephalalgia 2018;38(5):815–32.
49. Reed KL, Black SB, Banta CJ, et al. Combined occipital and supraorbital neurostimulation for the treatment of chronic migraine headaches: Initial experience. Cephalalgia 2010;30(3):260–71.
50. Hann S, Sharan A. Dual occipital and supraorbital nerve stimulation for chronic migraine: a single-center experience, review of literature, and surgical considerations. Neurosurg Focus 2013;35(3):E9.

51. Carayannopoulos A, Beasley R, Sites B. Facilitation of percutaneous trial lead placement with ultrasound guidance for peripheral nerve stimulation trial of ilioinguinal neuralgia: A technical note. Neuromodulation 2009;12(4):296–301.
52. Shaw A, Sharma M, Zibly Z, et al. Sandwich technique, peripheral nerve stimulation, peripheral field stimulation and hybrid stimulation for inguinal region and genital pain. Br J Neurosurg 2016;30(6):631–6.
53. Rosendal F, Moir L, De Pennington N, et al. Successful treatment of testicular pain with peripheral nerve stimulation of the cutaneous branch of the ilioinguinal and genital branch of the genitofemoral nerves. Neuromodulation 2013;16(2):121–4.

Intrathecal Pumps

Tyler Ericson, MD[a], Priyanka Singla, MD[a], Lynn Kohan, MD[b],*

KEYWORDS

- Intrathecal pumps • Chronic pain • Intrathecal • Intrathecal drug

KEY POINTS

- Intrathecal pumps are a well-established method of pain control in cancer and noncancer pain states.
- Intrathecal pumps allow for the local administration of analgesics resulting in lower systemic concentrations and side effects.
- Intrathecal pumps are starting to be used earlier in pain management pathways.
- Intrathecal pumps have been shown to improve pain scores and quality of life in numerous large studies.

INTRODUCTION

Intrathecal (IT) pumps are a well-established method of pain control in cancer and noncancer chronic pain states. The first IT delivery of an anesthetic was demonstrated in 1898 with the "cocainization of the spinal canal" by Bier and the first reported implantable drug delivery system (IDDS) was in 1981 by Onofrio and colleagues.[1] A standard IDDS consists of a surgically implanted, refillable reservoir and pump that delivers medications through a catheter directly into the IT space. Percutaneous catheters with an external pump are sometimes used in patients with limited life expectancy.

The direct delivery of medication into the cerebrospinal fluid (CSF) allows it to act on the receptor-rich dorsal horn of the spinal column without having to cross the blood-brain barrier.[2] The advantage of targeted drug delivery is that lower systemic levels of medication are needed to achieve a desired effect with reduced systemic side effects.[3] Moreover, recent advances in CSF flow dynamics have informed the understanding of IT drug delivery (IDD) and advancements in device manufacturing and design have resulted in more sophisticated systems that are smaller, safer, and allow for more patient feedback than the original systems. New developments in pharmacology have also broadened the availability of medications to be administered through IDDS.

[a] Department of Anesthesiology, University of Virginia, Charlottesville, VA, USA; [b] Pain Medicine Fellowship, Pain Management Center, Fontaine Research Park, Third Floor, 545 Ray C Hunt Drive, Charlottesville, VA 22908, USA
* Corresponding author.
E-mail address: LRK9G@hscmail.mcc.virginia.edu

Phys Med Rehabil Clin N Am 33 (2022) 409–424
https://doi.org/10.1016/j.pmr.2022.01.004

Traditionally, IDDS has been a treatment option of last resort for patients who have failed almost all available less-invasive modalities. Current consensus, however, is moving toward earlier implementation of IDDS in the treatment of various pain states because of its proven effect on quality of life. Regardless, given the invasive nature of the implantation procedure and the risks associated with having a permanent device, proper patient selection and screening should be performed before pursuing this treatment modality. In this article we discuss patient selection criteria, medication selection, risks, complications, supporting data, and future directions of IDDS.

Patient Selection

A large body of clinical evidence supports the efficacy and safety of IT therapies in a variety of pain states. Reduced pain, use of systemic opioids, and drug-related toxicities have been reported in several IDDS trials.[3] IDDS has been recommend as an option for select patients requiring long-term management of refractory pain states by the Polyanalgesic Consensus Conference (PACC) and others.[4,5]

It is important to carefully select patients for implantation who have been appropriately diagnosed with pain types that have been shown to benefit from IDDS. First, a patient should be diagnosed with moderate to severe chronic pain that has no reversible anatomic causes. IDDS has been shown to be more successful in the treatment of nociceptive rather than neuropathic pain; however, patients with neuropathic and mixed pain states can still benefit.[4–6] Before the implementation of IDDS the patient should have failed a trial of reasonable conservative therapies. The patient should be evaluated for history of prior systemic opioid trials and any history of improper handling of opioids. Furthermore, it is important to establish realistic expectations that IDDS may help to reduce pain and quality of life but does not "take away" all pain. A detailed conversation regarding what defines success or failure of a trial should be undertaken. Additionally, insurance should be confirmed for approval of the therapy.[2] It is also important to assess for absolute or relative contraindications including evaluating for comorbidities (see later).

A trial of IDD therapy is useful because it can emulate the patient's response to the medications that will be used during therapy. The PACC recommends that a trial be performed whenever ziconotide or baclofen is used and when using opioids in patients at increased risk of respiratory depression.[7] Alternatively, the PACC does not consider a trial period to be required in cases of advanced disease with limited survival and in patients who have a high likelihood of trial success and a high risk of trial-associated bleeding or infection. A single-shot IT trial is often used when it is primarily nociceptive pain. If the pain is mixed or neuropathic consider either an epidural or IT morphine infusion. If the patient is not able to tolerate an infusion for trial then a bolus injection of morphine is used. A reasonable dose for a single-shot trial is 0.15 mg of morphine, 0.04 mg of hydromorphone, or 25 μg of fentanyl. If the appropriate risk stratification justifies an outpatient opioid trial, the patient should be observed for at least 6 to 8 hours.[7]

There is strong consensus by the PACC that a bolus trial of ziconotide is preferred over a continuous trial and that the patient should be monitored in a clinical setting for at least 6 hours after the trial. Bolus trialing with IT ziconotide should start at 1 to 2 μg. A continuous infusion trial of ziconotide should not be increased by more than 1.2 μg per day, and trialing with short-term continuous IT infusion does require inpatient admission.[7]

The recommended starting doses for bupivacaine and clonidine bolus trials are 0.5 to 2.5 mg and 5 to 20 μg, respectively. Bolus trialing with bupivacaine or clonidine is done in an outpatient setting with at least 6 hours of observation afterward. Trialing with a continuous infusion of bupivacaine or clonidine should be done as an inpatient with frequent heart rate and blood pressure monitoring.[7]

A complete evaluation of the patient must be made before considering IDD therapy. Failure of IDD therapy seems higher in patients maintained on large amounts of systemic opioids before starting IT therapy.[2] Thus, consideration to weaning systemic opioids before IT therapy should be considered.

Specific indications for IDDS include patients with axial neck or back pain that is not amenable to surgical correction secondary to numerous compression fractures, discogenic disease, spinal stenosis, severe spondylosis, and postlaminectomy syndrome. Patients with abdominal and pelvic pain may also be candidates for IDDS. Additional indications for IDDS include complex regional pain syndrome, postherpetic neuralgia, postthoracotomy syndrome, and efficacy with systemic opioids but intolerable side effects. Finally, cancer pain from direct tumor invasion and chemotherapy-related pain are indications for IDDS.[7]

Acceptable indications for the general usage of IDDS are as follows[7,8]:

1. Patients with moderate to severe pain.
2. Failure of conservative treatments to adequately treat pain or inability to tolerate oral administration of analgesics.
3. Testing phase provides adequate pain control, with tolerable side effects and functional improvement.
4. Patient's anatomy is conducive to implantation.
5. Presence of appropriately trained implantation and maintenance infrastructure.
6. Free of contraindications to implantation.

Nonmalignant pain

Pain that lasts longer than 6 months that is not associated with a cancer condition is defined as chronic nonmalignant pain. One prospective study assessed the efficacy of IT morphine in patients with various noncancer-related chronic pain including failed back surgery syndrome, chronic low back pain, and peripheral neuropathy. Therapy was shown to reduced visual analog scale pain scores by more than 25% after 24 months in more than half of the subjects.[9]

IDDS is used for the treatment of a variety of noncancer pain–related chronic pain states (**Box 1**).

Cancer pain

IT therapy is increasingly being considered earlier in the treatment of cancer-related pain. It has been shown to be effective in treating cancer pain, but also has been

---

Box 1
Noncancer chronic pain indications

Noncancer pain indications for IDDS
    Axial low back pain (compression fractures, discogenic pain, multilevel spondylosis)
    Neuropathic pain (diabetic neuropathy, postherpetic neuralgia, spinal cord injury, thalamic syndrome)
    Radicular pain from failed back surgery syndrome
    Complex regional pain syndrome
    Spinal stenosis
    Pancreatitis
    Phantom limb pain
    Extremity pain

associated with improved functionality and mood, and prolonged survival when compared with medical management.[7] More than 33% of patients with advanced cancer grade their pain as moderate or severe, and of those 10% to 30% do not have adequate pain relief with traditional management.[8] In one study of patients with refractory cancer pain, IT analgesics have been shown to decrease the prevalence of severe pain from 86% to 17% in the 8-week study period.

Patients with cancer are classified into three different categories: category one includes patients with short life expectancy with palliation as primary objective; category two includes patients whose disease is stable or slow to progress, but have high likelihood of recurrence of progression; and category three includes patients with cancer in partial remission or in whom cancer has been cured, however they are left with residual chronic pain.[7] These categories are used to help guide patient selection (ie, an external pump is used in patients with short life expectancies).

Candidates for IDDS include patients with high tumor burden and chronic postsurgical.[10] Hypothetically, because of the increased potential of respiratory depression IDDS is better for more localized pain below the neck.[11–13]

Patient assessment. IT medications have several systemic adverse effects. In addition, implantation is a surgical procedure under general anesthesia or monitored anesthesia care. It is important to have a comprehensive assessment of comorbidities and the ability to tolerate potential adverse effects of the drugs used in IT solution. Because of the risk of respiratory depression, a careful cardiopulmonary assessment should be performed before considering IT treatment with opioids. Patient's age, kidney, and liver function should also be evaluated given their effect on drug clearance.[12] Comorbidities to consider before the implementation of an IT opioid are sleep apnea; pulmonary disease, such as chronic obstructive pulmonary disease; and cardiac disease. The use of other systemic medications that may also because respiratory depression should be reviewed. Trials have shown creatinine kinase levels can rise two- or three-fold with the use of ziconotide so creatinine kinase levels should be monitored during therapy.[13]

A thorough review of concomitant medications is advised. Medication that may interfere with IT medications include benzodiazepines, antidepressants, anticonvulsants, muscle relaxants, and alcohol consumption.[14]

The PACC of 2017 recommends that before IT therapy, patients should have a psychological evaluation that includes an assessment of coping skills and to confirm that the patient is free of cognitive issues that may interfere with IT therapy.[13] Many patients with chronic pain suffer from psychiatric comorbidities that have been shown to decrease the long-term response to treatment.[14] In patients with cancer with short life expectancy where IDDS is being implemented as a form of palliation, the PACC also recommends that psychological evaluation should not delay the implementation of treatment. Moreover, because of the logistical requirements involved with an IDDS, such as maintaining a refilling schedule, the patient's socioeconomic situation and reliability for follow-up are all important factors to consider when selecting patients for therapy.[3]

Medication selection. The pharmacokinetics of IT delivery are better understood now that more is known about CSF flow dynamics. It is now understood that bulk flow and spread within the IT space is limited around the catheter tip.[15] The implications of this are that location of catheter placement, hydrophilicity, and rate of infusion of medication are all influential factors.[15]

Morphine and ziconotide are the only two Food and Drug Administration (FDA)-approved medications for IT therapy for the treatment of pain; however, many other medications are frequently used. In fact, most clinicians in the United States use off-label IT medications.[16] However, according to the PACC guidelines off-label monotherapy or combination therapy should only be considered after FDA-approved medications are tried and failed or are contraindicated.[7] According to the PACC guidelines, for nonmalignant pain there is level Ia evidence for the monotherapy use of morphine or ziconotide; level II-3 evidence for the use of monotherapy hydromorphone or combination morphine or hydromorphone and bupivacaine; and level III-C evidence for hydromorphone or morphine with combined clonidine, fentanyl combined with bupivacaine, or ziconotide combined with either morphine or hydromorphone. The evidence for other combinations of IT medications is considered weak.[7] Medication selection relies on many factors including pain characteristics, patient comorbidities, and drug availability.[7] For instance, the 2017 PACC states that neuropathic pain generally responds to opioids with local anesthetic combined, ziconotide, clonidine, and clonidine plus opioids. Nociceptive pain generally responds more to ziconotide, local anesthetics alone or in combination with opioids, or opioids alone.[7] Patient comorbidities also influence drug selection largely based on the knowledge of the drug side effects, which are elaborated on in the section on the individual drug side effects.

Morphine, hydromorphone, and fentanyl are all common opioid IT medications, but morphine is the only that is FDA opioid-approved for treating chronic pain.[15] The bioavailability of IT opioids is heavily determined by their lipid solubility. Opioids act to reduce pain by binding to mu-opioid receptors (**Tables 1** and **2**) that are concentrated in the substantia gelatinosa of the spinal cord.[17] Hydrophilic drugs, such as morphine and hydromorphone, have greater bioavailability at the dorsal horn than hydrophobic drugs, which include fentanyl and sufentanil.[18]

Although IT trialing with opioid medications is common, the process is complicated by lack of standard equianalgesic conversion doses from systemic to IT opioids.[19]

COMMON INTRATHECAL MEDICATIONS AND RECOMMENDED STARTING DOSES
Opioids

A variety of different opioids are used in IDDs, and they are discussed in the literature.[20–25]

Nonopioids

Bupivacaine is an amide local anesthetic and has high lipid solubility. It is often used off label in IT therapy.[26] Continuous dose is 0.01 to 4 mg/d; bolus dose is 0.5 to 2.5 mg.[22]

Local anesthetics, such as bupivacaine, are commonly used with opioids because of their synergistic activity. Coadministration of IT bupivacaine and an opioid decreased the rate of opioid dose escalation by 65% in one retrospective review.[26]

Table 1 Intrathecal drugs and receptors	
Medication	**Target Receptor**
Morphine, fentanyl, sufentanil, methadone, hydromorphone	Mu opioid
Ziconotide	Calcium channel
Baclofen, benzodiazepines	γ-Aminobutyric acid
Local anesthetics	Sodium channel
Ketamine	N-methyl-D-aspartate
Clonidine, dexmedetomidine	α_2

Table 2
Opioids used in IDD

		Opioids Used in Intrathecal Drug Delivery		
Opioid	Mechanism	Line of Usage	Side Effects	Dosage
Morphine	Morphine is a mu opioid receptor agonist.	Data support the use of morphine as a first-line therapy.[20]	Morphine has been demonstrated to have a propensity for IT granuloma formation in preclinical trials.[21]	Continuous dose 0.1–0.5 mg/d; bolus dose 0.1–0.5 mg.[22]
Hydromorphone	Hydromorphone is a mu opioid receptor agonist.	Hydromorphone is considered a first- and second-line treatment according to the PACC guidelines.[12]	It has been associated with granuloma formation at higher concentrations and is generally more expensive than morphine.[23]	Continuous dose 0.01–0.15 mg/d; bolus dose 0.025–0.1 mg.[22]
Fentanyl	Fentanyl is a lipophilic mu opioid agonist.[24]	For localized pain, fentanyl is considered a first-line therapy. Preclinical studies have not demonstrated granuloma formation even at high doses.[25]	Preclinical studies have not demonstrated granuloma formation even at high doses.[25]	Continuous dose 25–75 μg/day; bolus dose 15–75 μg.[22]

Ziconotide is a novel nonopioid analgesic that acts by selectively blocking N-type calcium channels located in the spinal cord.[27] Ziconotide should be considered if the patient is already receiving a high dose of opioids that cannot be weaned before implantation or if the patient has opioid intolerance.[28] It also has a first-line indication for neuropathic and nociceptive pain.[7]

A benefit of ziconotide is that it is not associated with issues of tolerance, withdrawal, or granuloma formation; however, it is contraindicated in patients with a history of psychosis and is expensive.[29] Continuous dose is 0.5 to 2.4 μg/day; bolus dose is 1 to 5 μg.[22]

Baclofen is an agonist of the β subunit of γ-aminobutyric acid receptors that inhibits the release of excitatory neurotransmitters with resultant relief of spasticity.[30] Although it is FDA-approved for IT administration in spastic disorders, baclofen is generally not considered early in the drug selection for patients with chronic pain.[7] As the use of IT baclofen has expanded the number of adverse events has increased including toxicity or withdrawal. Careful attention to patient history, vital sign abnormalities, and physical examination are paramount to establish the diagnosis. Generally, hypotonia and flaccid paralysis are signs of baclofen overdose, whereas increased spasticity and hyperreflexia are signs of withdrawal. Both toxicity and withdrawal are life threatening.[31]

Clonidine is an α_2-agonist that exerts its antinociceptive effects by inhibiting the activation of nuclear factor-κB and p38, which are both associated with neuropathic pain pathways.[32] The PACC guidelines provided guidance on the use of clonidine. The panel reports grade Ia evidence that IT clonidine decreases pain scores over time in patients with complex regional pain syndrome.[7] Continuous dose is 20 to 100 μg/day; bolus dose is 5 to 20 μg.[22]

RISKS AND CONTRAINDICATIONS

Complication of IDDS are divided into pharmacologic, device, and surgical complications. In a retrospective review by Kamran and Wright,[33] 77% of adverse events were caused by the IT medications themselves, 16% were from catheter malfunctions, and 5% were from infections. Mortality rates with IT opioid therapy are 0.088%, 0.39%, and 3.89% at 3 days, 1 month, and 1 year after implementation.[34]

Surgical Complications

Surgical-related complications include those seen with any surgical procedure, such as bleeding and infection, in addition to complications relating specifically to IDDS implantation and maintenance including CSF leakages and pocket fills.

- Bleeding: Bleeding is most likely to present in the immediate postoperative period. A superficial hematoma may form, and these are usually self-resolving. A more worrisome complication is a pump pocket hematoma. Obtaining adequate hemostasis during pocket formation can mitigate this risk but if one does occur an abdominal binder can help prevent further fluid buildup.[7] Significant bleeding into the epidural space can present as a rapid increase in back pain, decreased sensory and motor function, or even the loss of bowel and bladder control.[34] This presentation justifies immediate imagining with an MRI and emergent surgical decompression.
- Infection: As with any procedure there is a risk of infection. Most common infections are superficial but serious infections, such as meningitis, may still occur. The PACC guidelines provide essential guidance on preventing infection including use of proper sterile technique and perioperative antibiotics, optimizing

glucose control, smoking cessation, use of electric clippers to remove hair immediately before surgery, and avoidance of routine use of vancomycin.[35] In addition the use of appropriate agents for skin antisepsis, maintenance of positive pressure ventilation in the operating room, keeping operating room doors closed during the procedure, and limiting operating room traffic are also identified as measures to decrease risk of infection. Postoperatively, the use of an occlusive dressing for 4 to 48 hours is advised.[7] Anemia, smoking, cancer, malnutrition, and cardiovascular disease increases the risk.[7] If any deep infection involving the pump or pocket occurs then the IDDS must be removed, cultures obtained, and antibiotics initiated.[24]

- Pump migration: In the presence of a seroma or oversized pocket, there is an increased risk of pump migration or flipping. Placing a manufacturer-provided sock over the pump promotes the formation of scar tissue that helps anchor the pump in place.[36]
- CSF leakage: In the case of a dural puncture a postdural puncture headache is likely and a blood patch may be required to alleviate symptoms.

Device Complications

IDDS are small devices with many different potential sources of malfunctions (**Box 2**).

- Catheter malfunction is reported to be the most common point of malfunction with an incidence of up to 25%. The abrupt cessation of medication flow initially presents as a loss of analgesia and can result in dangerous withdrawals if such medications as baclofen and clonidine are used.[37,38]
- A pocket fill can occur during IDDS refilling if drugs are inadvertently administered subcutaneously. This can result in a dangerous bolus of highly concentrated medications. Proper filling technique, including the use of manufacturer-provided template, ultrasonography, or even fluoroscopy, is used to mitigate the risk of pocket fills from occurring. Swelling at the injection site, reported burning or stinging sensation during drug injection, technical difficulties during the refill, and signs of overdose may be indicators of pocket fill. If pocket fill is suspected, but the patient is not exhibiting symptoms, an observation period of at least 2 hours is recommended because late overdose can occur. The patient should be hospitalized during this time. Ultrasound may be used to assess for the presence of fluid around the pump. Attempts should be made to aspirate the pocket around the IDDS, rinse with saline, and aspirate again.[39]
- MRI: IDDS has been shown to be completely safe when specified pre- and post-MRI protocols are followed.[40] For example, Medtronic pumps should be interrogated after an MRI to make sure that its motor has resumed. Flowonix pumps need to be emptied before an MRI because of previous instances of fatal IT boluses in the setting of the failure of the device gate to close.[41]

Box 2
Types of device malfunctions

Device Malfunction
   Catheter pump misconnection
   Loss of pump propellant
   Gear shaft wear and motor stall
   Leakage of administered agent
   Intrathecal kinking

Pharmacologic Complications

Because of the direct administration of medications into the IT space, complications can arise that are similar to elevated systemic drug levels in addition to IT administration-related complications. The various pharmacologic complications should be considered when implementing treatment with these medications.

- As the longest used IT medication, morphine, has some of the most understood side effect profiles. Similarly, to oral morphine, pruritus, nausea, urinary retention, constipation, and respiratory depression are common.[42] IT administration of morphine has also been shown to decrease libido in up to 96% of men and 69% of women and one study demonstrated the development of hypogonadotropic hypogonadism in most subjects that was refractory to hormone supplementation.[43] Because of the risk of respiratory depression, IT morphine should be used with caution in patients with kyphoscoliosis or paralysis of the phrenic nerve. Because the effects of respiratory depression from morphine can last for up to 24 hours, the patient should be monitored after administration of a test dose.[44]
- Ziconotide has a narrow therapeutic window and therefore requires careful dosing. With rapid titration, ziconotide is associated with psychosis. Central nervous system side effects include nystagmus, nausea, dizziness, ataxia, and hallucinations.[45]
- Local anesthetics: If given at high doses, fatigue, urinary retention, and paresthesia can occur.[46]
- Clonidine: variations in blood pressure, with hypotension at low doses and hypertension at high doses.[47] Sudden withdrawal and hypertensive crisis can occur if it is suddenly discontinued.[38]
- Baclofen: weight gain in children and dangerous withdrawal if flow stops.[37,40] Risks of IT baclofen include toxicity and withdrawal, both of which are life threatening. Signs and symptoms of toxicity include hypothermia, hyporeflexia, agitation, mania, confusion, tremor, seizures, coma, prolonged QTc, respiratory failure, nausea and vomiting, and death. Signs and symptoms of withdrawal include pruritus, hyperthermia, organ failure, hyperreflexia, delirium, seizures, rhabdomyolysis, cardiac arrest, and death.[31]

Granulomas

A granuloma (**Figs. 1** and **2**) is a sterile mass of inflammatory cells and fibroblasts that develops near the IT catheter with a prevalence of 8%.[7] Granulomas mostly form in the thoracic region between the spinal cord and the dura and are thought to be caused by a reaction to the catheter tip or the infused medication. In fact, there is a direct correlation between the drug concentration and granuloma formation. Morphine is involved in most granuloma formations; however, they have also been seen with sufentanil, clonidine, baclofen, and tramadol.[41,42]

The most recent consensus guidelines on granulomas by Deer and colleagues[48,49] suggest using the lowest effective concentration and dose of IT opioids, especially morphine, to decrease the risk of granuloma formation. Other recommendations included the use of bolus dosing instead of continuous infusions, placing the tip in the lumbar thecal sac instead of above the consensus medullaris, the implementation of adjuvant therapy with nonopioid analgesics if concerned about granuloma formation, and switching from opioid therapy to ziconotide if concerned about granuloma recurrence. The most recent panel did not address compounding formulations of IT medication but the groups earlier opinion did not believe that compounding played a role in the development of granulomas; however, they advocated for meticulous evaluation of quality control for any compounded medications used.[48,49]

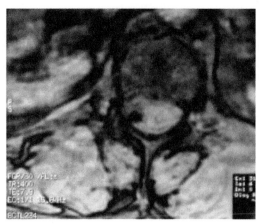

Fig. 1. Intrathecal granuloma depicted on MRI (axial view). (*From* Matthew T. Ranson Reducing Risks and Complications of Interventional Pain Procedures.)

Clinical presentation of a granuloma can present as spinal cord compression with sensorimotor impairment, radicular pain, or failure of analgesia because the drugs are not able to reach their target tissue. Granuloma formation should be considered anytime that there is a new-onset pain or neurologic finding. MRI or high-resolution computed tomography myelogram are the imaging modalities of choice in these cases.

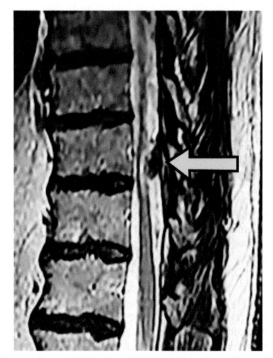

Fig. 2. Intrathecal granuloma depicted on MRI (sagittal view). (*From* Matthew T. Ranson Reducing Risks and Complications of Interventional Pain Procedures.)

If there are no neurologic deficits but a granuloma is suspected, then the pump medications are changed to a lower concentration with close monitoring of the granuloma, or the medication is completely replaced with saline.[43] If the latter occurs, it is important to watch for medication withdrawal, in particular with baclofen or clonidine because both are fatal. If neurologic deficits are present, then the system should be surgically removed, and serial MRIs should be obtained to observe regression of the granuloma.[43]

OUTCOME DATA

In a long-term follow-up study for 13.5 years, Duarte and colleagues, monitored 20 patients receiving IT drug therapy. They reported statistically significant improvements in pain relief and coping and quality of life.[9,44]

In a study of patients with cancer with chronic pain, nociceptive pain responded better than neuropathic pain to IT opioids.[46] Patients with severe chronic noncancer pain who underwent a successful epidural morphine infusion trial, had good to excellent satisfaction and improved quality of life after IT pump placement.[47,50] Patients on high initial opioid consumption have lower likelihood of long-term pain relief with IT opioids.[47,51]

In a case series, IT ziconotide decreased pain intensity by 47.5% at an average follow-up duration of 3.1 years.[52,53] In a retrospective review of long-term efficacy of IT therapy in patients with CRPS, Herring and colleagues studied the effect of IT therapy on pain intensity and oral opioid intake.[53] Decrease in oral opiod intake was reported in patients with IT ziconotide but not in patients with IT opioids.[53] A low starting dose and slow titration can help improve safety profile of the ziconotide.[52,53] Typical starting continuous doses for ziconotide are 0.5 to 2.4 μg/day; bolus dose 1 to 5 μg.[22]

In patients with refractory chronic cancer pain, benefits of IDDS extend beyond significant pain relief. In a randomized controlled trial of IDDS compared with comprehensive medical management, patients with cancer with IDDS had greater survival at 6 months because of reduced pain and significant decrease in drug toxicities.[47,50] In a prospective review of a multicenter registry of 1403 patients with IDDS, Stearns and colleagues reported adequate and improved pain control in patients with cancer along with improvement in quality of life, even in advanced stages.[52] In a double-blind placebo-controlled multicenter randomized controlled trial involving patients with cancer or chronic AIDS pain, Staats and colleagues reported 53% improvement in mean visual analog scale scores with IT ziconotide as compared with 18% with placebo.[53]

DISCUSSION

IT drug therapy has been used for many years with good efficacy. Chronic pain has an immense negative impact on patients' quality of life along with increased 10-year mortality.[9,44,45] Patients with chronic and refractory malignant and nonmalignant pain respond well to IDDS. It is, however, important to choose an appropriate patient and pain condition as outlined previously.

The effectiveness of IT therapy depends on the mechanism of pain and the drug used.[45] IDDS is effective for many nociceptive, neuropathic, and mixed-type chronic pain syndromes in cancer and noncancer pain conditions.[45] Discrete pain presentations respond better than vague, generalized chronic pain.[46]

IT ziconotide is effective as a sole agent or combination therapy to treat refractory neuropathic pain.[52] In patients with refractory chronic cancer pain, benefits of IDDS extend beyond significant pain relief to include improvements in quality of life.

Despite the reported benefits for IDDS therapy, there are several limitations that restrict the use of this therapy to tertiary centers with advanced therapies. These include, complications and their management, requirement of adequate infrastructure and specialized personnel for refills, and the time investment needed for drug titration.[54,55]

Infection is the most common complication with incidence varying from 3% to 15%.[45,52,56–58] A retrospective review of FDA Manufacturer and User Facility Device Experience database over 2.5 years reported infection in about 15% and adverse medication reaction in about 11% patients.[56] For safety reasons, dose changes in outpatient setting should not exceed more than 10% to 15% of the daily dose.[54]

Future Directions

Recently, trials using a combination of IT ketamine and pregabalin have been shown to reduce neuropathic pain in animals.[59] A selective noradrenaline transport inhibitor called Xen 2174 has been shown to decrease allodynia in rats when administered intrathecally.[60] The capsaicin analogue, resiniferatoxin, produces analgesia in animals.[61] CGX-1260 is an effective agent for the treatment of pain after spinal cord injury.[62] Advancements in nanoparticles could potentially allow for an even more selective distribution of IT-administered medications.

New developments in IDDS, such as piezoelective membrane pumps, are reducing size and energy requirements. The development of biofeedback loops that communicate, record, and respond to feedback from organs and tissue can theoretically be developed soon. These advancements paired with the recent recommendation of earlier intervention with IT pumps for patients with chronic pain leave a lot of exciting opportunities for the future of IDDS.

SUMMARY

IDDs are an established method of targeted drug delivery that allows for reduced side effects[3] and increased pain control as demonstrated by multiple studies.[7,9,44,47,50] Given advancements in the actual systems themselves and novel drug developments, IDDS are now being considered earlier in chronic pain treatments.[5] Given the risks associated with the device implantation procedure, device malfunctions, and pharmacologic side effects, IDDS should only be used after the proper patient is selected. Because of the expanding impact of chronic pain on patients, consensus is that IDD should be used earlier in pain management treatments, and pharmacologic and device advancements, the understanding of IT pumps is essential for anyone treating chronic pain.

CLINICS CARE POINTS

- Proper patient selection is critical to successful intrathecal drug therapy.
- Appropriate implantation and maintenance should be had to minimize the risk of therapy failure or complications.
- In a study of patients with cancer with chronic pain, nociceptive pain responded better than neuropathic pain to intrathecal opioids.
- Patients with severe chronic noncancer pain who underwent a successful epidural morphine infusion trial had good to excellent satisfaction and improved quality of life after intrathecal pump placement.
- Patients on high initial opioid consumption have lower likelihood of long-term pain relief with intrathecal opioids.

DISCLOSURE

The authors have nothing to disclose.

REFERENCES

1. Onofrio BM, Yaksh TL, Arnold PG. Continuous low-dose intrathecal morphine administration in the treatment of chronic pain of malignant origin. Mayo Clin Proc 1981;56:516–20.
2. Stearns L, Boortz-Marx R, Du Pen S, et al. Intrathecal drug delivery for the management of cancer pain: a multidisciplinary consensus of best clinical practices. J Support Oncol 2005;3(6):399–408.
3. Centers for Disease Control (CDC). Vital signs: overdoses of prescription opioid pain relievers—United States, 1999-2008. Morb Mortal Wkly Rep 2011;60:1–6.
4. Deer TR, Smith HS, Burton AW, et al. Center for pain relief, Inc. Pain Physician 2011;14(3):E283–312.
5. Deer TR, Prager J, Levy R, et al. Polyanalgesic Consensus Conference 2012: recommendations for the management of pain by intrathecal (intraspinal) drug delivery: report of an interdisciplinary expert panel. Neuromodulation 2012;15(5): 436–64 [discussion: 464-6].
6. Paice JA, Penn RD, Shott S. Intraspinal morphine for chronic pain: a retrospective, multicenter study. J Pain Symptom Manage 1996;11(2):71–80.
7. Deer TR, Hayek SM, Pope JE, et al. The Polyanalgesic Consensus Conference (PACC): recommendations for trialing of intrathecal drug delivery infusion therapy. Neuromodulation 2017;20:133–54.
8. Van den Beuken-van Everdingen MH, de Rijke JM, Kessels AG, et al. Prevalence of pain in patients with cancer: a systematic review of the past 40 years. Ann Oncol 2007;18:1437–49.
9. Duarte RV, Raphael JH, Sparkes E, Southall JL, LeMarchand K, Ashford RL. Long-term intrathecal drug administration for chronic non[1]malignant pain. J Neurosurg Anesthesiol 2012;24(1):63–70.
10. Brian M, Bruel MD, Allen W, Burton MD. Intrathecal therapy for cancer-related pain. Pain Med 2016;17(12):2404–21.
11. Bruel BM, Burton AW. Intrathecal therapy for cancer-related pain. Pain Med 2016; 17:2404–21.
12. Gulati A, Puttanniah V, Hung J, et al. Considerations for evaluating the use of intrathecal drug delivery in the oncologic patient. Curr Pain Headache Rep 2014;18(2):391.
13. Wallace M, Rauck R, Fisher R, et al. Intrathecal ziconotide for severe chronic pain: safety and tolerability results of an open-label, long-term trial. Anesth Analg 2008;106(2):628–37.
14. Rauck R, Webster L, Wallace M, et al. Effect of concomitant antidepressant and anti-convulsant use on adverse events in patients receiving intrathecal ziconotide in long-term extension study. Poster Resented West Va Soc Interv Pain Physicians 2014.
15. Jose de A, Luciano P, Vicente V, Juan Marcos AS, Gustavo FC. Role of Catheter's Position for Final Results in Intrathecal Drug Delivery. Analysis Based on CSF Dynamics and Specific Drugs Profiles. Korean J Pain 2013 Oct;26(4):336–46. https://doi.org/10.3344/kjp.2013.26.4.336. Epub 2013 Oct 2. PMID: 24155999; PMCID: PMC3800705.
16. Consent Decree of Permanent Injunction. United States of America vs. Medtronic, Inc., and S. Omar Ishrak and Thomas M. Teft. United States District Court for the

District of Minnesota. April 2015. 5. Pope J, Poree L, McRoberts WP, Falowski S, Deer T Consent decree: physician and institution ramifications?. Neuromodulation 2015;18:653–6.

17. Duarte RV, Raphael JH, Eldabe S. Editorial (Thematic selection: spinal neuropharmacological agents for the management of pain). Curr Neuropharmacol 2017; 15(2):196–7.

18. Bujedo BM. Spinal opioid bioavailability in postoperative pain. Pain Pract 2014; 14(4):350–64.

19. Shaheen PE, Walsh D, Lasheen W, et al. Opioid equianalgesic tables: are they all equally dangerous? J Pain Symptom Manage 2009;38(3):409–17.

20. Deer TR, Prager J, Levy R, et al. Polyanalgesic Consensus Conference 2012: recommendations for the management of pain by intrathecal (intraspinal) drug delivery: report of an interdisciplinary expert panel. Neuromodulation 2012;15:436–64 [discussion: 464–436].

21. Michael A, Buffen E, Rauck R, et al. An in vivo canine study to assess granulomatous responses in the MedStream Programmable Infusion System (TM) and the SynchroMed II Infusion SystemVR. Pain Med 2012;13:175–84.

22. Deer TR, Hayek SM, Pope JE, et al. The Polyanalgesic Consensus Conference (PACC): recommendations for trialing of intrathecal drug delivery infusion therapy. Neuromodulation 2017;20(2):133–54.

23. Johansen MJ, Satterfield WC, Baze WB, et al. Continuous intrathecal infusion of hydromorphone: safety in the sheep model and clinical implications. Pain Med 2004;5:14–25.

24. Hatheway JA, Caraway D, David G, et al. Systemic opioid elimination after implantation of an intrathecal drug delivery system significantly reduced healthcare expenditures. Neuromodulation 2015;18:207–13 [discussion: 213].

25. Yaksh TL, Allen JW, Veesart SL, et al. Role of meningeal mast cells in intrathecal morphine-evoked granuloma formation. Anesthesiology 2013;118(3):664–78.

26. Veizi IE, Hayek SM, Narouze S, et al. Combination of intrathecal opioids with bupivacaine attenuates opioid dose escalation in chronic noncancer pain patients. Pain Med 2011;12:1481–9.

27. McGivern JG. Ziconotide: a review of its pharmacology and use in the treatment of pain. Neuropsychiatr Dis Treat 2007;3(1):69–85.

28. Walker MJ, Webster LR. Opioid-induced hyperalgesia and monotherapy intrathecal ziconotide: experience with four cases. J Pain Manag 2013;6(3):257–64.

29. Elan Corporation. Prialt (ziconotide) [prescribing information] San Diego (CA): 2004.U.S. Food and Drug Administration website n21060 AP Ltr 12 2004.doc (fda.gov)Revised December 23rd 2004. Accessed February 15, 2022.

30. Munro G, Ahring PK, Mirza NR. Developing analgesics by enhancing spinal inhibition after injury: GABA-A receptor subtypes as novel targets. Trends Pharmacol Sci 2009;30:453–9.

31. Romito JW, Turner ER, Rosener JA, et al. Baclofen therapeutics, toxicity, and withdrawal: a narrative review. SAGE Open Med 2021. https://doi.org/10.1177/20503121211022197.

32. Zhao Y, He J, Yu N, et al. Mechanisms of dexmedetomidine in neuropathic Pain. Front Neurosci 2020;14:330.

33. Kamran S, Wright BD. Complications of intrathecal drug delivery systems. Neuromodulation 2001;4(3):111–5.

34. Coffey RJ, Owens ML, Broste SK, et al. Mortality associated with implantation and management of intrathecal opioid drug infusion systems to treat noncancer pain. Anesthesiology 2009;111:881–91.

35. Deer TR, Provenzano DA, Hanes M, et al. The Neurostimulation Appropriateness Consensus Committee (NACC) recommendations for infection prevention and management. Neuromodulation 2017;20(1):31–50.

36. Vender JR, Hester S, Waller JL, et al. Identification and management of intrathecal baclofen pump complications: a comparison of pediatric and adult patients. J Neurosurg 2006;104(1 Suppl):9–15.

37. Mohammed I, Hussain A. Intrathecal baclofen withdrawal syndrome: a life-threatening complication of baclofen pump: a case report. BMC Clin Pharmacol 2004;4:6.

38. Lee HM, Ruggoo V, Graudins A. Intrathecal clonidine pump failure causing acute withdrawal syndrome with 'stress-induced' cardiomyopathy. J Med Toxicol 2016; 12(1):134–8.

39. Maino P, Perez RSGM, Koetsier E. Intrathecal pump refills, pocket fills, and symptoms of drug overdose: a prospective, observational study comparing the injected drug volume vs. the drug volume effectively measured inside the pump. Neuromodulation 2017;20(7):733–9.

40. De Andres J, Villanueva V, Palmisani S, et al. The safety of magnetic resonance imaging in patients with programmable implanted intrathecal drug delivery systems: a 3-year prospective study. Anesth Analg 2011;112(5):1124–9.

41. Andrés J De, Tatay Vivò J, Palmisani S, et al. Intrathecal granuloma formation in a patient receiving long-term spinal infusion of tramadol. Pain Med 2010;11(7): 1059–62.

42. Gupta A, Martindale Ty, Christo PJ. Intrathecal catheter granuloma associated with continuous sufentanil infusion. Pain Med 2010;11(6):847–52.

43. Rauck R. Management of intrathecal pump complications. ASRA Conference Proceedings; 2005 Nov 17-20; Loews Miami beach Hotel, Miami, FL; USA.Alternative reference: Knight KH, Brand FM, Mchaourab AS, Veneziano G. Implantable intrathecal pumps for chronic pain: highlights and updates. Croat Med J. 2007;48(1):22–34.

44. Cummings A, Orgill BD, Fitzgerald BM. Intrathecal morphine. In: StatPearls. Treasure Island (FL): StatPearls Publishing; 2021.

45. Abd-Elsayed A, Karri J, Michael A, et al. Intrathecal drug delivery for chronic pain syndromes: a review of considerations in practice management. Pain Physician 2020;23(6):E591–617.

46. Belverud SA, Mogilner AY, Schulder M. Intrathecal bupivacaine for head and neck pain. Local Reg Anesth 2010;3:125–8.

47. Deer TR, Pope JE, Panchal SJ, et al. Intrathecal therapy for cancer and non-cancer pain. Pain Physician 2011;14(3):219–48.

48. Deer T, Krames ES, Hassenbusch S, et al. Management of intrathecal catheter-tip inflammatory masses: an updated 2007 consensus statement from an expert panel. Neuromodulation 2008;11(2):77–91.

49. Deer TR, Prager J, Levy R, et al. Polyanalgesic Consensus Conference—2012: consensus on diagnosis, detection, and treatment of catheter-tip granulomas (inflammatory masses). Neuromodulation 2012;15:483–95.

50. Duse G, Davià G, White PF. Improvement in psychosocial outcomes in chronic pain patients receiving intrathecal morphine infusions. Anesth Analg 2009; 109(6):1981–6.

51. Atli A, c c, Loeser JD. Intrathecal opioid therapy for chronic nonmalignant pain: a retrospective cohort study with 3-year follow-up. Pain Med 2010;11(7):1010–6.

52. Stearns LM, Abd-Elsayed A, Perruchoud C, Spencer R, Hammond K, Stromberg K, Weaver T. Intrathecal Drug Delivery Systems for Cancer Pain: An Analysis of a

Prospective, Multicenter Product Surveillance Registry. Anesth Analg. 2020 Feb;130(2):289-297. doi: 10.1213/ANE.0000000000004425. PMID: 31567325; PMCID: PMC6948791.

53. Staats PS, Yearwood T, Charapata SG, et al. Intrathecal ziconotide in the treatment of refractory pain in patients with cancer or AIDS: a randomized controlled trial. JAMA 2004;291(1):63–70.

54. Delhaas EM, Huygen FJPM. Complications associated with intrathecal drug delivery systems. BJA Educ 2020;20(2):51–7.

55. Huntoon MA. Intrathecal drug therapy for cancer pain: time for a boost! Pain Pract 2009;9(5):325–6.

56. Goel V, Yang Y, Kanwar S, et al. Adverse events and complications associated with intrathecal drug delivery systems: insights from the manufacturer and user facility device experience (MAUDE) database. Neuromodulation 2020;24(7): 1181–9.

57. Taira T, Ueta T, Katayama Y, et al. Rate of complications among the recipients of intrathecal baclofen pump in Japan: a multicenter study. Neuromodulation 2013; 16(3):266–72 [discussion: 272].

58. Spader HS, Bollo RJ, Bowers CA, et al. Risk factors for baclofen pump infection in children: a multivariate analysis. J Neurosurg Pediatr 2016;17(6):756–62.

59. Lim HS, Kim JM, Choi JG, et al. Intrathecal ketamine and pregabalin at sub-effective doses synergistically reduces neuropathic pain without motor dysfunction in mice. Biol Pharm Bull 2013;36(1):125–30.

60. Nielsen, Carsten & Lewis, Richard & Alewood, Dianne & Drinkwater, Roger & Palant, Elka & Patterson, Margaret & Yaksh, Tony & McCumber, Damon & Smith, Maree. (2005). Anti-allodynic efficacy of the X-conopeptide, Xen2174, in rats with neuropathic pain. Pain. 118. 112-24. 10.1016/j.pain.2005.08.002.

61. Brown DC, Agnello K, Iadarola MJ. Intrathecal resiniferatoxin in a dog model: efficacy in bone cancer pain. Pain 2015;156(6):1018–24.

62. Sang, C.N., Barnabe, K.J. and Kern, S.E. (2016), Phase IA Clinical Trial Evaluating the Tolerability, Pharmacokinetics, and Analgesic Efficacy of an Intrathecally Administered Neurotensin A Analogue in Central Neuropathic Pain Following Spinal Cord Injury. Clinical Pharmacology in Drug Development, 5: 250-258. https://doi.org/10.1002/cpdd.253.

Vertebroplasty and Kyphoplasty

Sherief Boss, MD[a], Vidhan Srivastava, MD[b], Magdalena Anitescu, MD, PhD[c],*

KEYWORDS

- Vertebroplasty • Kyphoplasty • Vertebral augmentation procedures

KEY POINTS

- Vertebroplasty and kyphoplasty are minimally invasive procedures that collectively are named vertebral augmentation procedures (VAPs).
- VAPs are used to restore height and reduce fractures in vertebral body compression fractures.
- In osteoporotic fractures, height restoration is achieved with kyphoplasty or equivalent procedures.
- In metastatic vertebral compression fractures (VCFs), tumor burden may be reduced by bone radiofrequency ablation (RFA) performed before the kyphoplasty portion of the procedure.

INTRODUCTION

Every year, more than 700,000 vertebral compression fractures (VCFs) occur in the United States, which is more than the number of hip and ankle fractures combined.[1] The financial impact of these fractures is immense. By some estimates, VCFs from osteoporosis alone are estimated to reach $25 billion by 2025.[2] VCFs also reduce the quality of life and increase patient morbidity. VCFs occur secondary to bone weakening from osteoporosis, metastatic disease, and other pathologic processes. Managing VCFs varies widely. On the conservative side, providers recommend rest, back braces, over-the-counter analgesics, and physical therapy. More invasive techniques include surgical fixation and fusion. In between these 2 options is an alternative therapeutic approach: vertebral augmentation.

Vertebroplasty and kyphoplasty are percutaneous, minimally invasive vertebral augmentation procedures (VAPs) that aim to strengthen weakened vertebral bodies

[a] Department of Neurology, University of Chicago, 5841 S. Maryland Avenue, Chicago, IL 60637, USA; [b] Department of Anesthesia and Critical Care, University of Chicago, 5841 S. Maryland Avenue, Chicago IL, 60637, USA; [c] Division of Pain Management, Pain Medicine Fellowship Program, Department of Anesthesia and Critical Care, University of Chicago Medical Center, 5841 S. Maryland Avenue, MC 4028, Chicago, IL 60637, USA
* Corresponding author.
E-mail address: manitescu@dacc.uchicago.edu

Phys Med Rehabil Clin N Am 33 (2022) 425–453
https://doi.org/10.1016/j.pmr.2022.01.008
1047-9651/22/© 2022 Elsevier Inc. All rights reserved.

and improve pain. During these procedures, cement, most commonly polymethylme-thacrylate (PMMA), is injected into the fracture under image guidance.[3]

Vertebroplasty involves the direct injection of cement into the trabecular vertebral body, whereas kyphoplasty involves deploying an inflatable balloon before cement injection. The first vertebroplasty was performed by Galibert (et al) in 1984 for a case of vertebral hemangioma. Since then, the role of vertebral augmentation has expanded to include the management of vertebral tumors and osteoporotic fractures.[3] In 1988, kyphoplasty was introduced to help restore vertebral body height and assist with spinal alignment.[1] VAPs are considered common interventions for vertebral body compression fractures. Despite this trend, some earlier studies by Buchbinder et all and Kallmes et all, were not entirely supportive of vertebroplasty as a successful procedure in treating pain, mainly having significant limitations such as reduced sample size and using only vertebroplasty and no other techniques.[4,5] More recent evidence, however, shows VAPs to be effective up to 1 year in treating pain and restoring the functional status of patients treated.[6]

ANATOMY AND PHYSIOLOGY

The human spine consists of 33 vertebrae stacked on one another. Vertebrae consist of a vertebral body, pedicles, transverse processes, laminae, and spinous processes from anterior to posterior. In between the vertebrae are shock-absorbing intervertebral discs. The vertebrae articulate superiorly and inferiorly at facet joints. The vertebral column is supported by 3 main ligaments: anterior longitudinal ligament, posterior longitudinal ligament, and ligamentum flavum. All 3 help to maintain the structure of the spine. Vertebral physiology changes based on the location. Cervical vertebrae are capable of rotating and translating in the sagittal plane and can rotate in the coronal plane. In contrast, lumbar vertebrae are well designed for axial loading but are limited in their rotation due to the posterior elements.[7] The thoracic region is more rigid than the lumbar region and 60%–75% of VCFs occur in the thoracolumbar region because of these mechanical differences.[8]

VCFs occur when the weight of the upper body exceeds the ability of the vertebral body to support the load, resulting in a fracture within the vertebral body.[9] The spinal column is traditionally divided into 3 columns: anterior (anterior vertebral body, anterior annulus, anterior longitudinal ligament), middle (posterior vertebral body, posterior annulus, posterior longitudinal ligament), and posterior (structures posterior to the posterior longitudinal ligament) (**Fig. 1**).

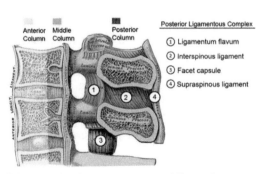

Fig. 1. 3 columns of the spinal column: anterior, middle, and posterior. H. Dexter Barber, Michael P. Powers, Robert V. Walker, David E. Frost, Raymond J. Fonseca, Oral and Maxillo-facial Trauma, Fourth Edition, 2013, 978-1-4557-0554-2. Elsevier Inc.

If a fracture involves 2 or more columns, it is unstable and the patient may require surgery.[10] VCFs are considered stable fractures as they only involve the anterior column of the vertebral body. Fractures that extend beyond the anterior column are termed burst fractures (see **Figs. 1**; **2** and **3**).[10]

CAUSES OF VERTEBRAL COMPRESSION FRACTURES

VCFs may occur due to myriad pathologic conditions. The most common cause is osteoporosis, a condition of reduced bone mineral density. Fragility fractures are a hallmark of osteoporosis and VCFs are the most common form of fragility fractures. Nearly 25% of women over age 50 have at least one VCF. Forty to fifty percent of patients over age 80 have suffered a VCF either acutely or have been diagnosed with a VCF incidentally.[10] Osteoporosis is formally diagnosed with a dual-energy X-ray absorptiometry (DEXA) scan. A T-score of −2.5 or less on a DEXA scan, is an osteoporosis diagnosis, whereas a score from −1 to −2.5 is osteopenia. Risk factors for osteoporosis are categorized as modifiable or nonmodifiable. Nonmodifiable risk factors include advanced age, female gender, Caucasian race, presence of dementia, susceptibility to falls, history of fractures in adulthood, and history of fractures in a first-degree relative. Potentially modifiable risk factors include abusive relationships, alcohol and/or tobacco abuse, presence of estrogen deficiency, early menopause or bilateral oophorectomy, premenopausal amenorrhea for greater than 1 year, frailty, impaired eyesight, insufficient physical activity, low body weight, and low dietary calcium and/or vitamin D deficiency.[9] The amount of force required to cause a fracture varies depending on the severity of a patient's osteoporosis. In moderate osteoporosis, picking up a heavy object or falling off a chair may cause a fracture. In severe osteoporosis, lighter forces may be equally damaging. Nearly 30% of compression fractures occur while patients are in bed.[9]

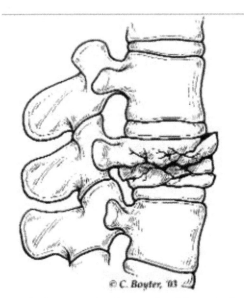

© C. Boyter, '03

Fig. 2. Example of a vertebral compression fracture involving only the anterior column and causing a wedge-shaped deformity. (*From* Solène Prost, Sébastien Pesenti, Stéphane Fuentes, Patrick Tropiano, Benjamin Blondel, Treatment of osteoporotic vertebral fractures, Orthopaedics & Traumatology: Surgery & Research, Volume 107, Issue 1, Supplement, 2021102779, ISSN 1877-0568, https://doi.org/10.1016/j.otsr.2020.102779.).

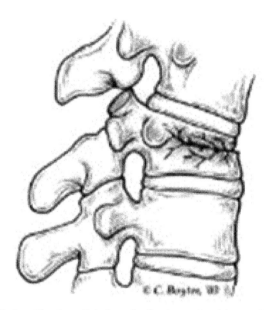

Fig. 3. Example of a burst fracture. Note how the fracture extends beyond the anterior column. (*From* Solène Prost, Sébastien Pesenti, Stéphane Fuentes, Patrick Tropiano, Benjamin Blondel, Treatment of osteoporotic vertebral fractures, Orthopaedics & Traumatology: Surgery & Research, Volume 107, Issue 1, Supplement, 2021102779, ISSN 1877-0568, https://doi.org/10.1016/j.otsr.2020.102779.).

VCF may also be caused by malignant pathology. Up to 30% of advanced cancers metastasize to the spine.[11] Metastasis occurs through one of the 3 routes—hematologic, lymphatic, or direct invasion. Cancers most likely to metastasize to the spine are breast, lung, and prostate. Rates of metastasis with these cancers can reach 70%. Multiple myeloma is another malignancy that spreads to the spine but originates in bone marrow. Not infrequently, patients receive their first cancer diagnosis when they present with a vertebral fracture. Unfortunately, the median survival for patients diagnosed with spinal metastasis is 7 months.[11] Spinal cord compression (SCC) causing neurologic deficits is the most feared complication of malignant spinal lesions.

Spinal hemangioma is the most common primary tumor of the spine. Hemangiomas are vascular tumors that involve a proliferation of capillaries and venous structures. Although generally benign and incidentally found in 11% of autopsies, spinal hemangiomas have the potential to cause significant pain.[12] Approximately 0.9% to 1.2% of hemangiomas will become symptomatic. These tumors may extend into the spinal canal or neural foramina causing neurogenic pain. They may also cause vertebral pain from vertebral fractures.[12]

PRESENTATION AND EVALUATION

VCFs have a significant impact on patients' health. Acute and chronic pain from a VCF may cause physical limitations, and place emotional and psychosocial stress on elderly patients struggling to maintain independent function.[9] If multiple adjacent VCFs are present, they can cause kyphosis of the thoracic spine and lead to secondary complications, including restrictive pulmonary disease, abdominal pain, crowding of internal organs, constipation, and loss of height.[8]

Initial evaluation of patients suspected of having VCFs begins with a history and physical. Patients with acute trauma should be stabilized, followed by a thorough back and neurologic examination. Patients presenting with VCF thought to be secondary to osteoporosis or a malignant process should also undergo a history and physical. Up to one-third of VCFs are not diagnosed as patients often ascribe their symptoms to other pathologies, such as normal aging and arthritis. Patients with VCF may describe their symptoms as acute or chronic back pain. They may have evidence of kyphosis. Pain from a VCF is typically localized to the site of pathology. Pain worsens by standing or walking and decreases when lying flat.[13] A physical examination will reveal tenderness at the site of injury; the straight leg raise test and neurologic examination should be normal.[6] However, in some cases, especially in comminuted, retropulsed fractures, displaced bone fragments may potentially compress the cord and present with signs of cord compression. Percussion over the spinous process with fist closed has been the principal provocative test for diagnosis of a VCF as the projection of the pressure into the broken bone elicits pain; however, more recently, an auscultatory percussion test seems to be more sensitive in identifying those conditions.[14,15]

VCFs are best evaluated by radiographical imaging, with plain frontal and lateral X-rays as the initial radiographical studies of choice. Because 20% to 30% of VCFs are multiple, the entire spine should be imaged. Compression fractures will seem as narrowing of the anterior segment of the vertebral body creating a wedge shape. A 20% or 4 mm loss in vertebral height is considered positive for VCF.[9] Computed tomography (CT) scans are indicated to evaluate fracture stability, other causes of back pain, and more complex fractures observed on a plain radiograph. If neurologic deficits exist, magnetic resonance imaging (MRI) should be used for evaluation. Other advantages of MRI include differentiating between malignancy and osteoporosis and determining the age of a fracture. Bone marrow signaling indicates an acute fracture and can help guide clinical management.[8] If an MRI is contraindicated, a CT myelogram can be used instead. For patients whose symptoms do not improve despite conservative therapy, additional films or a CT/MRI should be obtained.

Treatment

Initial management of a stable VCF is conservative, including bed rest, over-the-counter analgesics, short-term opioids, physical therapy, and back bracing. Bed rest should be limited to a few days to minimize deconditioning. Pharmacologic treatments should be monitored for medication side effects. Nonsteroidal anti-inflammatory drugs (NSAIDS) may increase the risk of gastrointestinal bleeding, particularly in elderly patients.[9] Opioid medications may cause constipation, respiratory depression, urinary retention, and confusion.[11] Back bracing is for patient comfort rather than stability to the spine and can be used for 4 to 12 weeks (or until MRI radiographic proof of healing occurs) as most patients will have significant improvement after 6 to 12 weeks.[13]

For patients who do not respond to conservative treatment, intervention with VAPs is an option. For unstable fractures or when neurologic injury is threatened, surgery is required.[8] While more invasive techniques exist, such as decompression and stabilization with hardware, they are more difficult to perform in osteoporotic bone. Absolute contraindications to both vertebroplasty and kyphoplasty include the infection of the vertebral bone, patient refusal, coagulopathy, bone fragment retropulsion, and allergy to any of the procedure's materials.[8]

Both conservative and surgical treatment will address the immediate fracture. The risk of any type of fracture substantially increases for patients who have suffered already a VCF.[9] Patients with osteoporosis should continue their treatments with preventative measures including regular weight-bearing exercises, calcium, and Vitamin D as well as treatments with bisphosphonates, raloxifene, and calcitonin.[8]

If fractures occur secondary to a malignant process, the patient should be evaluated by a multidisciplinary team. These fractures may require multiple interventions, including surgical, medical, and radiation therapies.[12] Vertebral augmentation treatment of a malignancy-induced fracture will not treat underlying cancer. Unfortunately, most therapies are not curative; rather they focus on meeting goals such as maintaining the quality of life, restoring, or preventing worsening neurologic function, and pain relief. If patients develop SCC, they may require surgical decompression, high-dose steroids, and/or radiotherapy.[13]

In 2010, the Spine Oncology Study Group, a multidisciplinary team of physicians, developed the Spine Instability Neoplastic Score (SINS) to assess the degree of spine stability in metastatic disease of the spine.[16] This scoring system helps guide physicians in determining the appropriate sorting priority of treatments for patients as many individuals will require multiple treatments, such as radiation therapy, surgery, or VAPs to help with pain relief. Some recent studies raised the question of timing of VAPs in relation to radiation as well as the indication of spine surgery.[17] (**Table 1**)

PATIENT SELECTION CRITERIA (INDICATIONS)

Between the 2 most frequent causes of VCF, osteoporosis or malignancy, osteoporotic fractures are by far the more common of the two, usually presenting after minor events, such as a strong cough, a sneeze, carrying an object, or sometimes simply turning in bed.[8,18]

The incidence of VCFs per year for those 50 to 79 years of age is 1.21% for women and 0.68% for men. The percentages increase with age.[14] Risk factors for osteoporotic fractures include smoking, early menopause, alcohol, frailty, dementia, and vitamin D deficiency.[19]

Routine course of a VCF shows a response to conservative regimen (medication, gentle physical therapy, and wearing support braces) over 3 to 4 weeks. In a best-case scenario, the fracture heals within 3 months and pain gradually decreases. In some cases, patients may become severely disabled, with uncontrolled pain and developing major side effects to opioids, such as constipation, urine retention, respiratory distress, and severe nausea. It is in those situations when an acute intervention with VAPs should be considered[20–22]

Malignant infiltration and pathologic fracture of vertebral bodies are associated with significant pain without a natural healing progression. In these cases, intervention is considered earlier in the treatment algorhythm and is intended to control the pain. In a study of 57 patients with malignancy complicated by pathologic fractures, 84% of patients with kyphoplasty or vertebroplasty had total or marked resolution of pain that lasted up to 1 year after the procedure.[23] Bone biopsy can also be performed during the procedure if the type of cancer diagnosis is uncertain. Additionally, tumor burden can be decreased by radiofrequency ablation (RFA) of the metastatic process before cement injection. RFA can be performed via conventional RFA with uni and/or bipedicular cannulas, or via water-cooled RFA using bipedicular cannulas. MRI can distinguish an osteoporotic fracture from a malignant compression fracture with 100% sensitivity and 93% specificity for diagnosing metastatic compression fractures.[24]

Another indication for vertebral augmentation interventions is axial fibrous dysplasia (FD), a benign, genetic, noninherited disease in which bone is replaced with fibrous

Table 1
Spine Instability Neoplastic Index (SINS), Binary scale: stable 0-6 points, unstable 7-18 points; Tertiary scale: stable 0-6 points, impending/potentially unstable 7-12 points, unstable 13-18 points

SINS Component	Score
Location	
Junctional (occiput-C2, C7-T2, T11-L1, L5-S1)	3
Mobile segment (C3-C6, L2-L4)	2
Semirigid (T3-T10)	1
Rigid (S2-S5)	0
Pain	
Yes	3
Occasional pain but not mechanical	1
Pain-free lesion	0
Bone lesion	
Lytic	2
Mixed (lytic/blastic)	1
Blastic	0
Spinal alignment	
Subluxation/translation	4
De novo deformity (kyphosis/scoliosis)	2
Normal alignment	0
Body collapse	
> 50% collapse	3
< 50% collapse	2
No collapse with > 50% body involved	1
None of above	0
Posterolateral involvement of spinal element	
Bilateral	3
Unilateral	1
None	0

From Kim, Y.R., Lee, CH., Yang, S.H. et al. Accuracy and precision of the spinal instability neoplastic score (SINS) for predicting vertebral compression fractures after radiotherapy in spinal metastases: a meta-analysis. Sci Rep 11, 5553 (2021). https://doi.org/10.1038/s41598-021-84975-3.

connective tissue, occurring due to a mutation of guanine nucleotide stimulatory protein on chromosome 20. The result is the widening of the affected bone secondary to ineffective remodeling, resulting in pain and fractures. It is a rare disease that occurs in both males and females equally and reportedly affects 200,000 US citizens per year.[25–29]

The initial treatment is conservative and includes disease monitoring, pain control, and bisphosphonates.[26] VAPs remain a good option for cases with refractory pain nonresponsive to conservative treatments. When indicated, surgical procedures restore spinal stability, correct fractures or severe deformities, and address pain.[30]

Multiple myeloma is a condition often associated with pathologic compression fractures. In this subgroup of patients, kyphoplasty has shown significant improvements, including marked decreases in need for walking aids and oral pain medication after vertebral augmentation surgeries. In another study, more than 80% of patients treated with kyphoplasty reported pain relief.[31,32]

A rare indication for kyphoplasty is vertebral fracture secondary to vertebral angiomas causing intractable pain without neurological symptoms.[33] Additionally, VCFs can sometimes be associated with trauma. However, unless these fractures are displaced, unstable, or osteoporotic in nature, bracing and conservative measures may be sufficient to control pain.

Equipment for Vertebral Augmentation Procedures

VAPs are usually performed on patients in prone positions and under monitored anesthesia care. In some situations, for example, when patients cannot tolerate positioning due to pain or comorbidities (respiratory insufficiency), procedures can be conducted under regional anesthesia (neuraxial such as spinal or epidural anesthesia) or general anesthesia. However, in all situations, the need for local anesthetic and radiographic imaging (whether CT or fluoroscope) is necessary. In all cases, a working cannula, bone cement, cement delivery device, and the balloon tamp in kyphoplasty are necessary.[33]

Cement Type

Injectable PMMA, composite bone cement, biodegradable bone cement, calcium phosphate cement (CPC), and acrylic cement are the commonly used cement materials.[34,35]

Cement should be injected when it has a toothpaste-like consistency to decrease complications from extravasation, as the flow characteristics of the cement change over time. Also, cement injection should be stopped when the anterior two-thirds of the vertebral body are filled and cement is homogenously distributed between both endplates (usually about 2.5–4 mL) under continuous fluoroscopic monitoring.[34,36]

Silicone as an augmentation material has biomechanical properties similar to bone; one study shows that silicone can be used as an alternative to PMMA.[37]

RISKS AND CONTRAINDICATIONS

The American Society of Bone and Mineral Research recommends not using kyphoplasty or vertebroplasty in acute osteoporotic compression fractures.[38]

Another contraindication of kyphoplasty is severe vertebral fracture or when the facet joint has been involved in the fracture.[39] Similarly, kyphoplasty should be reconsidered in vertebral body fracture with posterior cortical breach is due to concern of a higher chance of cement extravasation and neurologic injury.[40] As noted above other absolute contraindications for VAPs are: complete vertebral body collapse (very high chance of cement extravasation,[41,42] coagulopathy, unstable fracture, allergy to cement, tumor mass with the involvement of the spinal canal, and infection, locally, in the vertebral column or systemic infection.[33,41]

The most common and feared complications of VAPs are cement leak with extravasation of the cement. Most of those incidents occurring in almost 40% of the procedures are asymptomatic. Less than 1% of the patients suffer from devastating cement leaks. Cement extravasation can present by the leak of the polymethyl methacrylate in paravertebral soft tissue and muscles, the intervertebral disc, the track of the needle, the veins in the epidural and paravertebral area, the neural foramina, and the spinal canal. More aggressive cement leakage to the inferior vena cava, the heart, and the kidney has been reported with fatal consequences.[43–46]

Cement extravasation may cause pulmonary embolism, which is among the most feared and fatal complications of the procedure.[47–49] Recompression of the augmented vertebrae is a common postoperative complication, which is defined as an increase of local kyphosis angle more than or equal to 10° or loss of vertebral height more than or equal to 15%.[50–52] New fractures of the adjacent vertebrae can be caused by cement leakage within the intervertebral disc.[53]

Thermal damage to the nearby soft tissue, spine, and/or spinal nerves can happen either due to cement polymerization at 85°C or during RFA of vertebral tumor if the probe is too close to the posterior vertebral wall.[54] Bone necrosis secondary to cement injection has been reported [55] and so did infection as an infrequent but serious complication.[56]

In a case report, cerebellar stroke and leptomeningeal carcinomatosis occurred after cervical vertebroplasty from a metastatic osteolytic bone lesion from breast cancer. It occurred after extravasation of the cement and tumor to the vertebral artery.[57]

Other extremely rare complications include gall bladder necrosis and pneumothorax with cardiac perforation, which was described in a couple of case reports following a vertebroplasty procedure.[58,59]

Technical Description of Procedures Techniques

As mentioned, VAP aims toward reducing and immobilization of the fracture within the vertebral body, subsequently decreasing pain and at times re-establishing height.[60]

Of the VAPs available, vertebroplasty is the VAPs that allows the injection of the cement through a needle into the cancellous bone, without the use of the balloon; as such, the consistency of the cement may be more fluid (**Fig. 4**).[61]

The initial small case series of vertebroplasty used in the treatment of cervical hemangioma was conducted by Galliber and colleagues in Europe in 1984. It took almost 9 more years before the first vertebroplasty was performed in the United States by Jensen and colleagues. Since then, vertebroplasty has gained widespread popularity, mainly owing to its high success rate, low complications, less sedation requirement, and the short to no hospital stay.[62]

Vertebroplasty is best performed using both biplanar fluoroscopy and CT scans for the accurate evaluation of needle location and cement distribution. Monitoring cement distribution under direct fluoroscopic control is a very important aspect of the procedure to reach the lowest complication rate. This is because in vertebroplasty the consistency of the cement is more fluid and injected under higher pressure. As such, it is more likely to leak through vertebral clefts often present in fractured vertebrae.[60]

Usually, vertebroplasty is conducted under local anesthesia or with conscious sedation, which is preferred in patients at high risk of general anesthesia.[63] The access path depends on the level of the vertebral segment. In the lumbar spine, transpedicular access is used. In the thoracic vertebrae, an extrapedicular, intercostovertebral approach is recommended. In the cervical vertebrae, anterolateral access is used.[64]

Vertebroplasty is preferred if the MRI spine has shown suspicion of bone marrow swelling and edema caused by osteoporotic compression fracture with minimal underlying compression.[65] Depositing the cement in compressed vertebrae with minimal height loss will stabilize the fracture and cement all fractured portions together.

Hardware to perform vertebroplasty is also important as steps must be taken to reduce possible complications of the procedure. As such, in one cohort study, 2 types of cannulas, one with a front opening and one with a side opening, were evaluated for the rate of cement leak. Charts of 811 patients who underwent vertebroplasty were analyzed between March 2016 and September 2018. The study found that the side-opening cannula decreased the rate and severity of D type and S type leaks compared

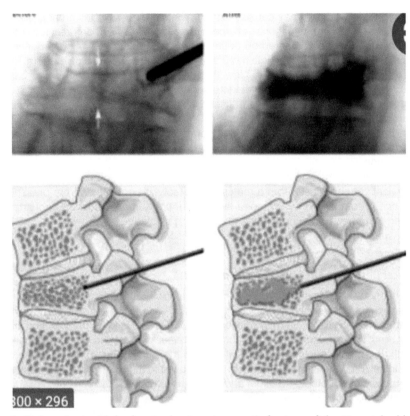

Fig. 4. Male patient with back pain due to osteoporotic fracture of the L1 vertebral body, frontal and the lateral fluoroscopy view—needles were placed in the posterior third of L1 vertebral body and cement injection was finished under continuous fluoroscopy. (*From* Denoix E, Viry F, Ostertag A, et al. What are the predictors of clinical success after percutaneous vertebroplasty for osteoporotic vertebral fractures? Eur Radiol 2018 287. 2018;28(7):2735 to 2742. https://doi.org/10.1007/S00330-017-5274-1).

with the front-opening cannula.[66] Similarly, in a retrospective study, a new generation of robotic-assisted vertebroplasty was reviewed, showing the safety and efficacy of the procedure.[67,68]

Kyphoplasty

Balloon kyphoplasty is a procedure in which fluoroscopic guidance is used to insert a trocar into the vertebral body. Unlike vertebroplasty, an inflatable balloon is then placed in the vertebral body to compress the bone and create a cavity for subsequently injecting cement under low pressure. This process decreases the chances of extravasation (**Fig. 5**).[61]

Kyphoplasty has gained more use in recent years as multiple observational studies indicate that it seems to provide more pain control—both short term and long term—than vertebroplasty.[69] However, kyphoplasty is technically more challenging and may potentially be more painful for the patient during balloon inflation.[70]

Access is usually a mono- or bilateral trans- or extrapedicular approach using biplanar fluoroscopy or CT guidance. The working cannula is placed into the

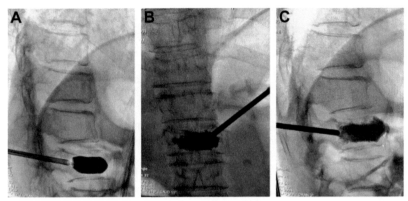

Fig. 5. (*A*) The balloon was inflated to restore the height of the fractured vertebra and to create a cavity within the vertebra. (*B*) Frontal fluoroscopy view when bone cement was injected into the fractured vertebra. (*C*) Lateral fluoroscopy view when bone cement was injected into the fractured vertebra. (*From* Yang H, Chen L, Zheng Z, et al. Therapeutic effects analysis of percutaneous kyphoplasty for osteoporotic vertebral compression fractures: A multicentre study. J Orthop Transl. 2017;11:73. https://doi.org/10.1016/J.JOT.2017.04.003).

posterior aspect of the vertebral body and from here a drill is advanced under a direct lateral fluoroscopy view to 2 to 3 mm behind the anterior vertebral wall; this step is essential to creating a small cavity whereby the balloon will subsequently be inflated. The balloon is inflated using visual volume and pressure controls to reduce the fractured vertebra and to produce a cavity that is monitored under fluoroscopic control. Usually, inflation stops when one of the following is achieved or noticed: pressure is above 250 psi, balloon contacts the cortical surface of the vertebral body or expands beyond the border of the vertebral body, or height of the vertebra is restored. Successively, balloons are retracted and cement polymethyl methacrylate (PMMA) is injected using a blunt cannula under continuous fluoroscopic control to prevent cement leakage.[34]

If the compression fracture occurs due to metastatic disease, a RFA probe is inserted after the drill; this allows for decreased tumor burden locally before kyphoplasty. Several systems will provide RFA energy to control local tumor burden.

The DFINE spinal tumor ablation with radiofrequency (STAR) system and the Osteo-Cool RFA system are minimally invasive techniques for the palliative treatment of painful metastatic spinal lesions. The STAR ablation system received US Food and Drug Administration (FDA) 510(k) clearance in 2012. OsteoCool was cleared in November 2015 and then introduced into clinical practice in January 2016. Thoracic, lumbar, and sacral vertebral body lesions are ideal targets for treatment, although pedicle lesions also can be treated. The devices cannot be used in patients with cardiac pacemakers or other electronic device implants. The use of these devices is contraindicated in patients with cervical (C1–C7) vertebral lesions. This procedure may be particularly useful for patients with radioresistant tumors, recurrent pain after radiation therapy, or posterior vertebral body metastatic tumors, and in patients who have reached the maximum limit of radiation dose.

When the unipedicular system is used, conventional RFA can be achieved via the StabiliT, DFine system. As only 1 cannula is placed, possible less fluoroscopic exposure of the proceduralist can occur.[71,72]

Navigation toward the tumor lesion is conducted via the curved tip that has steering capabilities and is performed from one side (unipedicular)(see **Figs. 1** and **2**).

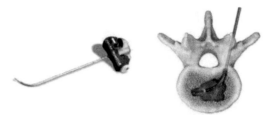

Fig. 6. Cannula and radiofrequency probe; curved probe allows unipedicular approach to treat vertebral metastases (from DFINE). Used with permission of ©2021 Merit Medical Systems.

Fig. 6 Cannula and radiofrequency probe; curved probe allows the unipedicular approach to treat vertebral metastases (from DFINE). A bipedicular approach can also be used depending on the size and location of the lesion. Once the STAR ablation instrument is positioned within the center of the lesion, the ablation electrode is extended and radiofrequency energy is delivered. Two thermocouples within the ablation system monitor the temperature within the tumor in real-time. An ablation zone can be 3 × 2 cm or 2 × 1.5 cm. The zone depends on the location of the thermocouples (10/15 mm from the center of the ablation zone or 5/10 mm) (see **Fig. 3**). Once the temperature reaches 50°C in the proximal thermocouple (the temperature at the most peripheral point of the ablation zone), delivery of energy is discontinued. As with conventional RFA, repositioning the ablation instrument may be needed to target another component of the lesion. Multiple ablation zones are typically created to cover the lesion as much as safely possible (**Fig. 7**).

After DFINE ablation, vertebral augmentation can be performed with the direct deposit of cement through the cannula as per routine vertebroplasty. After the cavity is created, the procedure of the DFINE StabiliT Vertebral Augmentation system is deployed. An Ultra-high viscosity StabiliT ER^2 Bone Cement fills the cavity and permeates the surrounding bone to stabilize the fracture. Several studies suggest a lower cement leakage rate with this system (**Figs. 8–10**).[73–75]

RFA systems work when alternating currents flow through probes inside the lesion resulting in coagulation necrosis and tissue death.[76]

The OsteoCool system has 2 internally water-cooled bipolar probes that are heated to 70°C to prevent charring. Because of the 2 probes, heat synergistically extends into the tumor and creates a spherical lesion bigger than the one created by a conventional

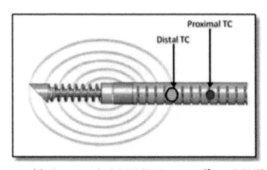

Fig. 7. Radiofrequency ablation zone in DFINE STAR system (from DFINE). Used with permission of ©2021 Merit Medical Systems.

A
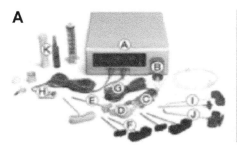

B
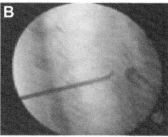

Fig. 8. (*A*) radiofrequency device and application system: (A) multiplex controller, (B) hydraulic assembly, (C) master syringe, (D) activation element, (E) locking delivery cannula, (F) StabiliT introducer-working cannula and stylet, (G) activation element cable, (H) handswitch cable, (I) straight line osteotome, (J) power curve navigating osteotome, and (K) StabiliT ER2 bone cement. (*B*) Intraoperative X-ray of L1 vertebra (lateral view) using RFK. (*From* Yang H, Chen L, Zheng Z, et al. Therapeutic effects analysis of percutaneous kyphoplasty for osteoporotic vertebral compression fractures: A multicentre study. J Orthop Transl. 2017;11:73. https://doi.org/10.1016/J.JOT.2017.04.003).

probe. As the probes are continuously cooled, the temperature is constant around them and, thus, char formation is reduced (**Fig. 11**).

Heat from the probes ablates most of the metastatic vertebral tumor which, in some cases, involves the entire vertebral body. Specificity in heat lesioning time and intensity through the OsteoCool system depends on probe size (7 mm, 10 mm, 15 mm, or 20 mm).

With OsteoCool, the procedure starts in a prone patient under mild to moderate conscious sedation and with extensive local anesthetic infiltration of the subcutaneous tissue and periosteum. To access the vertebral bone requires the OsteoCool bone access kit. The kit has Kyphon-equivalent sizes (8G, 10G, 13 G) for the location of the

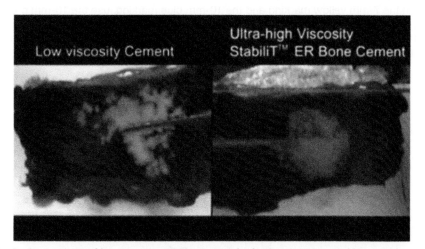

Fig. 9. Comparison of low viscosity Cement versus high viscosity Cement.((*From* Robertson S.C. (2011) Percutaneous Vertebral Augmentation: StabilitiT A New Delivery System for Vertebral Fractures. In: Alexandre A., Masini M., Menchetti P. (eds) Advances in Minimally Invasive Surgery and Therapy for Spine and Nerves. Acta Neurochirurgica Supplementum, vol 108. Springer, Vienna. https://doi.org/10.1007/978-3-211-99370-5_29).

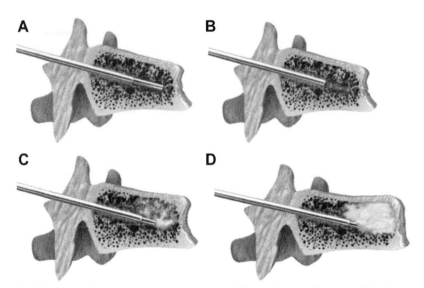

Fig. 10. (*A*) VectecoR cement staging osteotome, (*B*) vertebral cavity created by the osteotome, (*C*) placement of delivery cannula, (*D*) StabiliT ER cement delivery. (*From* Robertson S.C. (2011) Percutaneous Vertebral Augmentation: StabilitiT A New Delivery System for Vertebral Fractures. In: Alexandre A., Masini M., Menchetti P. (eds) Advances in Minimally Invasive Surgery and Therapy for Spine and Nerves. Acta Neurochirurgica Supplementum, vol 108. Springer, Vienna. https://doi.org/10.1007/978-3-211-99370-5_29).

lesion. After routine drilling and bone biopsy, radiofrequency probes are placed in the 2 trocars. For convenience, the drill in the OsteoCool bone access kit is marked at the level of exit from the trocar and color coded to correspond to the intended lesion. The company recommends upgrading to the bigger size: If the color-coded drill falls between the 7-mm yellow marking and the 10-mm blue marking, use the 10-mm probe. We, however, downgrade to a smaller size if the tumors treated are too close to vertebral body walls. A thermocouple probe can be placed via a transforaminal approach at the level of fracture to monitor the temperature around the spinal nerves (**Fig. 12**).

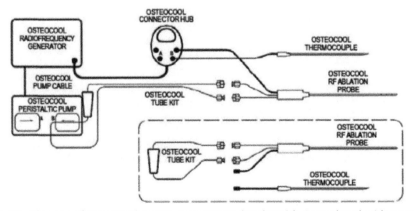

Fig. 11. Diagram of OsteoCool system connections (Medtronic). Reproduced with permission of Medtronic, Inc.

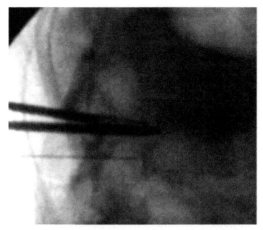

Fig. 12. Thermocouple placed via transforaminal approach at the posterior border of the vertebral border allows the monitoring of the spinal canal (personal image).

Because of the built-in safety features, a physician can identify the optimal position for ablation from anteroposterior and lateral views. Thus, once placed in the vertebral body, the tip of the styletted trocar ensures a safe posterior margin of the lesion during ablation; the tip of the probe ensures the anterior margin of the lesion (**Fig. 13**).

Once the probes are placed and the water-cooled system is connected, a single application of radiofrequency at 70°C ablates the tumor. Ablation success depends on time, probe size, and destruction of local nociceptors. A cavity is created that is subsequently filled with cement via routine kyphoplasty. No additional repositioning or cleaning of char from the probe is necessary. Pain relief is immediate, and patients are discharged home the same day. The temperature close to the electrodes, often placed in the middle of the tumor, can be 20°–25° higher than the temperature recorded at the thermocouple tip (**Fig. 14**).

The main benefit of the bipolar probe is the presence of grounding and active electrodes on the same probe. This minimizes manipulations and decreases side effects with increasing the efficacy in addition to decreasing the ablation power and time with less of a heat sink effect.[76,77]

Implantable Systems for Vertebral Augmentation Procedures

While both kyphoplasty and vertebroplasty have been successful procedures in decreasing pain and stabilizing fractures, the presence of the cement may, theoretically, predispose subsequent vertebrae to additional fractures especially in

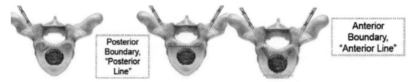

Fig. 13. Distal tip of the stylet provides the posterior boundary beyond which the lesion does not extend. Similarly, the most distal tip of the drill provides the anterior boundary above which the lesion does not extend (Medtronic). Reproduced with permission of Medtronic, Inc.

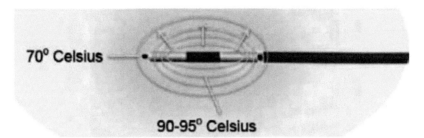

Fig. 14. OsteoCool probe is temperature controlled reaching 70° centigrade at the tip and 90 to 95 centigrades within the lesion (Medtronic). Reproduced with permission of Medtronic, Inc.

osteoporotic conditions. As such, several procedures were developed with the preservation of vertebrae elasticity in mind. These procedures use various surgical grade plastic (PEEK) or metal implants to decrease the amount of cement used in fracture stabilization of the VAPs.

The SpineJack Implant System

The SpineJack Implant System consists of a Vexim SpineJack expandable titanium implant and acrylic cement. Recently approved by the FDA to treat VCFs, SpineJack is mainly designed to restore the height of the vertebral body. However, US-based outcome data are lacking (**Fig. 15**).[35,72,78]

The device includes a mechanical working system (unlike a hydraulic system) that helps in controlled, progressive reductions of the vertebral fracture. The benefits of this feature include providing 3D support and facilitating the restoration of the injured vertebrae (**Fig. 16**).[79]

A retrospective study to evaluate the efficacy and safety of the SpineJack System included analyses of 30 patients with VCFs between November 2018 and February 2020. The patients underwent 53 vertebral augmentations with 106 SpineJack implants; every vertebrae treated had 2 devices deployed. The results: markedly decreased pain scores, improved local kyphotic angle, and regained vertebral height without marked adverse effects.[78]

THE KIVA SYSTEM

The Kiva System is an alternative surgical approach to treat osteoporotic VCFs. A nitinol Osteo Coil guidewire is advanced through a cannula percutaneously until the nitinol coil is appropriately located in the cancellous portion. Next, a polyether ether ketone (PEEK) (containing 15% barium sulfate for radiopacity to form a nesting,

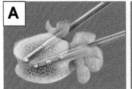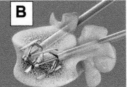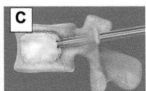

Fig. 15. Stryker Spine Jack System. (*A*) closed system. (*B*) opened system. (*C*) cemented implant. Used with permission of © Stryker 1998-2022.

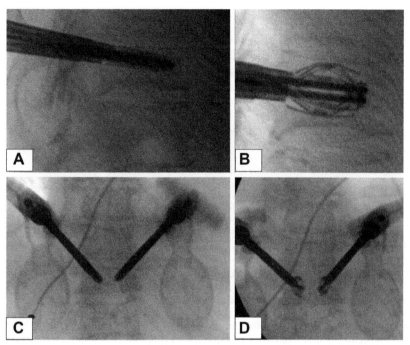

Fig. 16. Spinal fixation in vertebral compression fracture with spine jack. A and C lateral and posteroanterior view of deployed and closed spine jack system. B and D lateral and posteroanterior view of deployed and opened spine jack system. Used with permission of © Stryker 1998-2022.

cylindrical column) is implanted incrementally over the coil until the desired restoration of the fractured vertebral height is achieved. The guidewire is removed and bone cement is injected and deployed within the implanted cage. One comparative study of Kiva to regular balloon kyphoplasty showed identical outcomes, including the effective relief of pain (**Fig. 17**).[72,80,81]

SKyphoplasty

Sky Kyphoplasty is a Sky bone expander polymer device.[82] While less used in the US, it involves the deployment of stiff polymer "accordioned" into a crenelated configuration by rotating the device handle. A disadvantage is that cannula, unlike kyphoplasty, cannot be repositioned (**Fig. 18**).

THE OSSEOFIX SYSTEM

The Osseofix System (Alphatec Spine Inc., Carlsbad, California, USA) is an expandable titanium mesh cage that is placed in the anterior third of the vertebra with osteoporotic compression fracture. It prevents kyphotic deformity by compacting the surrounding trabecular bone and re-establishes the vertebral height by the cage; cement is then injected into the cage. A major benefit of this system is that it uses far less cement than regular balloon kyphoplasty, thus decreasing the possibility of a cement leak. This system provides immediate and long-term benefits in reducing kyphotic deformity and pain (**Fig. 19**).[83,84]

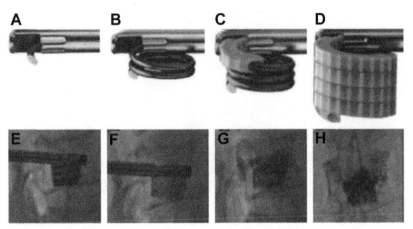

Fig. 17. A percutaneous nitinol coil guidewire (*A*) is coiled within the cancellous portion of the fractured vertebral body. (*B*) Afterward, a radiopaque PEEK implant is delivered incrementally via the nitinol coil guidewire (*C*) and then a nesting, cylindrical column is formed that provides vertical displacement, which may restore the height of the fractured vertebra (*D*) [10]. Fluoroscopic images illustrate the procedure using the Kiva VCF treatment system (*E*). After removing the coil, a radiopaque PEEK implant was implanted (*F*) to provide structural support to the vertebral body, and bone cement was injected through the implant, as shown by lateral (*G*) and anteroposterior (*H*) fluoroscopic images. (*From* Yang H, Chen L, Zheng Z, et al. Therapeutic effects analysis of percutaneous kyphoplasty for osteoporotic vertebral compression fractures: A multicentre study. J Orthop Transl. 2017;11:73. https://doi.org/10.1016/J.JOT.2017.04.003).

VERTEBRAL BODY STENTING

Vertebral body stenting is an expandable, titanium, intrasomatic device used for percutaneous vertebral augmentation. It is designed to use the balloon of regular kyphoplasty to achieve an expansion ratio of 400%. By using ligamentotaxis, it reduces the fracture size of the spine, with good recovery of the vertebral height by injecting the PMMA. After the expansion phase, the balloon is deflated and then removed without the previous risk of losing vertebrae height. Indications for VBS: osteoporotic VCFs from T10-L5 without the involvement of the posterior vertebral edge classified after Genant, grade 2 and grade 3 with a kyphotic angulation of greater than 15 (**Fig. 20**).[85–89]

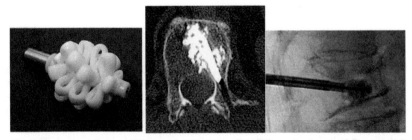

Fig. 18. Appearance of the stiff polimer, photography, CT scan image, and fluoroscopic image. (*From* Rashid R, Munk PL, Heran M, Malfair D, Chiu O. SKyphoplasty. Can Assoc Radiol J. 2009;60(5):273 to 278. https://doi.org/10.1016/J.CARJ.2009.07.004).

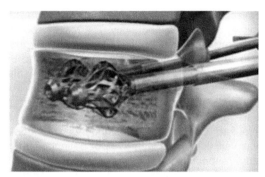

Fig. 19. Osseofix devise Courtesy of https://clinicaltrials.gov/ct2/show/NCT00961714.

OUTCOME DATA

Conservative measures, at least in some osteoporotic fractures, have shown relatively good outcomes, which means debates about early use of VAPs will be ongoing. The main disadvantage of postponing the procedure is decreased functional ability, which is especially prevalent in the elderly population and primarily due to pain.

As many techniques and systems are currently available, several studies have evaluated these procedures—comparing them on short- and long-term outcomes for pain relief, maintaining and improving functional status, and reducing fractures.

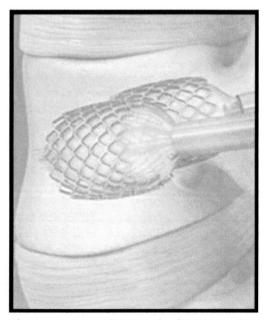

Fig. 20. Vertebral Body stenting System. (*From* England RW, Gong A, Li T, et al. Clinical outcomes and safety of the SpineJack vertebral augmentation system for the treatment of vertebral compression fractures in a United States patient population. J Clin Neurosci. 2021;89:237 to 242. https://doi.org/10.1016/J.JOCN.2021.04.031).

One large, randomized control trial compared conservative medical nonsurgical care—including medication versus kyphoplasty. The results show statistically significant improved pain scores and quality of life scores in the kyphoplasty group after 1 month of therapy. However, the benefits were lost at 1-year and 2-year end points.[90]

Three systematic review studies assessed the efficacy and safety of kyphoplasty and vertebroplasty for the management of VCFs.

The first study was a systematic literature review to evaluate patient pain relief, regaining mobility and vertebral body height, complication rate, and occurrence of new adjacent vertebral fractures when patients underwent kyphoplasty and vertebroplasty. Pain relief was very satisfying with 87% of patients with vertebroplasty and 92% with kyphoplasty, respectively, reporting excellent pain relief. Vertebral height restoration was possible using kyphoplasty and for a group of patients using vertebroplasty when decreased height was not significant (<20%). Cement leakage occurred in 41% of vertebroplasty and 9% of patients with kyphoplasty. New fractures occurred in both groups at a rate similar to the general osteoporotic population that previously suffered vertebral fractures.[1]

The second study evaluated the safety and efficacy of balloon kyphoplasty and vertebroplasty in indirect comparisons from case series; the authors concluded that kyphoplasty showed better pain relief and better quality of life.[91]

The third study evaluated vertebroplasty adverse effects in osteoporotic VCFs. Among 1136 interventions performed on 793 patients, the most common complication was cement leak outside of the vertebral body ranging from 3.3% to 75.6%; most patients were asymptomatic but a few were serious.[92]

DISCUSSION

Among the VAPs, direct comparison between vertebroplasty and kyphoplasty have shown comparable results for long term pain relief and functional outcomes; however, differences do exist in particular related to the cement leak outside the vertebral body (**Table 2**).[93]

Several early studies were not enthusiastic about VAPs[4,5] and at times recommended vertebroplasty versus kyphoplasty for the treatment of symptomatic osteoporotic VCFs refractory to conventional medical therapy is, at best, a level III.[91] Many of the early studies cited here had somewhat questionable designs and had some difficulty recruiting[4]; as those early data, current data are supporting the use of kyphoplasty in the treatment of VCFs [6]

Table 2
Direct comparison between kyphoplasty and vertebroplasty

	Vertebroplasty	Kyphoplasty
Long-term pain relief	Comparable	Comparable
Short-term pain relief	Inferior	Inferior
Functional outcome	Comparable	Comparable
New adjacent vertebral compression fracture	Comparable	Comparable
Injected cement volume	Higher	Lower
Improvement kyphotic angle	Inferior	Superior
Cement extravasation rate	Higher	Lower
Procedure rime	Shorter	Longer
Material cost	Lower	Higher

Table 3
Comparison of radiofrequency kyphoplasty (RFK) and balloon kyphoplasty (BKP) in the treatment of vertebral compression fractures

	RFK	BKP
Pain relief	Better after operation and up to 1 y	Inferior
Vertebral Height	Better initially then decreases over time	Stays the same but may decrease with increased tumor burden
Decreased Kyphotic angel	Better immediately and at 6 mo	Inferior
Cement	High viscosity	Low viscosity
Cement Leakage	Less	More with no major significance
Operation Time	More	Less

VAPs are used in malignant lesions of the vertebral body either alone or accompanied by RFA. Given that tumor burden is reduced with RFA, reported pain is favorable at 1 year when compared with the simple kyphoplasty; **Tables 3** and **4**[94–98] summarizes this finding.[94,95]

Exothermic reaction during the deployment of cement used with the peek implant during Kiva procedure may contribute to the pain relief in the absence of RFA in patients with osteolytic metastatic lesions.[98]

VAPs have incorporated many techniques that contribute to the treatment of pain in VCFs. A direct comparison between those can be found in **Table 5**.[83]

Another big metanalysis reviewed the 7 most commonly used treatments of osteoporotic VCFs, including vertebroplasty (VP), kyphoplasty (KP), SpineJack system (SJ), radiofrequency kyphoplasty (RFK), kiva system (Kiva), SKyphoplasty system (SK), and conservative treatment. In a review of 56 studies with 6974 patients, the results showed that the SK was the best intervention in decreasing VAS scores and recovering middle vertebral height. Radiofrequency Kyphoplasty was the best intervention to improve ODI scores and decrease the incidence of new fractures. SpineJack was the best intervention to restore kyphosis angle, and Kiva was the best intervention to reduce the incidence of bone cement leakage. In general, SK may be the most effective treatment in relieving pain, improving quality of life, and recovering vertebral body height and kyphotic angle, while RFK may be the safest intervention.[99]

Table 4
Comparison of Kiva implant and balloon kyphoplasty (BKP) in treating osteolytic metastasis of the spine in 23 patients with Osteolytic lesions.

	Kiva Implant with PMMA	BKP
Pain Relief	Same	Same
Vertebral Body Height	Same	Same
Gardner Angle	Same	Same
Visual Analog Scale	Same	Same
Oswestry Disability Index	Same	Same
Cement Leak	Less	More

Table 5
Characteristics of third-generation vertebral augmentation devices

Percutaneous Device	Indications	Mechanism	Working Components	Type	Material
Kyphon	VBF due to Recent trauma, osteoporosis, metastasis	Fracture reduction Cavity creation Space filled with cement	Balloon	Not permanent	Elastomer
Vertebral body stenting (VBS)	VBF due to Recent trauma, osteoporosis, metastasis	Fracture reduction Cavity creation Space inside stent filled with cement	Balloon + deformable metallic component	Permanent	Titanium
Spine Jack	VBF due to Recent and not recent trauma, osteoporosis metastasis	Fracture reduction Cavity creation Space around jack filled with cement	Deformable metallic component	Permanent	Titanium
OsseoFix	VBF due to Osteoporotic collapse	Fracture reduction Cavity creation Titanium mesh cavity filled with cement	Deformable metallic component	Permanent	Titanium

Abbreviation: VBF, vertebral compression fracture.

SUMMARY

VCFs whether osteoporotic or metastatic are a relatively common appearance in elderly populations. Left untreated, severe pain from fractures predisposes patients to immobility and functional decline. VAPs offer the advantage of treating acute pain, stabilizing fracture and, in some cases, vertebral re-expansion. In addition, RFA in vertebral metastases is able to locally control tumor burden. Yet, effective as they are, these procedures may be associated with some complications; however, only a few are serious with most adverse effects being asymptomatic.

CLINICS CARE POINTS

- More than 700,000 vertebral fractures occur in the United States, which is more than the number of hip and ankle fractures combined.
- Health care costs of vertebral fractures from osteoporosis alone will reach $25 billion by 2025.
- The most common indication for vertebral augmentation procedures (VAPs) is vertebral compression fractures (VCFs) most likely secondary to osteoporosis versus malignancy.
- Cement leakage and cement extravasation are the most common and feared complications of VAPs.
- All VAPs improved pain in a statistically significant way.
- Every procedure has its benefits, and treatments should be tailored for each patient. In general, SKyphoplasty is the best intervention to decrease VAS scores and recover middle vertebral height; Radiofrequency Kyphoplasty is the best intervention to improve ODI scores and decrease the incidence of new fractures; SpineJack is the best intervention to restore kyphosis angle; and Kiva is the best intervention to reduce the incidence of bone cement leakage.

DISCLOSURE

M. Anitescu: Advisory Board: Medtronic, Boston Scientific, Funded Research: Abbott, Boston Scientific, Fellowship Grant: Abbott, Boston Scientific, Medtronic.

REFERENCE

1. Hulme PA, Krebs J, Ferguson SJ, et al. Vertebroplasty and kyphoplasty: a systematic review of 69 clinical studies. Spine (Phila Pa 1976) 2006;31(17): 1983–2001.
2. Chandra RV, Maingard J, Asadi H, et al. Vertebroplasty and kyphoplasty for osteoporotic vertebral fractures: what are the latest data? AJNR Am J Neuroradiol 2018;39(5):798.
3. Armsen N, Boszczyk B. Focus on vertebroplasty and kyphoplasty. Eur J Trauma 2005;5:433–41.
4. Kallmes DF, Comstock BA, Heagerty 4. PJ, et al. A randomized trial of vertebroplasty for osteoporotic spinal fractures. New Engl J Med 2009;361(6):569–79.
5. Buchbinder R, Osborne RH, Ebeling PR, et al. A randomized trial of vertebroplasty for painful osteoporotic vertebral fractures. New Engl J Med 2009; 361(6):557–68.
6. Beall DP, Chambers MR, Thomas S, et al. Prospective and multicenter evaluation of outcomes for quality of life and activities of daily living for balloon kyphoplasty

in the treatment of vertebral compression fractures: the EVOLVE trial. Neurosurgery 2019;84(1):169–78.

7. Bogduk N. Functional anatomy of the spine. Handb Clin Neurol 2016;136:675–88.

8. Alexandru D, So W. Evaluation and management of vertebral compression fractures. Perm J 2012;16(4):46.

9. Old JL, Calvert M. Vertebral compression fractures in the elderly. Am Fam Physician 2004;69(1):111–6. Accessed. www.aafp.org/afp. [Accessed 25 October 2021]. Available at:.

10. Donnally CJ III, DiPompeo CM, Varacallo M. Vertebral compression fractures. StatPearls 2021. Accessed. https://www.ncbi.nlm.nih.gov/books/NBK448171/. [Accessed 15 November 2021]. Available at:.

11. Mattie R, Brar N, Tram JT, et al. Vertebral augmentation of cancer-related spinal compression fractures: a systematic review and meta-analysis. Spine 2021; 46(24):1729–37.

12. Tafti D, Cecava ND. Spinal Hemangioma. StatPearls 2021. Accessed. https://www.ncbi.nlm.nih.gov/books/NBK532997/. [Accessed 25 October 2021]. Available at:.

13. Whitney E, Alastra AJ. Vertebral Fracture. StatPearls 2021. Accessed. https://www.ncbi.nlm.nih.gov/books/NBK547673/. [Accessed 25 October 2021]. Available at:.

14. Dai L, Zeng R. Physical examination of the musculoskeletal system. In handbook of clinical diagnostics. Singapore: Springer; 2020. p. 241–53.

15. Dydyk AM, Das JM. Vertebral Augmentation. StatPearls 2021. Accessed. https://www.ncbi.nlm.nih.gov/books/NBK547726/. [Accessed 25 October 2021]. Available at:.

16. Fisher CG, Dipaola CP, Ryken TC, et al. A novel classification system for spinal instability in neoplastic disease: an evidence-based approach and expert consensus from the spine oncology study group. Spine (Phila Pa 1976 2010; 35(22):E1221–9.

17. Kim YR, Lee CH, Yang SH, et al. Accuracy and precision of the spinal instability neoplastic score (SINS) for predicting vertebral compression fractures after radiotherapy in spinal metastases: a meta-analysis. Sci Rep 2021;11(1):5553.

18. Felsenberg D, Silman AJ, Lunt M, et al. Incidence of vertebral fracture in europe: results from the European Prospective Osteoporosis Study (EPOS). J Bone Miner Res 2002;17(4):716–24.

19. Old JL, Calvert M. Vertebral Compression Fractures in the Elderly. Am Fam Physician 2004;69(1):111–6. Accessed. www.aafp.org/afp. [Accessed 21 September 2021]. Available at:.

20. Park SY, Modi HN, Suh SW, et al. Epidural cement leakage through pedicle violation after balloon kyphoplasty causing paraparesis in osteoporotic vertebral compression fractures - a report of two cases. J Orthop Surg Res 2010;5(1):54.

21. Lee HM, Park SY, Lee SH, et al. Comparative analysis of clinical outcomes in patients with osteoporotic vertebral compression fractures (OVCFs): conservative treatment versus balloon kyphoplasty. Spine J 2012;12(11):998–1005.

22. Hide I, Gangi A. Percutaneous vertebroplasty: history, technique and current perspectives. Clin Radiol 2004;59(6):461–7.

23. Fourney DR, Schomer DF, Nader R, et al. Percutaneous vertebroplasty and kyphoplasty for painful vertebral body fractures in cancer patients. J Neurosurg 2003;98(1 Suppl):21–30.

24. Jung H-S, Jee W-H, McCauley TR, et al. Discrimination of Metastatic from Acute Osteoporotic Compression Spinal Fractures with MR Imaging1. Radiographics 2003;23(1):179–87.

25. Chapurlat RD, Orcel P. Fibrous dysplasia of bone and McCune–Albright syndrome. Best Pract Res Clin Rheumatol 2008;22(1):55–69.

26. DiCaprio MR, Enneking WF. Fibrous dysplasia. Pathophysiology, evaluation, and treatment. J Bone Joint Surg Am 2005;87(8):1848–64.

27. Kashima TG, Nishiyama T, Shimazu K, et al. Periostin, a novel marker of intramembranous ossification, is expressed in fibrous dysplasia and in c-Fos–overexpressing bone lesions. Hum Pathol 2009;40(2):226–37.

28. Treatment results of 5 patients with fibrous dysplasia and review of the literature. Case Rep Endocrinol 2015;2015:1–7.

29. Mancini F, Corsi A, DeMaio F, et al. Scoliosis and spine involvement in fibrous dysplasia of bone. Eur Spine J 2009;18(2):196.

30. Fitzpatrick KA, Taljanovic MS, Speer DP, et al. Imaging findings of fibrous dysplasia with histopathologic and intraoperative correlation. AJR Am J Roentgenol 2012;182(6):1389–98.

31. McDonald RJ, Gray LA, Cloft HJ, et al. The effect of operator variability and experience in vertebroplasty outcomes. Radiology 2009;253(2):478–85.

32. Dudeney S, Lieberman IH, Reinhardt MK, et al. Kyphoplasty in the treatment of osteolytic vertebral compression fractures as a result of multiple myeloma. J Clin Oncol 2002;20(9):2382–7.

33. Dydyk AM, Das JM. Vertebral Augmentation. StatPearls 2021. Accessed. https://www.ncbi.nlm.nih.gov/books/NBK547726/. [Accessed 20 September 2021]. Available at:.

34. Armsen N, Boszczyk B. Vertebro-/kyphoplasty history, development, results. Eur J Trauma 2005;31(5):433–41. https://doi.org/10.1007/S00068-005-2103-Z.

35. Diallo M, Kouitcheu R, Touta A, et al. [Percutaneous kyphoplasty using expandable SpineJack® implant for the treatment of osteoporotic vertebral fractures]. Pan Afr Med J 2020;35:1–8.

36. Chavali R, Resijek R, Knight SK, et al. Extending polymerization time of polymethylmethacrylate cement in percutaneous vertebroplasty with ice bath cooling. Am J Neuroradiol 2003;24(3):545–6.

37. Schulte TL, Keiler A, Riechelmann F, et al. Biomechanical comparison of vertebral augmentation with silicone and PMMA cement and two filling grades. Eur Spine J 2013;22(12):2695–701.

38. Ebbeling PR, Akesson A, Bauer DC, et al. The efficacy and safety of vertebral augmentation: a second ASBMR task force report. J Bone Miner Res 2019; 34(1):3–21.

39. Molloy S, Sewell MD, Johnson P, et al. Is balloon kyphoplasty safe and effective for cancer-related vertebral compression fractures with posterior vertebral body wall defects? J Surg Oncol 2016;113(7):835–42.

40. Fessl R, Roemer FW, Bohndorf K. Perkutane vertebroplastie der osteoporotischen wirbelkörperfraktur: Erfahrungen und prospektive ergebnisse bei 26 patienten mit 50 frakturen. RoFo 2005;177(6):884–92.

41. Denaro V, Maffulli N, Longo UG, et al. Vertebroplasty and kyphoplasty. Clin Cases Miner Bone Metab 2009;6(2):125 /pmc/articles/PMC2781232/. Accessed September 21, 2021.

42. Dydyk AM, Das JM. Vertebral Augmentation. StatPearls 2021. Accessed. https://www.ncbi.nlm.nih.gov/books/NBK547726/. [Accessed 22 October 2021]. Available at:.

43. Kim MH, Lee AS, Min SH, et al. Risk factors of new compression fractures in adjacent vertebrae after percutaneous vertebroplasty. Acta Radiol 2004;45(4):440–5.

44. Chung SE, Lee SH, Kim TH, et al. Renal cement embolism during percutaneous vertebroplasty. Eur Spine J 2006;15(Suppl 5):590.

45. Barragán-Campos HM, Vallée J-N, Lo D, et al. Percutaneous vertebroplasty for spinal metastases: complications. Radiology 2006;238(1):354–62.

46. Kim SY, Seo JBS, Do KH, et al. Cardiac perforation caused by acrylic cement: a rare complication of percutaneous vertebroplasty. AJR Am J Roentgenol 2005; 185(5):1245–7.

47. Quesada N, Mutlu GM. Pulmonary embolization of acrylic cement during vertebroplasty. Circulation 2006;113(8):295–6.

48. Kim YJ, Lee JW, Park KW, et al. Pulmonary cement embolism after percutaneous vertebroplasty in osteoporotic vertebral compression fractures: incidence, characteristics, and risk factors. Radiology 2009;251(1):250–9.

49. Choe DH, Marom EM, Ahrar K, et al. Pulmonary embolism of polymethyl methacrylate during percutaneous vertebroplasty and kyphoplasty. AJR Am J Roentgenol 2012;183(4):1097–102.

50. An Z, Chen C, Wang J, et al. Logistic regression analysis on risk factors of augmented vertebra recompression after percutaneous vertebral augmentation. J Orthop Surg Res 2021;16(1):374.

51. Yu W, Liang D, Yao Z, et al. Risk factors for recollapse of the augmented vertebrae after percutaneous vertebroplasty for osteoporotic vertebral fractures with intravertebral vacuum cleft. Medicine (Baltimore) 2017;96(2):e5675.

52. Kim Y-Y, Rhyu K-W. Recompression of vertebral body after balloon kyphoplasty for osteoporotic vertebral compression fracture. Eur Spine J 2010;19(11):1907.

53. Uppin AA, Hirsch JA, Centenera LV, et al. Occurrence of new vertebral body fracture after percutaneous vertebroplasty in patients with osteoporosis. Radiology 2003;226(1):119–24.

54. Radev BR, Kase JA, Askew MJ, et al. Potential for thermal damage to articular cartilage by PMMA reconstruction of a bone cavity following tumor excision: a finite element study. J Biomech 2009;42(8):1120–6.

55. Huang KY, Yan JJ, Lin RM. Histopathologic findings of retrieved specimens of vertebroplasty with polymethylmethacrylate cement: case control study. Spine (Phila Pa 1976 2005;30(19):E585–8.

56. Walker DH, Mummaneni P, Rodts GE. Infected vertebroplasty: report of two cases and review of the literature. Neurosurg Focus 2004;17(6):1–3.

57. Bing F, Dandache J, Mettey L, et al. Cerebellar stroke and leptomeningeal carcinomatosis following cement leakage into the vertebral artery during cervical vertebroplasty. J Vasc Interv Radiol 2021;0(0). https://doi.org/10.1016/J.JVIR.2021.09.013.

58. Yu H, Peng Y, Tuo H, et al. Gallbladder gangrene after percutaneous vertebroplasty, an uncommonpresentation of vascular complication: a case report and analysis of the causes. J Int Med Res 2021;49(3):1–8.

59. Kim SJ, Kim KH. Unusual pneumothorax with cardiac perforation by bone cement after percutaneous vertebroplasty. Am J Respir Crit Care Med 2021;203(8): E29–30.

60. Laredo JD, Hamze B. Complications of percutaneous vertebroplasty and their prevention. Skeletal Radiol 2004;33(9):493–505.

61. McCall T, Cole C, Dailey A. Vertebroplasty and kyphoplasty: a comparative review of efficacy and adverse events. Curr Rev Musculoskelet Med 2008;1(1):17.

62. Multimodality imaging guidance in interventional pain management - Google Books. Available at: https://books.google.com/books?hl=en&lr=&id=FGT0DAAAQBAJ&oi=fnd&pg=PA331&dq=d-fine+kyphoplasty&ots=jlo5_rVNOA&sig=4XvOB-hRtGZc1P-7Hw0T-uzD7BM#v=onepage&q=d-fine kyphoplasty&f=true. [Accessed 25 October 2021]. Accessed.

63. Gangi A, Guth S, Imbert JP, et al. Percutaneous vertebroplasty: indications, technique, and results. Radiographics 2003;23(2):e10.

64. Mathis JM. Percutaneous vertebroplasty: complication avoidance and technique optimization. AJNR Am J Neuroradiol 2003;24(8):1697 /pmc/articles/PMC7973982/. Accessed September 22, 2021.

65. Goz V, Errico TJ, Weinreb JH, et al. Vertebroplasty and kyphoplasty: national outcomes and trends in utilization from 2005 through 2010. Spine J 2015;15(5):959–65.

66. Zixian W, Linqiang Y, Mo L, et al. Comparison of cement leakage rate and severity after percutaneous vertebroplasty for osteoporotic vertebral compression fractures using front-opening versus side-opening cannulas. Orthopedics 2021;44(3):134–40.

67. Shi B, Hu L, du H, et al. Robot-assisted percutaneous vertebroplasty under local anaesthesia for osteoporotic vertebral compression fractures: a retrospective, clinical, non-randomized, controlled study. Int J Med Robot Comput Assist Surg 2021;17(3):e2216.

68. Boonen S, Meirhaeghe J Van, Bastian L, et al. Balloon kyphoplasty for the treatment of acute vertebral compression fractures: 2-year results from a randomized trial. J Bone Miner Res 2011;26(7):1627–37.

69. Yang H, Chen L, Zheng Z, et al. Therapeutic effects analysis of percutaneous kyphoplasty for osteoporotic vertebral compression fractures: A multicentre study. J Orthop Transl 2017;11:73.

70. Buchbinder R, Johnston RV, Rischin KJ, et al. Percutaneous vertebroplasty for osteoporotic vertebral compression fracture. Cochrane Database Syst Rev 2018;2018(11). https://doi.org/10.1002/14651858.CD006349.PUB4.

71. Reißberg S, Lüdeke L, Fritsch M. Comparison of radiation exposure of the surgeon in minimally invasive treatment of osteoporotic vertebral fractures – Radiofrequency kyphoplasty versus balloon kyphoplasty with cement delivery systems (CDS). RöFo 2019;192(01):59–64.

72. Long Y, Yi W, Yang D. Advances in vertebral augmentation systems for osteoporotic vertebral compression fractures. Pain Res Manag 2020;2020:3947368.

73. Study Suggests lower cement leakage rate with DFINE radiofrequency targeted vertebral augmentation™ (RF-TVA) in the treatment of vertebral compression fractures | business wire. Accessed. https://www.businesswire.com/news/home/20110705006194/en/Study-Suggests-Cement-Leakage-Rate-DFINE-Radiofrequency. [Accessed 25 October 2021]. Available at:.

74. Robertson SC. Percutaneous vertebral augmentation: StabilitiT a new delivery system for vertebral fractures. Acta Neurochir Suppl 2011;108(108):191–5.

75. Mattyasovszky SG, Kurth AA, Drees P, et al. Minimal-invasive Zementaugmentation von osteoporotischen Wirbelkörperfrakturen mit der neuen Radiofrequenz-Kyphoplastie. Oper Orthop Traumatol 2013;26(5):497–512.

76. Saravana-Bawan S, David E, Sahgal A, et al. Palliation of bone metastases—exploring options beyond radiotherapy. Ann Palliat Med 2019;8(2):168–77.

77. Pezeshki PS, Woo J, Akens MK, et al. Evaluation of a bipolar-cooled radiofrequency device for ablation of bone metastases: preclinical assessment in porcine vertebrae. Spine J 2014;14(2):361–70.

78. England RW, Gong A, Li T, et al. Clinical outcomes and safety of the SpineJack vertebral augmentation system for the treatment of vertebral compression fractures in a United States patient population. J Clin Neurosci 2021;89:237–42.

79. Vanni D, Pantalone A, Biggosi F, et al. New perspective for third generation percutaneous vertebral augmentation procedures: Preliminary results at 12 months. J Craniovertebral Junction Spine 2012;3(2):47–51.

80. Tutton SM, Pflugmacher R, Davidian M, et al. KAST study: the kiva system as a vertebral augmentation treatment-A safety and effectiveness trial: a randomized, noninferiority trial comparing the kiva system with balloon kyphoplasty in treatment of osteoporotic vertebral compression fractures. Spine (Phila Pa 1976 2015;40(12):865–75.

81. Olivarez LMR, Dipp JM, Escamilla RF, et al. Vertebral augmentation treatment of painful osteoporotic compression fractures with the Kiva VCF treatment system. SAS J 2011;5(4):114.

82. Tong SC, Eskey CJ, Pomerantz SR, et al. SKyphoplasty": a single institution's initial experience. J Vasc Interv Radiol 2006;17(6):1025–30.

83. Vanni D, Galzio R, Kazakova A, et al. Third-generation percutaneous vertebral augmentation systems. J Spine Surg 2016;2(1):13.

84. Eschler A, Ender SA, Ulmar B, et al. Cementless fixation of osteoporotic VCFs using titanium mesh implants (OsseoFix): preliminary results. Biomed Res Int 2014; 2014:853897.

85. Disch AC, Schmoelz W. Cement augmentation in a thoracolumbar fracture model: reduction and stability after balloon kyphoplasty versus vertebral body stenting. Spine (Phila Pa 1976 2014;39(19):E1147–53.

86. Furderer S, Anders M, Schwindling B, et al. [Vertebral body stenting. A method for repositioning and augmenting vertebral compression fractures]. Orthopade 2002;31(4):356–61.

87. Klezl Z, Majeed H, Bommireddy R, et al. Early results after vertebral body stenting for fractures of the anterior column of the thoracolumbar spine. Injury 2011; 42(10):1038–42.

88. Joseph RN, Swift AJ, Maliakal PJ. Single centre prospective study of the efficacy of percutaneous cement augmentation in the treatment of vertebral compression fractures. Br J Neurosurg 2013;27(4):459–64.

89. Kruger A, Oberkircher L, Figiel J, et al. Height restoration of osteoporotic vertebral compression fractures using different intravertebral reduction devices: a cadaveric study. Spine J 2015;15(5):1092–8.

90. Wardlaw D, Cummings SR, Meirhaeghe J Van, et al. Efficacy and safety of balloon kyphoplasty compared with non-surgical care for vertebral compression fracture (FREE): a randomised controlled trial. Lancet 2009;373(9668):1016–24.

91. Taylor RS, Fritzell P, Taylor RJ. Balloon kyphoplasty in the management of vertebral compression fractures: an updated systematic review and meta-analysis. Eur Spine J 2007;16(8):1085.

92. Ploeg WT, Veldhuizen AG, The B, et al. Percutaneous vertebroplasty as a treatment for osteoporotic vertebral compression fractures: a systematic review. Eur Spine J 2006;15(12):1749–58.

93. Yu W, Liang D, Jiang X, et al. Comparison of effectiveness between percutaneous vertebroplasty and percutaneous kyphoplasty for treatment of osteoporotic vertebral compression fracture with intravertebral vacuum cleft. Zhongguo Xiu Fu Chong Jian Wai Ke Za Zhi 2016;30(9):1104–10.

94. Dalton BE, Kohm AC, Miller LE, et al. Radiofrequency-targeted vertebral augmentation versus traditional balloon kyphoplasty: radiographic and morphologic outcomes of an ex vivo biomechanical pilot study. Clin Interv Aging 2012;7:525–31.

95. Miller MA, Race A, Gupta S, et al. The role of cement viscosity on cement-bone apposition and strength: an in vitro model with medullary bleeding. J Arthroplasty 2007;22(1):109–16.

96. Baroud G, Crookshank M, Bohner M. High-viscosity cement significantly enhances uniformity of cement filling in vertebroplasty: an experimental model and study on cement leakage. Spine (Phila Pa 1976 2006;31(22):2562–8.

97. Anselmetti GC, Zoarski G, Manca A, et al. Percutaneous vertebroplasty and bone cement leakage: clinical experience with a new high-viscosity bone cement and delivery system for vertebral augmentation in benign and malignant compression fractures. Cardiovasc Intervent Radiol 2008;31(5):937–47.

98. Bornemann R, Jansen TR, Kabir K, et al. Comparison of radiofrequency-targeted vertebral augmentation with balloon kyphoplasty for the treatment of vertebral compression fractures: 2-year results. Clin Spine Surg 2017;30(3):E247–51.

99. Chang M, Zhang C, Shi J, et al. Comparison between 7 osteoporotic vertebral compression fractures treatments: systematic review and network meta-analysis. World Neurosurg 2021;145:462–70.e1.

Sympathetic Blocks for Sympathetic Pain

Melissa E. Phuphanich, MD, MS[a],*, Quinn Wonders Convery, PharmD, BCPS[a,b],
Udai Nanda, DO[a,c,d], Sanjog Pangarkar, MD[a,e,f]

KEYWORDS

- Sympathetic blocks • Sympathetic neurolysis • Sympathetic pain
- Sympathetically maintained pain • Neuropathic pain • Vascular pain

KEY POINTS

- The SNS has broad effects on pain perception that include suppressing or amplifying pain perception depending on disease state and chronicity.
- Sympathetic blockade can provide relief from pain secondary to vascular, and neuropathic pain states.
- Specific medications and techniques are described to achieve sympathetic blockade systemically, regionally, and locally.
- Sympathetic blocks with local anesthetic can serve diagnostic, prognostic, and therapeutic purposes. Neurolytic (chemical and thermal) techniques are selected for therapeutic effect.

INTRODUCTION

The sympathetic nervous system (SNS) is a division of the autonomic nervous system, which is responsible for involuntary localized responses to stress. Activation of this system has widespread effects involving the cardiac, integumentary, pulmonary,

[a] Physical Medicine and Rehabilitation Department (117), Veterans Administration Greater Los Angeles Healthcare System, 11301 Wilshire Boulevard, Los Angeles, CA 90073, USA; [b] Department of Pharmacy, VA Greater Los Angeles Health Care System, Los Angeles CA, USA; [c] Headache Center of Excellence, Department of Physical Medicine and Rehabilitation, Interventional Pain Service, VA Greater Los Angeles Health Care System, Los Angeles CA, USA; [d] Pain Medicine Fellowship Program, Division of Physical Medicine and Rehabilitation, Department of Medicine, University of California Los Angeles- UCLA, Los Angeles, CA, USA; [e] Inpatient and Interventional Pain Service, Department of Physical Medicine and Rehabilitation, VA Greater Los Angeles Health Care System, Los Angeles CA, USA; [f] Division of Physical Medicine and Rehabilitation, Department of Medicine, University of California Los Angeles- UCLA, Los Angeles, CA, USA
* Corresponding author. Physical Medicine and Rehabilitation Department (117), Veterans Administration Greater Los Angeles Healthcare System, 11301 Wilshire Boulevard, Los Angeles, CA 90073.
E-mail address: mphuphanich@gmail.com

Phys Med Rehabil Clin N Am 33 (2022) 455–474
https://doi.org/10.1016/j.pmr.2022.02.002
1047-9651/22/© 2022 Elsevier Inc. All rights reserved.

urinary, and digestive systems, among others. The attendant "fight-or-flight" reflex is coordinated with other systemic neural and hormonal responses to stress that modulate pain, behavior, and mood.

The Role of the SNS and Pain

The interplay between the SNS and pain is complex. In healthy individuals, the SNS acts to depress acute pain perception via descending inhibition of nociception through sympathetic cell bodies in the intermediolateral tracts of the spinal cord. Paradoxically, chronic activation of the SNS may augment pain and lead to sympathetically maintained pain (SMP), known as complex regional pain syndrome (CRPS). Evidence suggests the SNS modulates both nociceptive activation and peripheral inflammation, which is considered a causal agent for visceral pain.[1,2] As such, sympathetic blocks (SBs) are often performed to treat both SMP (ie, CRPS) and sympathetic independent pain (ie, visceral pain).

In addition, there is cortical interaction between pain and the SNS. The cortical areas of the brain that respond to nociceptive stimuli overlap with areas activated by the SNS via stressful stimuli.[3] This interaction is primarily mediated by the anterior cingulate cortex (ACC), insular cortex (IC), prefrontal cortex (PFC), and amygdala; fittingly, μ opioid receptors are abundant in these areas.[4] Moreover, functional MRI demonstrates distinct alterations in brain structure and activity that occur with chronic pain, suggesting that acute and chronic pain are processed differently by the SNS. In fact, neuroimaging studies in chronic pain demonstrate reductions in gray matter volume in the IC, ACC, and PFC, and abnormal activation in the ACC, PFC, and amygdala in response to pain.[5] Suitably, these findings are similar to areas commonly dysregulated in depressed patients.

Objective

SBs temporarily reduce the activity of the sympathetic nerves running parallel to the spine and are frequently used to treat vascular, visceral, and neuropathic pain conditions despite a lack of high-quality evidence.[3,4] This review aims to summarize the available evidence regarding the indications, contraindications, techniques, efficacy, and pharmacology of SBs for sympathetically maintained pain. This article will also focus on best practices for commonly performed SBs including (1) the stellate ganglion block (SGB) and (2) the lumbar sympathetic block (LSB).

USES OF SBs
Diagnostic SBs

Diagnostic blocks are commonly used to evaluate pain attributed to a sympathetic etiology. Local anesthetic is introduced adjacent to sympathetic neural structures, such as the stellate or lumbar ganglion, temporarily disrupting neural function to an affected limb or region.[4] A diagnostic injection should attempt to block the sympathetic chain without inadvertent somatic spread. For this reason, image guidance is used to confirm needle position and proximity to the sympathetic chain, often through fluoroscopy, ultrasound, or computerized tomography. False positives can occur due to unintentional spread of anesthetic to adjacent somatic nerves or epidural space, systemic absorption of anesthetic, or placebo effect.[3] As such, performing postprocedure assessment of sympathetic blockade is essential to confirm diagnostic accuracy.[5]

Techniques for diagnostic SBs include local anesthetic sympathetic blocks (LASBs), intravenous regional sympathetic blockade (IRSB), and systemic alpha-adrenergic blockade (SAAB).

Local anesthetic sympathetic blocks

Local anesthetics exert their action primarily by interrupting neural conduction via inhibition of voltage-gated sodium channels.[6] The concentrations of local anesthetics vary, commonly between 0.5% and 4%. The variation in potency is the result of the differences in lipid solubility that improves diffusion through neural membranes.

Local anesthetics differ in duration of effect due to variability in affinity for plasma proteins. Anesthetics with a higher affinity to plasma proteins have a higher affinity for sodium channels and a longer duration of action. Local anesthetics have the greatest efficacy on small, "fast" pain fibers (ie, Aδ- and Aγ-fibers).[6,7] The dosing of local anesthetics depends on several factors, including the type of procedure and the area injected. A general recommendation is to use the smallest dose necessary to achieve the desired effect.

Concerns with local anesthetics include potential for allergy, although true allergy is very rare.[7] Most reactions are thought to be related to preservatives or metabolites within the local anesthetic. Adverse effects include local ischemic necrosis of tissues and systemic toxicity that ranges from mild central nervous symptoms (ie, drowsiness) to seizure and cardiovascular collapse. Epinephrine is a common adjuvant to local anesthetics to prolong duration and decrease systemic absorption. **Table 1** reviews the pharmacology of the commonly used amide local anesthetics.

Intravenous regional sympathetic blockade

IRSB uses a tourniquet technique (ie, Bier Block) to administer medications from varying pharmacologic classes to an isolated limb. The technique used for tourniquet application differs between medical centers but is often similar to that used for intravenous regional anesthesia (IVRA) during surgery. Sedation may be used before tourniquet inflation for patient comfort if the limb is sensitive.[3]

Medications used in IRSB include guanethidine (not available in the United States due to availability at the time of writing), phentolamine, reserpine, lidocaine, prilocaine, clonidine, bretylium (not available in the United States), hydralazine, methyldopa, droperidol, ketorolac, and ketanserin (not available in the United States). In **Table 2**, the pharmacologic properties of common medications used in IRSB are provided in further detail.

IRSBs may be used for CRPS and other sympathetically mediated diseases but their use in diagnostic blocks has been limited.[5] The tourniquet itself can also cause relief of hyperalgesia and cause false positives. Concerns with IRSB include systemic circulation of medication with the sudden release of the tourniquet.[12,13] To decrease this risk a dual-bladder tourniquet or 2 cuffs may be used to provide additional control over release of tourniquet pressure. Some tourniquet systems also have an IVRA safety lockout to prevent unintentional deflating.

Systemic alpha-adrenergic blockade

SAAB uses the following medications: phentolamine, prazosin, phenoxybenzamine, nifedipine, clonidine, and pamidronate. In SAAB, there is systemic administration of medication without the use of a tourniquet. It is thought that the mechanism of SAAB is separate from cutaneous vasodilation and skin temperature changes.[5] One mechanism of pain relief from alpha-adrenergic blockers arises from the reduction of noradrenergic nociception.[17] Another potential mechanism of action is thought to be through immune modulation by reducing inflammatory cytokines, interleukin 1-beta, TNF-alpha, and prostaglandins that may be present in the neurons after nerve injury. Caution is advised for patients with hypotension. **Table 3** describes alpha-

Table 1
Local anesthetic pharmacology

Generic Name	Brand Names	Dosing	Onset of Effect	Protein Binding	Duration of Effect	How Supplied	Warnings
Bupivacaine hydrochloride[8]	Marcaine®, Sensorcaine®	Variable. • For example, sympathetic block using 0.25% bupivacaine: Inject 50–125 mg (20–50 mL) Maximum dose 90 mg/kg[6]	Variable. • Diagnostic nerve blocks: 15–20 min[6,9]	95%	• Elimination half-life (adults): 2.7 h • Duration of effect: 4–6 h	Injection Solution: 0.25%, 0.5%, 0.75%, 31.25 mg/1 mL, 40 mg/1 mL	BBW: • Buprenorphine 0.75% is not recommended for obstetric anesthesia due to reports of cardiac arrest with difficult resuscitation or death during epidural anesthesia. • Buprenorphine 0.75% concentration should be reserved for procedures when a high degree of muscle relaxation and prolonged effect are necessary Contraindicated in: • persons with sensitivity to product or to amide-like products • Contraindications for spinal injections: arrhythmias, local injection at the site, septicemia, severe hemorrhage, severe hypotension, and shock

Drug	Max individual dose		Onset/Tmax	Elimination half-life	Available solutions	Contraindications
Lidocaine hydrochloride[10]	Xylocaine®	Max individual dose 4.5 mg/kg; total dose, 300 mg	60%–80%	Variable • For example, infiltrative anesthesia onset is < 2 min • Diagnostic nerve blocks within 5 min[12]	Elimination half-life: 1.5–2 h	• Epidural solution: 1% • Injection solution: 0.5%, 1%, 1.5%, 2%, 4% • Intravenous solution: 2%	Contraindicated in: • persons with sensitivity to product or to amide-like products
Ropivacaine[11]	Naropin®	Variable: • Major nerve block (eg, brachial plexus block) using 0.5% solution: 175–250 mg (35–50 mL) dose must be adjusted to site of administration and patient status	94%	Variable. • Tmax, epidural block: 17–97 min (adult) • Tmax, plexus block: 54 min (adult)	Variable elimination half-life. • Epidural: 4.2–7.1 h (block and infusion; adult) • Plexus block: 6.8 h (adult) • Intravascular: 1.8 h (adult)	• Epidural solution: 0.5% • Injection solution: 1 gm/500 mL, 0.5%, 2 mg/1 mL, 200 mg/100 mL, 400 mg/200 mL, 5 mg/1 mL, 1000 mg/200 mL, 500 mg/100 mL, 7.5 mg/1 mL, 10 mg/1 mL	Contraindicated in: • persons with sensitivity to product or to amide-like products

Abbreviations: BBW, United States Food and Drug Administration Black Box Warning; Tmax, time of maximum concentration observed.

Table 2
Intravenous regional sympathetic blockade pharmacology

Generic Name	Brand Name	Mechanism of Action	Dosing	How Supplied	Warnings
Guanethidine monosulfate[14]	Ismelin®	Blocks the reuptake of NE and depletes stores in postganglionic nerve terminals	IV: 10–30 mg alone or in combination with heparin and lidocaine	—	Contraindications: • Hypersensitivity to guanethidine • MAOI therapy, concurrent or within 1 wk • Overt congestive heart failure • Pheochromocytoma
Phentolamine mesylate[15]	Regitine®	Alpha-adrenergic blocker that produces peripheral vasodilation and cardiac stimulation. The cardiovascular response is attributable to sympathomimetic, parasympathomimetic, and histamine-like actions	IV: variable • 1 mg/kg • 25–75 mg administered over 20 min	Injection Powder for Solution: 5 mg	Contraindications: • MI or history of MI, coronary insufficiency, angina, or other evidence suggestive of CAD • Hypersensitivity to phentolamine or related compounds
Reserpine[16]	—	Depletes NE stores and inhibits NE synthesis	IV: 0.5 mg in the upper extremity or 1 mg in the lower extremity in one study[17]	• Oral tablet: 0.1 mg, 0.25 mg. • Previously available in IV formulation	Contraindications: • Active peptic ulcer • Electroshock therapy • Known hypersensitivity • Depression, especially with suicidal tendencies • Ulcerative colitis

Abbreviations: CAD, coronary artery disease; IV, intravenous; MAOI, monoamine oxidase inhibitor; MI, myocardial infarction; NE, norepinephrine.

Table 3
Alpha-adrenergic blockade pharmacology

Generic Name	Brand Name	Mechanism of Action	Dose	How Supplied	Warnings
Prazosin hydrochloride[18]	Minipress®	A quinazoline derivative, causes reduction in total peripheral resistance that directly relaxes vascular smooth muscle that may be related to postsynaptic alpha adrenoreceptor blockade		• Oral capsule: 1 mg, 2 mg, 5 mg	Contraindication: • Hypersensitivity to prazosin, any other component of the product, or other quinazolines
Phenoxybenzamine hydrochloride[19]	Dibenzyline®	Binds covalently to smooth muscle in a nonselective, irreversible alpha-adrenergic blockade	IV: 5 mg with lidocaine in a solution of alcohol, propylene glycol, hydrochloric acid, and isotonic saline[20,21]	• Oral capsule: 10 mg • Injection solution: 50 mg/mL (not available in the United States)	Contraindication: • Any condition compromised by hypotension • Hypersensitivity to phenoxybenzamine
Nifedipine[22]	Procardia®, Adalat®, Afeditab®, Nifedical®	Selectively inhibits the transmembrane influx of calcium ions		• Oral capsule, liquid filled: 10 mg, 20 mg • Oral tablet, extended release: 30 mg, 60 mg 90 mg	Contraindications: • Cardiogenic shock • Concomitant use of strong CYP450 inducers • Hypersensitivity to nifedipine or any component of the medication
Clonidine hydrochloride[23]	Catapres®, Duraclon®, Kapvay®	Centrally acting alpha-agonist		• Epidural solution: 0.1 mg/mL, 0.5 mg/mL • Injection solution 5 mg/1 mL • Oral tablet: 0.1 mg, 0.2 mg, 0.3 mg • Oral tablet, extended release: 0.1 mg	Conditions: • Bleeding diathesis • Concurrent use with anticoagulant therapy • Epidural administration above the C4 dermatome • Hypersensitivity, sensitization, or allergic reaction to clonidine • Injection site infection

adrenergic blockade pharmacology. Note that at the time of publication, prazosin and nifedipine are only available in the United States in oral formulations (**Table 4**).

Prognostic SBs

Diagnostic SB techniques are used in a stepwise fashion to predict responses to more invasive procedures such as pulsed radiofrequency ablation (RFA) of sympathetic ganglion and surgical sympathectomy.[5] Generally, higher-risk neurolytic procedures are reserved for candidates who show consistent, but favorable short-term responses to the initial diagnostic and prognostic modalities.[3] Clinical practice guidelines for pain management of cancer generally recommend diagnostic and/or prognostic LASBs to determine efficacy as well as associated neurologic deficits before any neurolytic procedure.[24]

Therapeutic SBs

Although LASBs, IRSBs, and SAABs may be used as treatments, therapeutic SBs also include neurolytic and radiofrequency denervation techniques. Neurolytic blocks use solutions that denature neural tissue and can provide significant pain relief for months, but may lead to adverse events.

Chemical neurolytic pharmacology

Chemical neurolysis is a form of more permanent nerve blockade.[5,25] After a positive initial response to sympathetic nerve blockade, semipermanent methods of nerve damage including thermal neurolysis (ie, RFA), cryoablation, and chemical neurolysis can be used. Chemical neurolysis interrupts pain signal transmission by Wallerian degeneration distal to the injection site. Examples of chemical neurolytic agents include botulinum toxins, phenol 3% to 15% and ethyl alcohol 10% to 100%. For the latter, evidence suggests that a concentration of at least 35% to 60% is needed for efficacy (**Table 4**).[9,25–27]

Alcohol also works by denaturing proteins, fatty substance extraction, and precipitation of lipoproteins and mucoproteins.[26] Phenol diffuses into axon and perineural blood vessels within basal lamina tubes and denatures proteins. Phenol acts as a local anesthetic at lower concentrations, and a neurolytic at higher concentrations.

Table 4
Chemical neurolytic pharmacology

Generic Name	Dosing	Onset of Effect	Duration of Effect	How Supplied
Dehydrated alcohol (Ethanol, Ethyl alcohol)[29]	0.5–50 mL depending on concentration and location	Anesthetic effect occurs immediately, maximal neurolytic effect 24–48 h[9]	Variable, generally, 2–6 mo is expected[9]	Dehydrated alcohol injection; not <98% by volume, 5 mL
Phenol[30]	Safe practice suggests <1 g per treatment session, typical volumes are between 0.5 and 3 mL. 8.5 g is considered a lethal dose[9]	See above	See above	Injection kit: 6%, 5 mL

Alcohol is typically more painful upon injection. Alcohol is also water soluble and spreads rapidly from the site of injection; thus, neurolysis with alcohol requires larger volumes. Phenol can be formulated with either sterile water or glycerin and diffuses more slowly into the target tissues. There is little evidence comparing the efficacy of phenol and alcohol, but it is noted that alcohol may be associated with more neuritis. Typical duration of effect for phenol is between 8 to 12 weeks, whereas alcohol can last between 12 and 24 weeks.[27]

Alcohol should be avoided in patients prescribed disulfiram for alcoholism. There is a potential for accumulation of acetaldehyde which may cause tachycardia, nausea, and vomiting.[28] Complications of neurolysis can include deafferentation pain, bleeding, infection, and damage to nearby tissues. Should a neurolytic agent be administered intravascularly, systemic toxicity can occur (ie, seizures, central nervous system depression, and cardiovascular collapse), or if neurolysis of a motor nerve occurs, motor paralysis can be a consequence.[25,27]

PATIENT SELECTION FOR SBs

SBs are generally considered safe and well-tolerated procedures. Similar to other interventional pain procedures, SBs are contraindicated in the setting of infection, poor glycemic control, allergies to injectate, malignancy near treatment site, uncorrectable coagulopathy (INR > 1.5 or platelet count <50k), inability to lie prone or supine, patient refusal, or inability to provide informed consent. Before SBs, all imaging should be reviewed to assess anatomic alteration with neurologic deficits noted.

For each patient, the indication and physiologic effects of specific SBs must be considered. For example, SGBs are contraindicated in patients with severe emphysema given that unopposed parasympathetic activity may decrease respiratory compliance. In cancer patients, SBs are relatively contraindicated in the setting of neutropenia or antiblastic chemotherapy due to increased risk of infection.[24] Specific contraindications will be further discussed for each SB in the sections below.

SBs FOR SMP

SBs for SMP include the SGB and LSB. These blocks are first-line interventional procedures for CRPS of the upper and lower extremity, respectively.[31]

The Stellate Ganglion Block

Indications and specific contraindications for SGBs
The SGB was first trialed in the 1930s for angina pectoris and is now the most common SB performed. For pain practitioners, SGBs are primarily used to treat CRPS and peripheral vascular disease of the upper extremity; however, multiple case reports using SGBs for other conditions have been reported (**Table 5**).[32–37] Specific contraindications for SGBs are poorly controlled emphysema, recent myocardial infarction, preexisting counter lateral nerve palsy, or cardiac conduction blocks.[32]

Applicable anatomy of SGBs
The SGB with local anesthetic acts on the ipsilateral preganglionic and postganglionic fibers.[32] The preganglionic sympathetic fibers for the head, neck, heart, and upper extremities arise from the upper thoracic region (T1-6) of the spinal cord, ascend through the sympathetic chain, synapse in the cervical sympathetic trunk, and then exit as postganglionic fibers to supply sympathetic innervation to the upper extremities.

Table 5
Indications and complications of sympathetic blocks for sympathetic pain

Sympathetic Block	Specific Indications		Complications and Side Effects
Stellate Ganglion Block	Neuropathic pain	CRPS I and II Phantom limb pain Orofacial pain Tinnitus Meniere syndrome Postherpetic neuralgia Pain from acute herpes zoster of upper extremities and neck	Impaired vision Nasal congestion Temporary sensory and motor deficits in arm (due to anesthetic spread to brachial plexus) Temporary hoarseness, dysphagia, dyspnea (due to anesthetic spread to laryngeal nerve)
	Rheumatology-related pain Ischemic pain	Scleroderma Paget's disease Raynaud disease Vascular insufficiency Vasculitis Arterial embolism of face or upper extremities Vascular headache Cardiac arrythmias Atypical chest pain Chronic ulcerative colitis	Respiratory compromise in patients with preexisting lung disease (due to anesthetic spread to the phrenic nerve) Paralysis (due to accidental intrathecal/subdural/epidural injection) Hematoma (usually due to injury of inferior thyroid artery or thyrocervical trunk)
	Visceral pain Nonpainful conditions	Cancer pain PTSD Anxiety Hyperhidrosis Hot flashes	Thyroid injury Vascular air embolism Pneumocephalus Perforation of esophagus/trachea Chylothorax Pneumothorax Infection Seizures (due to intravascular injection, most common in vertebral artery)
Lumbar Sympathetic Block	Neuropathic pain	CRPS I and II Phantom limb pain Diabetic neuropathy Postherpetic neuralgia Chronic pelvic or perineal pain Recluse spider bites	Orthostatic hypotension Anterior thigh or groin pain (due to accidental injury to genitofemoral nerve or lateral femoral cutaneous nerve) Viscera puncture (most commonly kidney or urethra)
	Ischemic pain	Raynaud disease Vascular insufficiency Peripheral arterial disease Ischemic limb Vasculitis Frostbite	Hematoma Temporary sensory and motor deficits in leg (due to anesthetic spread to genitofemoral nerve)
	Visceral pain	Cancer pain Rectal tenesmus (from cancer) Intractable renal colic	Paralysis (due to accidental intrathecal/subdural/epidural injection) Impotence
	Nonpainful conditions	Plantar hyperhidrosis	Infection Muscle trauma (most commonly psoas injury)

The cervical sympathetic trunk is composed of 3 interconnected ganglia—the superior, middle, and inferior cervical ganglia. In 80% of people, the inferior cervical ganglia are fused with the first thoracic ganglia to form the cervicothoracic (stellate) ganglion. It is typically located anterior to the neck of the first rib and the C7 transverse process.[32] If cervical and thoracic ganglia are not connected, then the first thoracic ganglion is deemed the stellate ganglion.[38] If unfused, the stellate ganglion is more likely located adjacent to the anterior C7 tubercle.[32]

The SGB is not without significant associated adverse events given its proximity to numerous vital structures (see **Table 5**).[32–34] The stellate ganglion's anterior border includes the subclavian artery and carotid sheath, the posterior border includes the vertebral artery, the lateral border includes the first thoracic nerve, the medial border includes the esophagus, and the inferior border includes the pleural dome.[34] There has been an associated death reported due to a massive hematoma, and also a report of quadriplegia due to a cervical epidural abscess and discitis following an SGB.[39]

Although the stellate ganglion is most centrally located at C7, an image-guided approach at the C6 vertebral level was traditionally used to avoid pneumothorax or vertebral artery puncture.[32] Of note, C6 is the most inferior level where the vertebral artery runs within the transverse foramen; as opposed to C7, where the vertebral artery lies anterior to the transverse foramen.[33]

Techniques for SGBs
Fluoroscopic guidance is used to identify the C6 or C7 vertebral level and direct the needle with consideration of pertinent landmarks such as Chassaignac's tubercle (C6) and the junction of the vertebral body and the uncinate process. Contrast media is administered to confirm adequate superior and inferior spread and the absence of vascular access before injection of medication. Alternatively, an ultrasound-guided technique can offer increased safety, when performed by an experienced practitioner, due to direct visualization of structures in the path of the needle (**Figs. 1 and 2**).[40]

Postprocedure assessment of SGBs
Generally, an SB is considered successful when correct needle placement is confirmed on imaging, significant pain relief is achieved using limited amounts of anesthetic, and no signs of sensory or motor blockade are appreciated.[33] Patients may have suboptimal pain relief following the SGB if their pain is multifactorial or because sympathetic blockade is incomplete. To eliminate inadequate sympathetic blockade as a contributing cause, a postprocedure assessment using reliable signs of complete SB are necessary.

Signs of complete sympathetic blockade for the head
Horner syndrome (characterized by miosis, ptosis, and anhidrosis) is a sign of successful block of the cervical sympathetic trunk or head. Enophthalmos, conjunctival injection, unilateral nasal congestion (Guttman's sign), and hyperemia of the tympanic membrane are also associated findings.[34,38]

Signs of complete sympathetic blockade for the extremities
To reliably detect complete sympathetic blockage in the extremities, 2 tests can be used to evaluate (1) the adrenergic fiber activity—responsible for increased blood flow and resultant increased temperature, and (2) the sympathetic cholinergic fiber activity—responsible for the absence of sweating.[38] Most commonly, a combination of increased skin temperature and anhidrosis is used to confirm complete sympathetic blockage in the upper limb after SGB. Temperature increase, by at least 1°C, is widely

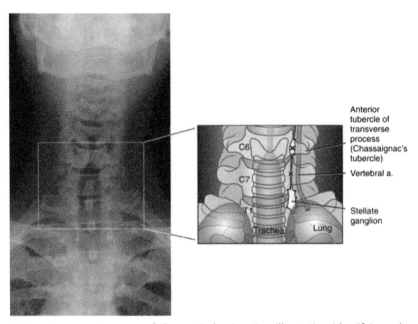

Fig. 1. Anterior-posterior x-ray of the cervical spine. See illustration identifying relevant anatomic structures. (*From* Janik JE, Hoeft MA, Ajar AH, et al. Variable osteology of the sixth cervical vertebra in relation to stellate ganglion block. *Reg Anesth Pain Med.* 2008;33[2]:102 to 108.)

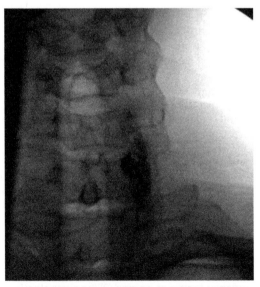

Fig. 2. Posterior-anterior fluoroscopic view of the cervical spine with contrast media administered at the location of the stellate ganglion. (*From* Sekhadia MP, Nader A, Benzon HT. Peripheral sympathetic blocks. In: Benzon HT, Raja SN, Fishman S, et al., eds. *Essentials of Pain Medicine.* 3rd ed. St. Louis: Saunders; 2011:621–628.)

used to assess sympathectomy success as it does not require additional specialized equipment. Sweat gland activity is evaluated by measuring skin conductance or using provocative sweat tests.[41–43]

Although temperature rise is the most commonly used clinical sign for sympathetic blockade, it is easily influenced by confounding variables such as clinical environment or location of temperature probe. For example, a more proximal temperature probe placed at the arm is more susceptible to elevated temperature measurements than a distally placed probe on the hand. Studies suggest ensuring the room temperature remains stable and measuring the affected limb temperature relative to core body temperature rather than the contralateral limb. Researchers have established that temperature measurements using the contralateral limb for comparison lead to higher rates of false positives.[5,41]

Furthermore, the magnitude of temperature increase after complete sympathetic blockade can vary with pathology. Patients with late-stage CRPS and subsequent vasoconstriction have lower preprocedure temperatures and respond to complete sympathetic blockade with greater rises in temperature than patients with early-stage CRPS and baseline vasodilation.[38] Also, if sympathetic blockade is done for claudication, temperature rise will be limited by peripheral vascular disease.

More objective but less convenient methods (rather than temperature) can be used to assess for increased skin perfusion. These techniques include laser Doppler flowmetry, skin plethysmography, and perfusion index change ratios.[44,45] Emerging data suggest finger blood flow that is maintained against postural changes may be a new indicator of sympathetic blockade in the upper limb.[41] Recent studies also suggest that increased pulse transit time (the amount of time it takes for a pulse wave to travel between 2 arterial sites) reflects increased blood flow, and may serve as an objective and easily-obtained marker for successful sympathetic blockade.[45]

SGB efficacy

Although SGBs are used for several conditions, CRPS is the most supported indication for SGBs presently. Typically, a series of injections is performed in combination with physical therapy; however, there is no consensus on the number of SGBs required for effective treatment.[31] Wie and colleagues recommend a trial of at least 2 blocks if the patient has not found clinical benefit, but other clinicians have suggested up to 3.[31]

Overall, moderate-quality evidence (ie, randomized control trials [RCTs] with limitations) supports the use of SGBs in the treatment of early-stage CRPS of the upper extremity; however, large RCTs and meta-analyses are still needed to demonstrate efficacy. Researchers have established that SGBs are significantly more effective when used earlier in the course of CRPS.[46,47] In a clinical trial by Ackerman and colleagues, SGBs are specifically shown to be more effective against early CRPS with decreased vasomotor activity, but less effective against late-stage CRPS with increased vasoconstriction.[47] Also, some research scientists favor blockade using local anesthetic over neurolysis given that studies on experimental animal models show extensive collateral DRG sympathetic sprouting following nerve ligation; however, this concern remains controversial.[47,48]

The Lumbar Sympathetic Block

Indications and specific contraindications for LSBs

The LSB is a first-line interventional treatment for CRPS of the lower extremity. It shares similar indications with SGBs, but for pathology of the lower extremities (see **Table 5**).[3,31,34,49] Poorly controlled heart disease is a contraindication specific to

LSBs.[49] The resultant hypotension with LSBs is more profound because vasculature of the pelvis and lower extremities is affected, rather than the arms.

Applicable anatomy of LSBs

The preganglionic sympathetic fibers that supply the lower extremities arise from the thoracolumbar region (T10-L3) of the spinal cord, descend through the sympathetic chain, and synapse in the appropriate ganglia, forming the lumbar sympathetic trunk. The lumbar sympathetic trunk is located along the anterolateral surface of the lumbar vertebrae (L2-L4) next to the psoas muscle. The majority of sympathetic innervation passes through the L2 and L3 sympathetic ganglia, creating the densest portion of the lumbar sympathetic trunk and the most common target for lumbar sympathetic blockade.[34,49] The postganglionic sympathetic fibers go on to contribute to the lumbosacral plexus, and accompany all major nerves to the lower extremities.[34] Complications from this procedure stem from proximity to nearby arteries and nerves (see **Table 5**).[33,49,50]

Techniques for LSBs

Fluoroscopic guidance is used to identify the L2 and L3 vertebral levels and direct the needle to the anterolateral margin of the appropriate vertebral bodies. Contrast media is administered to confirm adequate superior and inferior spread and the absence of vascular access before injection of medication (**Figs. 3** and **4**).

Postprocedure assessment of LSBs

Analogous to SGBs, signs of a successful LSB include decreased pain, improved function, improved range of motion, and increased limb temperature of 2 to 3°C.[45,49,51,52] Hypotension and a flushed appearance of the affected extremity are also common from the intense vasodilation that occurs in the pelvis and lower limb.[33,49] Like SGBs, increased skin perfusion and anhidrosis are used as markers of complete sympathetic blockade in the lower extremity following LSB.

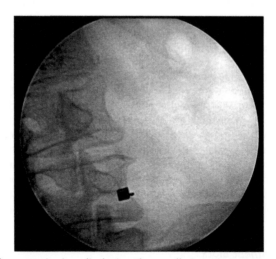

Fig. 3. Oblique fluoroscopic view displaying the needle in trajectory view aimed at the anterolateral vertebral body. (*From* Gofeld M, Shankar H, Benzon HT. Fluoroscopy and Ultrasound-Guided Sympathetic Blocks: Stellate Ganglion, Lumbar Sympathetic Blocks, and Visceral Sympathetic Blo. In: Benzon HT, Raja SN, Fishman S, et al., eds. *Essentials of Pain Medicine*. 4th ed. St. Louis: Elsevier; 2017:789–804.)

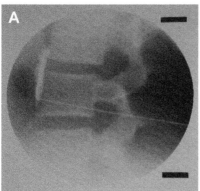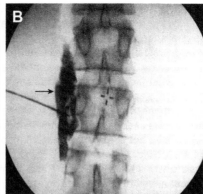

Fig. 4. Lateral fluoroscopic view (*A*) and anterior-posterior fluoroscopic view (*B*) demonstrate prevertebral spread of contrast media (*black arrow*). (*From* Gofeld M, Shankar H, Benzon HT. Fluoroscopy and Ultrasound-Guided Sympathetic Blocks: Stellate Ganglion, Lumbar Sympathetic Blocks, and Visceral Sympathetic Blo. In: Benzon HT, Raja SN, Fishman S, et al., eds. *Essentials of Pain Medicine.* 4th ed. St. Louis: Elsevier; 2017:789–804.)

LSB efficacy

Akin to SGBs, the literature largely supports the use of LSBs for CRPS of the lower extremity; however, there is a paucity of high-quality RCTs and systematic reviews to establish conclusive evidence. Many RCTs demonstrate positive outcomes but have limitations in study design. For example, a study of participants who developed CRPS after total knee arthroplasty reported 86% of patients experienced some pain relief following lumbar sympathetic blockade; however, a large injectate volume (20 mL of 0.375% bupivacaine) was used.[53] The larger the volume of anesthetic used, the greater the chance of obtaining false-positive results due to spread and blockade of nearby somatic sensory nerves.[33]

Another small study compared RFA to a neurolytic approach and found similar positive outcomes in both groups; but the study lacked a placebo arm, which limited the study's conclusions.[54] In the same way, a double-blind placebo-controlled crossover study in children was able to demonstrate significant pain reduction with LSBs but had a limited number of participants.[55] In summary, the SGB and LSB are considered first-line interventional treatments for CRPS; however, more research is needed to establish practice guidelines on when to perform them, the appropriate number of blocks, and sequencing of therapies for CRPS.[56]

DISCUSSION

Decision making regarding the treatment of SMP should incorporate current evidence, clinical experience, and a patient-centered approach. Although the evidence continues to grow, treatment modalities such as physical therapy, medication management, infusion therapies, SBs, neurolysis, and neuromodulation can be considered at various stages in the treatment algorithm.

LSBs and SGBs are often used for diagnostic and therapeutic purposes in the treatment of CRPS. These procedures may allow improved participation in physical therapy, reduction in pain medications, and increased mobility, especially when performed early in the treatment paradigm. To this end, LSBs and SGBs provide analgesia without impairing sensory or motor nerve fibers, confirming the diagnosis and providing a therapeutic target. In addition, the physician can readily verify successful block with physical examination without the need for diagnostic testing (ie, pupillary change, eyelid droop, temperature change).

The challenge for clinicians has been deciding which intervention to start with when managing presumed CPRS. The literature suggests controlling pain first with analgesics followed by SBs may be more effective than starting with injections.[57] If SBs fail to reduce pain sufficiently, neuromodulation has demonstrated promise. In fact, traditional SCS may provide 40% to 50% satisfactory pain relief with newer techniques, such as dorsal root ganglion stimulation, offering more benefit.[58,59] Although SBs and neuromodulation have separately shown promise in treating CPRS pain, success with SBs does not predict success with spinal cord stimulation.[60]

Wie and colleagues have suggested epidural infusions may be considered in cases of refractory or severe CRPS.[31] These treatments target the epidural space with opiates, local anesthetics, omega-conotoxin peptides, and/or clonidine with a catheter, which can potentially provide sustained sympathetic blockade.[31] Selecting the correct treatment paradigm for patients and which characteristics and symptoms respond best to a particular treatment will be the focus of future research but should improve outcomes.

CLINICS CARE POINTS

- SBGs and LSBs can be used as first-line interventional procedures for CPRS of the upper and lower limb, respectively.

- Image guidance is mandatory for performing sympathetic blocks in a safe and effective manner.

- There is limited evidence for timing, frequency, and total number of sympathetic blocks for most pain conditions. However, diagnostic/prognostic LASBs have been used to establish efficacy before advancing to neurolysis or RFA. Research suggests SGBs are more effective when used earlier in the course of CRPS.

- A dual-bladder tourniquet (or 2 cuffs) can be used during IRSBs to provide a controlled, graded reduction of tourniquet pressure to reduce the risk of releasing medications into systemic circulation when the tourniquet is released.

- Buprenorphine 0.75% should be reserved for procedures when a high degree of muscle relaxation and prolonged effect are necessary.

- Chemical neurolysis with alcohol should be avoided in patients taking disulfiram for alcohol use disorder. There is a risk of acetaldehyde accumulation, which may lead to tachycardia, nausea, and vomiting.

- A postprocedure assessment is necessary to evaluate SB efficacy. Increased skin perfusion and anhidrosis are used as markers of complete sympathetic blockade in the extremities. Horner syndrome is a sign of a successful block of the cervical sympathetic trunk or head.

- Severe emphysema is a contraindication specific to SGBs as unopposed parasympathetic activity can further decrease respiratory compliance.

- Poorly controlled heart disease is a relative contraindication specific to LSBs. The resultant hypotension with LSBs is more profound (compared with SGBs) because the vasculature of the pelvis and lower extremities is affected, rather than the arms.

SUMMARY

The SNS is an integral component of the body's response to stress. Once activated, the SNS has broad-reaching effects on multiple organ systems that modulate pain, behavior, and mood. Blockade of the system can improve pain associated with multiple etiologies, including vascular, visceral, and neuropathic pain. Multiple techniques are available to block the SNS and provide options that improve analgesia and can be individualized to a particular patient's needs and disease state.

DISCLOSURE

The authors have nothing to disclose.

REFERENCES

1. Schlereth T, Birklein F. The sympathetic nervous system and pain. Neuromolecular Med 2008;10(3):141–7.
2. Nagpal AS, Vydra D, Correa J, et al. Evidence analysis of sympathetic blocks for visceral pain. Curr Phys Med Rehabil Rep 2019;7(3):253–63.
3. Menon R, Swanepoel A. Sympathetic blocks. Contin Educ Anaesth Crit Care Pain 2010;10(3):88–92.
4. O'Connell NE, Wand BM, Gibson W, et al. Local anaesthetic sympathetic blockade for complex regional pain syndrome. Cochrane Database Syst Rev 2016;7:CD004598. https://doi.org/10.1002/14651858.CD004598.pub4.
5. Sharma A, Campbell JN, Raja SN. Sympathetic blocks for pain. Pain 2008;1: 227–35. Published online January.
6. Becker DE, Reed KL. Local anesthetics: review of pharmacological considerations. Anesth Prog 2012;59(2):90–101, quiz 102-103.
7. Lirk P, Hollmann MW, Strichartz G. The science of local anesthesia: basic research, clinical application, and future directions. Anesth Analg 2018;126(4): 1381–92.
8. Bupivacaine hydrochloride. Micromedex Solut Greenwood Village CO Truven Health Anal. Published online July 28, 2021. Available at: http://micromedex. com/. Accessed August 22, 2021.
9. Escaldi S. Neurolysis: a brief review for a fading art. Phys Med Rehabil Clin N Am 2018;29(3):519–27.
10. Lidocaine hydrochloride. Micromedex Solut Greenwood Village CO Truven Health Anal. Published online August 11, 2021. Available at: http://micromedex. com. Accessed August 22, 2021.
11. Ropivacaine hydrochloride. Micromedex Solut Greenwood Village CO Truven Health Anal. Published online February 4, 2021. Available at: http:// micromedex.com/. Accessed August 22, 2021.
12. Haghighi M, Mardani-Kivi M, mirbolook A, et al. A Comparison between single and double tourniquet technique in distal upper limb orthopedic surgeries with intravenous regional anesthesia. Arch Bone Jt Surg 2018;6(1):63–70.
13. AST guidelines for best practices for safe use of pneumatic tourniquets. Available at: https://www.ast.org/webdocuments/ASTGuidelineSafeUseofPneumaticTourniquets/ files/assets/common/downloads/publication.pdf. Accessed December 1, 2021.
14. Published online July 17Guanethidine monosulfate. *Micromedex solut greenwood village CO truven health anal.* Available at: http://micromedex.com/. Accessed August 22, 2021.
15. Phentolamine mesylate. Micromedex Solut Greenwood Village CO Truven Health Anal. Published online August 6, 2021. Available at: http://micromedex.com/. Accessed August 22, 2021.
16. Reserpine. Micromedex Solut greenwood village CO truven health anal. Published online July 17, 2020. Available at: http://micromedex.com/. Accessed August 22, 2021.

17. Carroll I, Mackey S, Gaeta R. The role of adrenergic receptors and pain: The good, the bad, and the unknown. Semin Anesth Perioper Med Pain 2007;26(1): 17–21. https://doi.org/10.1053/j.sane.2006.11.005.

18. Prazosin hydrochloride. Micromedex Solut Greenwood Village CO Truven Health Anal 2021. Published online August 25. http://micromedex.com/. [Accessed 26 August 2021].

19. Phenoxybenzamine hydrochloride. Micromedex Solut Greenwood Village CO Truven Health Anal 2021. Published online March 30. http://micromedex.com/. [Accessed 26 August 2021].

20. Malik VK, Inchiosa MA, Mustafa K, et al. Intravenous regional phenoxybenzamine in the treatment of reflex sympathetic dystrophy. Anesthesiology 1998;88(3): 823–7. https://doi.org/10.1097/00000542-199803000-00036.

21. Yoham AL, Casadesus D. Phenoxybenzamine. In: StatPearls. StatPearls Publishing. 2021. http://www.ncbi.nlm.nih.gov/books/NBK560667/. [Accessed 26 September 2021]. Accessed.

22. Nifedipine. Micromedex Solut greenwood village co truven health anal. Published online August 16, 2021. http://micromedex.com/. [Accessed 26 August 2021]. Accessed.

23. Clonidine hydrochloride. Micromedex Solut Greenwood Village CO Truven Health Anal 2021. Published online June 22. http://micromedex.com/. [Accessed 26 August 2021]. Accessed.

24. Bhatnagar S, Gupta M. Evidence-based clinical practice guidelines for interventional pain management in cancer pain. Indian J Palliat Care 2015;21(2):137–47. https://doi.org/10.4103/0973-1075.156466.

25. Tariq RA, Mueller M, Green MS. Neuraxial neurolysis. In: StatPearls. StatPearls Publishing; 2021. http://www.ncbi.nlm.nih.gov/books/NBK537157/. [Accessed 26 September 2021]. Accessed.

26. Koyyalagunta D, Engle MP, Yu J, et al. The effectiveness of alcohol versus phenol based splanchnic nerve neurolysis for the treatment of intra-abdominal cancer pain. Pain Physician 2016;19(4):281–92.

27. D'Souza RS, Hooten WM. Neurolytic blocks. In: StatPearls. StatPearls Publishing; 2021. http://www.ncbi.nlm.nih.gov/books/NBK537360/. [Accessed 26 September 2021]. Accessed.

28. Sachdev AH, Gress FG. Celiac plexus block and neurolysis: a review. Gastrointest Endosc Clin N Am 2018;28(4):579–86.

29. Ethanol Micromedex Solut Greenwood Village CO Truven Health Anal 2021. Published online January 21. http://micromedex.com/. [Accessed 28 August 2021]. Accessed.

30. Phenol. Micromedex Solut Greenwood Village CO Truven Health Anal Published Online 2021. Available at: http://micromedex.com/. Accessed August 28, 2021.

31. Wie C, Gupta R, Maloney J, et al. Interventional modalities to treat complex regional pain syndrome. Curr Pain Headache Rep 2021;25(2):10.

32. Piraccini E, Munakomi S, Chang KV. Stellate ganglion blocks. In: StatPearls. StatPearls Publishing; 2021. http://www.ncbi.nlm.nih.gov/books/NBK507798/. [Accessed 26 September 2021]. Accessed.

33. Doroshenko M, Turkot O, Horn DB. Sympathetic nerve block. In: StatPearls. StatPearls Publishing; 2021. http://www.ncbi.nlm.nih.gov/books/NBK557637/. [Accessed 26 September 2021]. Accessed.

34. Baig S, Moon JY, Shankar H. Review of sympathetic blocks: anatomy, sonoanatomy, evidence, and techniques. Reg Anesth Pain Med 2017;42(3):377–91.

35. Gunduz OH, Kenis-Coskun O. Ganglion blocks as a treatment of pain: current perspectives. J Pain Res 2017;10:2815–26.
36. Lipov E, Candido K. Efficacy and safety of stellate ganglion block in chronic ulcerative colitis. World J Gastroenterol 2017;23(17):3193–4.
37. Rastogi R, Agarwal S, Enany N, et al. Chapter 84 - SYMPATHETIC BLOCKADE. In: Smith HS, editor. Current therapy in pain. W.B. Saunders; 2009. p. 612–20.
38. Nader A, Benzon HT. Chapter 80 - peripheral sympathetic blocks. In: Benzon HT, Raja SN, Molloy RE, et al, editors. Essentials of pain medicine and regional anesthesia. Second Edition. Churchill Livingstone; 2005. p. 687–93.
39. Goel V, Patwardhan AM, Ibrahim M, et al. Complications associated with stellate ganglion nerve block: a systematic review. Reg Anesth Pain Med, 44, 6, 669, 678. Published online April 16, 2019:rapm-2018-100127. doi:10.1136/rapm-2018-100127
40. Aleanakian R, Chung BY, Feldmann RE, et al. Effectiveness, safety, and predictive potential in ultrasound-guided stellate ganglion blockades for the treatment of sympathetically maintained pain. Pain Pract Off J World Inst Pain 2020; 20(6):626–38.
41. Nakatani T, Hashimoto T, Sutou I, et al. Retention of finger blood flow against postural change as an indicator of successful sympathetic block in the upper limb. J Pain Res 2017;10:475–9.
42. Benzon HT, Cheng SC, Avram MJ, et al. Sign of complete sympathetic blockade: sweat test or sympathogalvanic response? Anesth Analg 1985;64(4):415–9.
43. Stevens RA, Stotz A, Kao TC, et al. The relative increase in skin temperature after stellate ganglion block is predictive of a complete sympathectomy of the hand. Reg Anesth Pain Med 1998;23(3):266–70.
44. Joo EY, Kong YG, Lee J, et al. Change in pulse transit time in the lower extremity after lumbar sympathetic ganglion block: an early indicator of successful block. J Int Med Res 2017;45(1):203–10.
45. Cañada-Soriano M, Priego-Quesada JI, Bovaira M, et al. Quantitative analysis of real-time infrared thermography for the assessment of lumbar sympathetic blocks: a preliminary study. Sensors 2021;21(11):3573.
46. Yucel I, Demiraran Y, Ozturan K, et al. Complex regional pain syndrome type I: efficacy of stellate ganglion blockade. J Orthop Traumatol Off J Ital Soc Orthop Traumatol 2009;10(4):179–83.
47. Ackerman WE, Zhang JM. Efficacy of stellate ganglion blockade for the management of type 1 complex regional pain syndrome. South Med J 2006;99(10): 1084–8.
48. Zhang JM, Strong JA. Recent evidence for activity-dependent initiation of sympathetic sprouting and neuropathic pain. Sheng Li Xue Bao 2008;60(5):617–27.
49. Alexander CE, De Jesus O, Varacallo M. Lumbar sympathetic block. In: StatPearls. StatPearls Publishing; 2021. http://www.ncbi.nlm.nih.gov/books/NBK431107/. [Accessed 26 September 2021]. Accessed.
50. Day M. Sympathetic blocks: the evidence. Pain Pract Off J World Inst Pain 2008; 8(2):98–109.
51. Park SY, Nahm FS, Kim YC, et al. The cut-off rate of skin temperature change to confirm successful lumbar sympathetic block. J Int Med Res 2010;38(1):266–75.
52. Tran KM, Frank SM, Raja SN, et al. Lumbar sympathetic block for sympathetically maintained pain: changes in cutaneous temperatures and pain perception. Anesth Analg 2000;90(6):1396–401.
53. Abramov R. Lumbar sympathetic treatment in the management of lower limb pain. Curr Pain Headache Rep 2014;18(4):403.

54. Manjunath PS, Jayalakshmi TS, Dureja GP, et al. Management of lower limb complex regional pain syndrome type 1: an evaluation of percutaneous radiofrequency thermal lumbar sympathectomy versus phenol lumbar sympathetic neurolysis–a pilot study. Anesth Analg 2008;106(2):647–9, table of contents.

55. Meier PM, Zurakowski D, Berde CB, et al. Lumbar sympathetic blockade in children with complex regional pain syndromes: a double blind placebo-controlled crossover trial. Anesthesiology 2009;111(2):372–80.

56. Zhu X, Kohan LR, Morris JD, et al. Sympathetic blocks for complex regional pain syndrome: a survey of pain physicians. Reg Anesth Pain Med 2019. Published online May 3. rapm-2019-100418.

57. Amr YM, Makharita MY. Comparative study between 2 protocols for management of severe pain in patients with unresectable pancreatic cancer: one-year follow-up. Clin J Pain 2013;29(9):807–13.

58. Kemler MA, de Vet HC, Barendse GA, et al. Effect of spinal cord stimulation for chronic complex regional pain syndrome Type I: five-year final follow-up of patients in a randomized controlled trial. J Neurosurg 2008;108(2):292–8.

59. Deer TR, Levy RM, Kramer J, et al. Comparison of paresthesia coverage of patient's pain: dorsal root ganglion vs. spinal cord stimulation. an ACCURATE study sub-analysis. Neuromodulation 2019;22(8):930–6.

60. Cheng J, Salmasi V, You J, et al. Outcomes of sympathetic blocks in the management of complex regional pain syndrome: a retrospective cohort study. Anesthesiology 2019;131(4):883–93.

Sympathetic Blocks for Visceral Pain

Kevin Vorenkamp, MD, FASA[a],*, Peter Yi, MD, MSEd[b], Adam Kemp, MD[b]

KEYWORDS

- Visceral pain • Sympathetic block • Neurolytic procedure • celiac plexus
- superior hypogastric plexus • ganglion impar

KEY POINTS

- Sympathetic blocks can be performed for patients with visceral pain of multiple etiologies.
- Sympathetic neurolysis, especially celiac plexus neurolysis, has demonstrated efficacy for patients with patients with cancer-related visceral pain.
- Superior hypogastric plexus and ganglion impar blocks may benefit patients with pain arising from the pelvic viscera.

INTRODUCTION

Pain emanating from the abdominal and pelvic viscera is often challenging to treat because of the complexity of multiple organ systems and overlapping symptom patterns of potential diagnoses. Even when a cause is identified, treatment of the underlying processes may be impossible, impractical, or incomplete in resolving pain. For more than 100 years, physicians have been pioneering methods to interrupt conduction of afferent pain signals from these structures as they course through sympathetic ganglia, which can be targeted for nerve block or chemoablation. Although these methods have been used to treat severe pain caused by many chronic noncancer pain syndromes, malignancy is the most common indication for these procedures.

Cancer-related pain often has mixed components of nociceptive, inflammatory, and/or neuropathic pain. Pain may be incited by pathologic processes, such as tumor mass effect; organ dysfunction; or obstruction and iatrogenic processes following radiation therapy, chemotherapy, or surgery. Often, pain is the most distressing symptom reported in these patients. Pharmacologic treatment of cancer-related pain

[a] Division of Pain Medicine, Duke Anesthesiology, Duke University, 2080 Duke University Road, Durham, NC 27708, USA; [b] Anesthesiology and Critical Care, Duke University, 2080 Duke University Road, Durham, NC 27708, USA
* Corresponding author.
E-mail address: kevin.vorenkamp@duke.edu

Phys Med Rehabil Clin N Am 33 (2022) 475–487
https://doi.org/10.1016/j.pmr.2022.01.010
1047-9651/22/© 2022 Elsevier Inc. All rights reserved.

according to the World Health Organization Analgesic Ladder is initiated with nonsteroidal anti-inflammatory drugs ± adjuvant medications and progresses to systemic opioids. Often, escalating doses are necessary with accompanying adverse effects that impair quality of life and limit efficacy of treatment.

The sympathetic nervous system spans the length of the axial skeleton and most of the plexuses and ganglia are readily accessible to percutaneous interruption. For patients with chronic pain or cancer-related pain, the most common indication for sympathetic block is to control visceral pain arising from malignancies or other alterations of the abdominal and pelvic viscera. Visceral pain is often described as a deep, squeezing pain that is difficult to localize and characterize. When it is recalcitrant to conservative care, or if the patient is intolerant to pharmacotherapy, consideration of sympathetic blocks or neurolytic procedures should be considered. Typically, neurolytic blocks are reserved for patients with cancer-related pain. Potential advantages of a neurolytic procedure, compared with spinal and epidural anesthetic infusions, include cost savings and avoidance of hardware (eg, catheters, tubes, pump), which are cumbersome, are subject to malfunction, and pose an infection risk. Interventional therapies that target afferent visceral innervation via the sympathetic ganglia can offer effective and durable analgesia and improve multiple metrics of quality of life.

ANATOMY

Typical visceral pain is described as poorly localized, aching, dull pain. These characteristics are attributable to the overlapping origination and conduction via afferent nerves that course along with sympathetic and parasympathetic fibers. This complex interplay and the resulting vague nature of pain are believed caused by viscerosomatic and viscerovisceral convergence of nerve signals.[1]

Anterolateral to the T1-L2 vertebral bodies lay the paired sympathetic ganglion. There are usually 22 to 23 pairs of these ganglia: three in the cervical region (cervical ganglia), 11 in the thoracic region (note the presence of the fused stellate cervicothoracic ganglia), four in the lumbar region, and four to five in the sacral region. The celiac plexus receives its primary innervation from the greater (T5-T9), lesser (T10-T11), and least splanchnic nerves (T12). These nerves, preganglionic in nature, traverse the posterior mediastinum and enter the abdomen through the crura of the diaphragm above L1. The plexus innervates most of the abdominal viscera, including the stomach, liver, biliary tract, pancreas, spleen, kidneys, adrenals, omentum, small bowel, and large bowel, to the level of the splenic flexure.

The superior hypogastric plexus receives contributions from the two lower lumbar splanchnic nerves (L3-L4), which are branches of the chain ganglia. They also contain parasympathetic fibers that arise from pelvic splanchnic nerve (S2-S4) and ascend from the inferior hypogastric plexus (**Fig. 1**). Fibers then course onward to innervate the pelvic visceral organs (**Table 1**).[2]

The ganglion impar (ganglion of Walther) is a single midline ganglion laying just anterior to the sacrum that consists of the terminal convergence of the sympathetic chains. From the ganglion impar, fibers continue as the sacral splanchnic nerves, which conduct sympathetic afferents that course along with spinal nerves of the sacrococcygeal levels. A small number of the fibers supply visceral branches to the inferior hypogastric plexus, whereas most provide innervation of the perineum.

Following with their embryologic origins, innervation of the subject anatomy predictably courses through one of three locations: (1) the celiac plexus, (2) the superior hypogastric plexus, or (3) the ganglion impar (see **Table 1**).

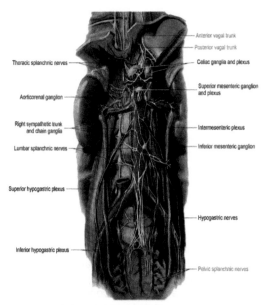

Fig. 1. Visceral innervation of the abdomen. (*From* Newaj Abdullah, Mark Abumoussa, Heena S. Ahmed, et. al. Interventional Management of Chronic Visceral Pain Syndromes, Elsevier, 2021, Pages v-vii, ISBN 9780323757751, (https://www.sciencedirect.com/science/article/pii/B9780323757751010023))

Table 1
Visceral innervation of the abdomen

Structure	Location	Origination	Structures Innervated
Celiac plexus (splanchnic nerves)	T12 and/or L1; periaortic around root of celiac and superior mesenteric arteries.	Sympathetic T5–T12; via greater, lesser, and least splanchnic nerves.	Upper abdominal; distal esophagus, diaphragm, liver, stomach, spleen, suprarenal glands, kidneys, ovaries/testes, small intestine, and ascending and transverse colon to splenic flexure.
Superior hypogastric plexus	Paired and anterolateral to the lower third L5–upper third S1 vertebral bodies. Anteromedial to psoas and inferior to the common iliac bifurcation.	Continuation of paravertebral sympathetic chain plus periaortic fibers.	All pelvic viscera except ovaries/testes and fallopian tubes.
Ganglion impar	First coccygeal vertebrae and sacrococcygeal junction. Midline structure.	Termination of sympathetic chain.	Lower rectum, anus, urethra, vagina, coccygeal ligaments (coccydynia), and perineum.

GENERAL PATIENT SELECTION

The methods described in later sections are fundamentally based on a common procedural sequence. Therapeutic blockade of the sympathetic ganglia involves directing a needle under imaging guidance to the respective target point, confirming placement with a low volume of contrast (when fluoroscopy or computed tomography [CT] is used), and injecting a local anesthetic (± corticosteroid) that is given several minutes to take effect. Pain severity is then reassessed. Several studies have used an improvement of 50% as the benchmark for a "successful" block; however, a range of values have been referenced. A neurolytic solution of phenol or alcohol is injected for durable effect.[3] Continuous and pulsed radiofrequency lesioning of these structures has been reported but requires further study before acceptance in common practice.[4]

CELIAC PLEXUS
Approaches

Celiac plexus block (CPB) is commonly performed using fluoroscopy, CT, or endoscopic ultrasound. Few studies have directly compared the efficacy of these different modalities.[5] In most settings, the modality and approach is determined by provider ability, patient preference, resource availability, concurrent procedures (ie, esophagogastroduodenoscopy, abdominal surgery), and disease processes. There are two different approaches for percutaneous fluoroscopy-guided procedures targeting the celiac plexus or the splanchnic nerves terminating in the celiac plexus. With the first approach, the classic CPB via an anterocrural approach, the target is the celiac plexus itself, which is typically located anterior to the aorta at the L1 level. Typically, a single needle approach is able to get appropriate bilateral spread. The second approach involves targeting the splanchnic nerves via a retrocrural approach at the T12 level. With this approach, typically bilateral needle placement and injection is required to provide appropriate analgesia. With both techniques, an anteroposterior view is used to identify the appropriate vertebral levels, then the view is rotated to an oblique view used to optimize visualization of the corresponding target area. A needle is introduced through anesthetized skin, then directed coaxially just medial to the lateral vertebral border on the image. Final positioning is performed in the lateral view.[6]

For the classic celiac plexus (anterocrural) approach, the fluoroscopic target is the upper third of the L1 vertebral body and anterior to the aorta. The target of the retrocrural approach is the anterior one-fifth of the T12 vertebral body on the lateral view (**Fig. 2**). Appropriate positioning for both is confirmed with live contrast injection (**Fig. 3**). If a neurolytic block is to be performed, it is highly recommended that digital subtraction angiography is used to better detect potential intravascular injection.

The aforementioned approaches can also be used under CT guidance with the potential advantage of performing anterocrural block with more reliably avoiding penetration of the aorta (**Fig. 4**). Transabdominal (anterior) approaches with CT or endoscopic ultrasound are performed in the supine position, which may be better tolerated by some patients.

Patient Selection Criteria

CPB is used as a therapeutic or diagnostic tool in the treatment of severe visceral pain involving the diaphragm, liver, stomach, spleen, suprarenal glands, kidneys, ovaries/testes, small intestine, and ascending and transverse colon to splenic flexure. General contraindications to these procedures should be considered (**Table 2**). Patients with painful malignancy involving these structures or associated lymphatics are likely to

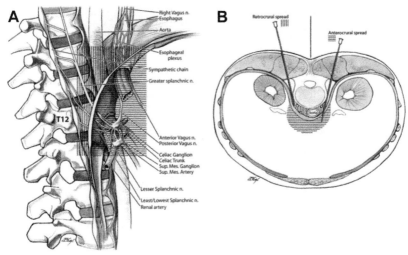

Fig. 2. (*A, B*) Approaches to celiac plexus block. (*From* Vorenkamp, K., & Dahle, N. (2011). Diagnostic celiac plexus block and outcome with neurolysis. *Techniques in Regional Anesthesia and Pain Management, 15*, 28–32).

benefit from a neurolytic CPB (NCPB). Because cancer pain likely involves multiple structures with somatic and visceral innervation, systemic opioid therapy is still usually required even with a successful block. A study of patients who received endoscopic ultrasound NCPB found that pancreatic tumors located in the body/tail of the pancreas rather than the head, and absence of metastatic disease were associated with better response to treatment.[7] Patients with advanced pancreatic cancer may be less appropriate candidates for CPB because of the likely presence of somatic

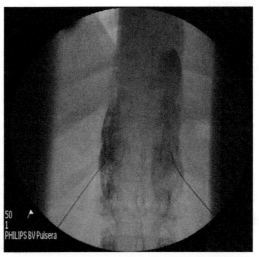

Fig. 3. Anteroposterior view of final bilateral needle placement for celiac plexus neurolysis. (*From* Vorenkamp, K., & Dahle, N. (2011). Diagnostic celiac plexus block and outcome with neurolysis. *Techniques in Regional Anesthesia and Pain Management, 15*, 28–32).

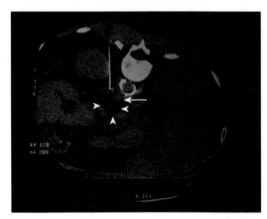

Fig. 4. CT-guided celiac plexus block. *Arrows* indicate celiac plexus. (*From* Benzon, H. T., Rathmell, J. P., Wu, C. L., Turk, D. C., Argoff, C. E., & Hurley, R. W. (2013). *Practical Management of Pain: Fifth Edition,* Figure 56.11. Elsevier Inc. https://doi.org/10.1016/C2009-0-64063-0)0020

pain from distal metastasis and likely medical fragility making them less tolerant should complications arise. Treatment earlier in the course of the disease may be particularly important for individuals likely to experience severe complication from escalating doses of systemic opioids.

For chronic nonmalignant pain, therapeutic CPB with local anesthetic is perhaps best used as a prognostic tool with the potential for repeat of therapeutic CPB or progression to NCPB later. However, duration of pain relief is typically limited to 2 to 3 months so realistic patient expectations and understanding of potential risks should be ensured.[5] Pain that is somatic rather than visceral is unlikely to benefit from sympathetic block.

Risks and Contraindications

General contraindications as discussed previously should be considered (see **Table 2**).

The most common complications of CPB are diarrhea (44%–60%), postural hypotension (10%–52%), and localized back pain (>90%). Diarrhea may be a desirable effect in patients experiencing constipation or obstipation secondary to opioids or obstructive tumor burden. The risk of diarrhea and postural hypotension varies depending on which approach is used. Splanchnic (retrocrural) block (10%–25%) is less likely to induce diarrhea compared with celiac (anterocrural) (65%). Block-induced diarrhea commonly resolves within 24 hours; however, there are reported

Table 2 General contraindications to sympathetic blocks	
Absolute Contraindications	**Relative Contraindications**
Systemic infection	Infection (other site)
Focal infection at procedure site	Hyperglycemia
Pregnancy	Hemodynamic instability
True contrast allergy; can consider gadolinium	Coagulopathy
	Comorbidities

cases of persistent diarrhea that is resistant to treatment.[8] Postural hypotension is less common with anterocrural (10%) block compared with retrocrural or splanchnic approaches (approximately 50%). However, for patients with severe cardiovascular conditions (ie, critical aortic stenosis), the effects of sudden vasodilation may be problematic. The severity and effects of postural hypotension are mitigated by preprocedural fluid bolus and/or holding noncritical antihypertensive medications before the procedure.[8–10]

Rare but potentially severe complications including pneumothorax, ileus, retroperitoneal hematoma, paraplegia, aortic dissection, and local anesthesia toxicity have been reported. One study examining 2730 NCPBs reported an incidence of these complications at "1 per 683 procedures."[10–12]

The destructive nature of neurolytic solutions can have unintended consequences. NCPB has rarely been associated with paraplegia or transient muscle weakness. The mechanism for this has been postulated as either direct injury caused by epidural spread of injectate or spinal cord ischemia secondary to reactive vasospasm induced by these agents (alcohol or phenol).[13] We are not aware of any reports of paralysis following neurolytic block of the celiac plexus or splanchnic nerves performed under fluoroscopic guidance with live contrast injection. Because these complications may occur even if the procedure is performed by an experience practitioner, it is appropriate to include discussion of these serious complications to the patient.

Outcome Data

There is a paucity of literature allowing for direct comparison of outcomes when using different imaging modalities and approaches for CPB. A 1995 meta-analysis of randomized controlled trials (RCTs) of NCPB for intra-abdominal tumors including pancreatic cancer showed significant improvement in pain at 3 months for 90% of patients with residual improvement until time of death in 70% to 90% of patients. The authors concluded that "1) NCPB has long-lasting benefit for 70%-90% of patients with pancreatic and other intraabdominal cancers, regardless of the technique used; 2) adverse effects are common but transient and mild; and 3) severe adverse effects are uncommon."[14]

A 2011 Cochrane Review of RCTs for pancreatic cancer pain found a significant decrease in opioid requirement at least 4 weeks following CPB. Improvement in pain severity was modest among these patient (visual analog scale [VAS] decreased by 0.42/10) but accompanied by a marked improvement in side effect profile including nausea and constipation.[15]

A 2014 meta-analysis of RCTs examining management of pancreatic cancer by medical management and/or CPB found durable pain improvement at 4 weeks that had waned by 8 weeks postprocedure. Opioid requirements were significantly lower for patients who had received CPB.[16]

A recent retrospective review of more than 507 patients who had fluoroscopy-guided celiac plexus neurolysis for visceral cancer-related pain demonstrated improved pain scores, daily opioid consumption, and quality of life with duration of benefit 4 to 6 months.[17]

Although some studies have demonstrated improved survival time in patients receiving plexus block compared with medical management alone, increased life expectancy is not an established benefit.[18]

Discussion

The numerous approaches and guidance techniques that have been described to perform CPB are evidence of its acceptance by a spectrum of medical specialties and common application for treatment of abdominal pain. The specific approach and treatment end point are determined by provider skills, medical resources, patient preference, and pathology. Although celiac plexus neurolysis offers a promising treatment of patients with visceral pain related to malignancy, there remains limited outcome data for use in patients with chronic visceral pain of nonmalignant origin.

SUPERIOR HYPOGASTRIC PLEXUS
Approaches

The paired anterolateral neural structures of the superior hypogastric plexus overly the L5 to S1 vertebrae (**Fig. 5**). In the classic approach using fluoroscopy, the patient is positioned prone and a bilateral paramedian dorsal approach is used, although cases are reported of lateral positioning in exceptional circumstances. The transdiscal approach is a less commonly used alternative with the proposed benefit of simplified needle placement by avoiding the need to navigate the needle past the transverse process of L5 and the iliac crest. For individuals with accentuated lumbar lordosis or high iliac crests, the classic approach may not be possible because of anatomic obstruction of the target.

Patient Selection Criteria

Superior hypogastric plexus block (SHPB) is used in treating pain emanating from anywhere in the pelvic viscera except the ovaries/testes and fallopian tubes. It is most often applied in the treatment of cancer-related pain but can also be used as a diagnostic tool for chronic noncancer-related pain.[19–22] Studies have yet to be performed evaluating the efficacy of SHPB in the treatment of nonmalignant chronic pelvic pain syndromes, such as endometriosis, uterine fibroids, or chronic genitourinary and chronic gastrointestinal conditions. There are case reports of success of SHPB in treating chronic penile pain following transurethral radical prostatectomy and interstitial cystitis.[22,23]

Risks and Contraindications

General contraindications as discussed previously should be considered (see **Table 2**).

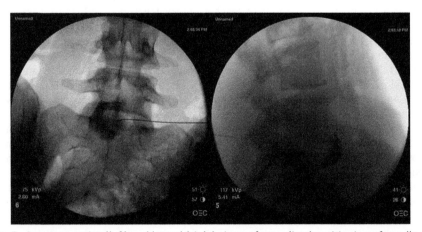

Fig. 5. Anteroposterior (*left*) and lateral (*right*) views of transdiscal positioning of needle at L5-S1 for superior hypogastric plexus block. (*From* Benzon, H. T., Rathmell, J. P., Wu, C. L., Turk, D. C., Argoff, C. E., & Hurley, R. W. (2013). *Practical Management of Pain: Fifth Edition*, Figures 59.6 and 59.5. Elsevier Inc. https://doi.org/10.1016/C2009-0-64063-0).

Particular to SHPB is the risk of retrograde spread of solution toward the nerve roots resulting in blockade or ablation of these structures. Reports of this complication are rare.[24] The transdiscal approach presents risks associated with compromise of the disk including diskitis and disk rupture.[25,26]

Outcome Data

SHPB has been reported to reduce VAS scores by about 70% and reduced opioid requirement by 67% with patient satisfaction with analgesia after neurolysis around 72%.[21,24] Although the same study defined successful block as a 50% decrease in opioid requirement, even patients falling below this threshold reported substantial (40%–45%) decreases in opioid consumption.[24]

Discussion

SHPB has been proven as an effective intervention for the treatment of pain for cancers involving the pelvic viscera. However, SHPB has not been well evaluated in the treatment of chronic nonmalignant conditions and is much less commonly performed for these indications. This is partly because chronic pelvic pain is known to be difficult to diagnose and treat with providers often unable to identify an inciting pathology. In some cases, SHPB may possibly provide therapeutic benefit and diagnostic utility.

GANGLION IMPAR
Approaches

The ganglion impar (Walther ganglion) is a single midline structure formed by the convergence of the distal terminations of the sympathetic chains. The original technique pioneered by Plancarte used surface landmarks to direct a needle through the anococcygeal ligament to the anterior surface of the sacrum with avoidance of bowel perforation assisted by tactile feedback via a digit inserted in the rectum (**Fig. 6**). Modern imaging tools have facilitated the development of more precise methods. Because the ganglion impar lies just anterior to the sacrococcygeal junction in the retroperitoneal space, it is accessed by a needle traversing the sacrococcygeal ligament in the aptly

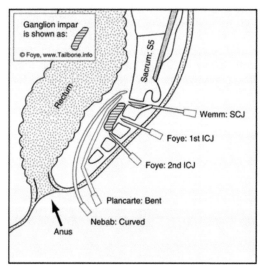

Fig. 6. Approaches to ganglion impar block. (*From* Furman, M. B., & Berkwits, L. (2018). *Atlas of image-guided Spinal procedures.* Figure 8A.9. Elsevier, Inc).

named transsacrococcygeal approach (**Fig. 7**). This is performed using fluoroscopic or CT guidance and low-volume contrast to confirm desirable spread of injectate. Ultrasound has been used to assist in location of the sacrococcygeal cleft, although lateral fluoroscopy remains necessary to confirm depth and contrast spread.[27]

Patient Selection Criteria

Ganglion impar blockade (GIB) is considered for treatment of visceral pain originating in the lower rectum, anus, distal urethra, vulva, and vagina (distal one-third), and coccygeal ligaments (coccydynia). Pain from these structures is often characterized as "poorly localized perineal pain with a burning character." Although GIB has most commonly been used for cancer-related pain, other pain syndromes have also been successfully treated using this technique.[28,29]

Small case series have demonstrated efficacy of GIB in treatment of chronic coccydynia and severe perineal pain (often described as vague and burning). In patients with chronic coccydynia, the degree of coccygeal mobility as measured on radiograph was not shown to influence treatment outcomes.[30]

Risks and Contraindications

General contraindications as discussed previously should be considered (see **Table 2**).

Because the rectum and distal sigmoid colon lay anterior to the sacrum, these structures are potentially at risk of perforation if the needle is advanced too far. However, there are no published reports of this complication occurring. A single case report describes spread of contrast into the epidural space but no therapeutic injectate was administered and no complication reported. Unguided injection of particulate steroid is reported to have resulted in conus infarction in one patient highlighting the utility of imaging guidance.[31]

Outcome Data

Quentin-Come and colleagues report their review of 83 patients with perineal or coccygeal pain treated with repeat (maximum of three) GIBs with 0.75% ropivacaine using CT guidance. Successful block was observed in 88% of injections with success defined as greater than 50% improvement in pain (VAS score) 30 minutes following the procedure. One month follow-up using the Patient Global Impression of Change demonstrated significant improvement in 41% of cases (43.6% for individuals treated with three blocks).[32,33]

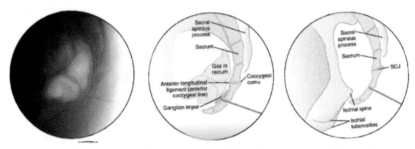

Fig. 7. Radiographic anatomy of ganglion impar block. (*From* Furman, M. B., & Berkwits, L. (2018). Atlas of image-guided Spinal procedures. Figure 8A.2. Elsevier, Inc).

A retrospective review of 29 patients with chronic coccydynia who underwent either diagnostic block alone or diagnostic block followed by pulsed radiofrequency ablation (RFA) demonstrated a durable improvement in VAS score at 3 to 6 months and 6 to 12 months for all but four patients. Although immediate postprocedure results were similar between groups, at 3- to 6-month follow-up the patients treated with combined diagnostic block plus pulsed RFA reported greater pain relief (72%) versus diagnostic block alone (40%).[34] However, a study comparing outcomes in patients with chronic perineal pain treated with pulsed RFA versus traditional (thermal) RFA found only thermal RFA improved patient VAS scores at follow-up.[35]

DISCUSSION

Patients presenting with pain emanating from the abdominal and pelvic viscera are often challenging to treat. Even when an underlying diagnosis is determined, benefits with conservative treatments may be limited. Additionally, pharmacologic treatments may contribute to side effects, such as constipation or nausea, that exacerbate the original presenting problem. Blockade of the sympathetic ganglia and nerves offers a promising approach for the diagnosis and treatment of patients with these pain conditions. Although there is supportive evidence for use of NCPB and splanchnic nerve block for visceral pain caused by abdominal malignancy, there is less robust evidence supporting use of neurolytic blockade of the superior hypogastric plexus and ganglion impar. Similarly, the role of sympathetic blocks for visceral pain of nonmalignant origin is less clearly defined.

CLINICS CARE POINTS

- The sympathetic ganglia is blocked or ablated for management of abdominal visceral pain. Duration of analgesia may be limited but may be used as a prognostic tool.

- Neurolysis should be reserved for carefully selected patients, most commonly those with cancer-related pain, because the duration of analgesia is typically limited to months.

- The celiac plexus and splanchnic nerves innervate most of the abdominal viscera. CPB is a widely performed and safe technique. It is most commonly used in the treatment of pancreatic cancer pain.

- The superior hypogastric plexus innervates much of the pelvic viscera. SHPB block is less commonly used and accepted than CPB.

- The ganglion impar provides visceral innervation of the lower vagina, rectum, and perineum. It is commonly used for treatment of cancer-related pain and to a lesser degree, perineal pain and chronic coccydynia.

REFERENCES

1. Bielefeldt K, Lamb K, Gebhart GF. Convergence of sensory pathways in the development of somatic and visceral hypersensitivity. Am J Physiol Gastrointest Liver Physiol 2006;291(4):G658–65.
2. Raizada V, Mittal RK. Pelvic floor anatomy and applied physiology. Gastroenterol Clin North Am 2008;37(3):493–509, vii.
3. Adams MCB, Benzon HT, Hurley RW. Chemical neurolytic blocks. Practical management of pain: Fifth edition. Published online January 1, 2014:784-793.e2. doi:10.1016/B978-0-323-08340-9.00058-X

4. Zacharias NA, Karri J, Garcia C, et al. Interventional radiofrequency treatment for the sympathetic nervous system: a review article. Pain Ther 2021;10(1):115–41.

5. Gress F, Schmitt C, Sherman S, et al. A prospective randomized comparison of endoscopic ultrasound- and computed tomography-guided celiac plexus block for managing chronic pancreatitis pain. Am J Gastroenterol 1999;94(4):900–5.

6. Atlas of image-guided intervention in regional anesthesia and pain medicine - James P. Rathmell. Available at. https://books.google.com/books?id=DZhSxcok 7poC&pg=PR4&lpg=PR4&dq=ISBN:+978-1-60831-704-2&source=bl&ots= uRZWlV4M6S&sig=ACfU3U2tItimGhJHDqRpFJvi-p7veAJN2Q&hl=en&sa=X& ved=2ahUKEwizotavzLf1AhXFHDQIHbLdBu4Q6AF6BAg4EAM#v=onepage&q= celiac&f=false. Accessed January 15, 2022.

7. Han CQ, Tang XL, Zhang Q, et al. Predictors of pain response after endoscopic ultrasound-guided celiac plexus neurolysis for abdominal pain caused by pancreatic malignancy. World J Gastroenterol 2021;27(1):69–79.

8. Gupta R, Madanat L, Jindal V, et al. Celiac plexus block complications: a case report and review of the literature. J Palliat Med 2021;24(9):1409–12.

9. Kibe H, et al. Pelvic and abdominal pain | principles and practice of pain medicine, 3e | AccessNeurology | McGraw Hill Medical. Accessed. https://neurology. mhmedical.com/content.aspx?sectionid=133687620&bookid=1845#133687623. [Accessed 12 January 2022]. Available at.

10. Sett SS, Taylor DC. Aortic pseudoaneurysm secondary to celiac plexus block. Ann Vasc Surg 1991;5(1):88–91.

11. Kaplan R, Schiff-Keren B, Alt E. Aortic dissection as a complication of celiac plexus block. Anesthesiology 1995;83(3):632–5.

12. Sample J, Hammad F, Ghazaleh S, et al. A rare complication of ileus following endoscopic ultrasound-guided celiac plexus neurolysis: a case report. Cureus 2020;12(10):e10963.

13. Kim SH, Jang KH, Cheon BK, et al. Paraplegia after celiac plexus neurolysis in a patient with pancreatic cancer: a case report and literature review. Anesth Pain Med 2019;14(1):85–90.

14. Eisenberg E, Carr DB, Chalmers TC. Neurolytic celiac plexus block for treatment of cancer pain. Anesth Analg 1995;80(2):290–5.

15. Arcidiacono PGG, Calori G, Carrara S, et al. Celiac plexus block for pancreatic cancer pain in adults. Cochrane Database Syst Rev 2011;2011(3):CD007519.

16. Zhong W, Yu Z, Zeng JX, et al. Celiac plexus block for treatment of pain associated with pancreatic cancer: a meta-analysis. Pain Pract 2014;14(1):43–51.

17. Rahman A, Rahman R, Macrinici G, et al. Low volume neurolytic retrocrural celiac plexus block for visceral cancer pain: retrospective review of 507 patients with severe malignancy related pain due to primary abdominal cancer or metastatic disease. Pain physician 2018;21(5):497–504.

18. Lillemoe KD, Cameron JL, Kaufman HS, et al. Chemical splanchnicectomy in patients with unresectable pancreatic cancer a prospective randomized trial. Ann Surg 1993;217(5):447–57.

19. Gofeld M, Shankar H. Peripheral and visceral sympathetic blocks. Practical management of pain: Fifth edition. Published online January 1, 2014:755-767.e2. doi:10.1016/B978-0-323-08340-9.00056-6

20. de Leon-Casasola OA, Kent E, Lema MJ. Neurolytic superior hypogastric plexus block for chronic pelvic pain associated with cancer. Pain 1993;54(2):145–51.

21. Plancarte R, de Leon-Casasola OA, El-Helaly M, et al. Neurolytic superior hypogastric plexus block for chronic pelvic pain associated with cancer. Reg Anesth 1997;22(6):562–8.

22. Rosenberg SK, Tewari R, Boswell M v, et al. Superior hypogastric plexus block successfully treats severe penile pain after transurethral resection of the prostate. Reg Anesth Pain Med 1998;23(6):618–20.
23. Kim JH, Kim E, Kim B il. Pulsed radiofrequency treatment of the superior hypogastric plexus in an interstitial cystitis patient with chronic pain and symptoms refractory to oral and intravesical medications and bladder hydrodistension. Medicine 2016;95(49):e5549.
24. LoDico MJP, de Leon-Casasola O. Neurolysis of the sympathetic axis for cancer pain management. Practical management of pain: Fifth edition. Published online January 1, 2014:794-801.e1. doi:10.1016/B978-0-323-08340-9.00059-1
25. Baig S, Moon JY, Shankar H. Review of sympathetic blocks: anatomy, sonoanatomy, evidence, and techniques. Reg Anesth Pain Med 2017;42(3):377–91.
26. Voiculescu LD, Chen QCC. Discitis following transdiscal approach for superior hypogastric plexus block. Challenging Cases Complication Management Pain Med undefined. Published online January 1, 2018:155-161. doi:10.1007/978-3-319-60072-7_26
27. Lin CS, Cheng JK, Hsu YW, et al. Ultrasound-guided ganglion impar block: a technical report. Pain Med 2010;11(3):390–4.
28. Lee CJ, Lee SC. Sympathetic nerve block and neurolysis. In: Minimally invasive percutaneous spinal techniques. Elsevier; 2010. p. 170–83. https://doi.org/10.1016/B978-0-7020-2913-4.00010-0.
29. Hong DG, Hwang SM, Park JM. Efficacy of ganglion impar block on vulvodynia. Medicine 2021;100(30):e26799.
30. Sencan S, Cuce I, Karabiyik O, et al. The influence of coccygeal dynamic patterns on ganglion impar block treatment results in chronic coccygodynia. Interv Neuroradiol 2018;24(5):580–5.
31. Kuek DKC, Chung SL, Zishan US, et al. Conus infarction after non-guided transcoccygeal ganglion impar block using particulate steroid for chronic coccydinia. Spinal Cord Ser Cases 2019;5(1):92.
32. Datir A, Connell D. CT-guided injection for ganglion impar blockade: a radiological approach to the management of coccydynia. Clin Radiol 2010;65(1):21–5. https://doi.org/10.1016/j.crad.2009.08.007.
33. le Clerc QC, Riant T, Levesque A, et al. Repeated ganglion impar block in a cohort of 83 patients with chronic pelvic and perineal pain. Pain physician 2017;20(6):E823–8.
34. Sagir O, Demir HF, Ugun F, et al. Retrospective evaluation of pain in patients with coccydynia who underwent impar ganglion block. BMC Anesthesiol 2020; 20(1):110.
35. Usmani H, Dureja GP, Andleeb R, et al. Conventional radiofrequency thermocoagulation vs pulsed radiofrequency neuromodulation of ganglion impar in chronic perineal pain of nononcological origin. Pain Med 2018;19(12):2348–56.

Peripheral Nerve Injections

Arti Ori, MD[a], Aparna Jindal, MBBS[b], Nenna Nwazota, MD[c],
Amy C.S. Pearson, MD[d],*, Bhavana Yalamuru, MBBS, MD[e]

KEYWORDS

- Peripheral nerve block • Chronic pain • Neuralgia • Interventional pain management

KEY POINTS

- Peripheral nerve injections can be considered for pain in the distribution of a peripheral nerve.
- These injections are typically performed under ultrasound guidance and occasionally via landmark or fluoroscopic guidance.
- Although published evidence for most peripheral nerve injections is limited to case series, there is renewed innovation in these injections and techniques as ultrasound and peripheral nerve stimulation technology advances.

INTRODUCTION

Peripheral nerve injections are used in acute pain management in the perioperative and postoperative period and following trauma. In addition, they have a role in diagnosing and treating chronic pain conditions.[1] In this article, we will discuss the anatomy, technical considerations, indications, and risks for nerve injections in the head and neck, upper extremity, trunk, and lower extremity. Although the common contraindications for any peripheral nerve injection are universal, such as patient refusal, patient inability to cooperate, severe local anesthetic allergy, and local infection at the injection site, we will elaborate on more specific contraindications that are applicable to each block based on the anatomy and likely complications. Similarly, certain complications are common to all peripheral nerve injections and include nerve injury or tissue damage, bleeding or hematoma formation, infection, allergy, and the risk of local anesthetic-induced systemic toxicity.

a Department of Anesthesiology and Perioperative Medicine, Pain Medicine Division, Brigham and Women's Hospital, 75 Francis Street, Boston, MA 02115, USA; b Department of Anesthesia, University of Iowa Hospitals and Clinics, 200 Hawkins Drive, Iowa City, IA 52242, USA; c University of Texas at Southwestern, 221 N Polk Street, Dallas, TX 75208, USA; d Department of Anesthesia, Pain Division, University of Iowa Hospitals and Clinics, 200 Hawkins Drive, Iowa City, IA 52242, USA; e Pain Division, Department of Anesthesiology, University of Virginia Health System, 475 Ray C Hunt Drive, Charlottesville, VA 22903, USA
* Corresponding author.
E-mail address: amy.schultz.pearson@gmail.com

Phys Med Rehabil Clin N Am 33 (2022) 489–517
https://doi.org/10.1016/j.pmr.2022.02.004
1047-9651/22/© 2022 Elsevier Inc. All rights reserved.
pmr.theclinics.com

General Comments

Unless otherwise stated in this article, peripheral nerve injections are commonly performed with sterile technique under real-time ultrasound guidance with injectate observed spreading perineurally as opposed to epineurally.[2] Local anesthetic is commonly used as an injectate with steroid sometimes chosen to extend the duration of relief. These injections can be used as therapeutic interventions or as diagnostic to aid in procedural planning, for example, to identify the painful nerve before peripheral nerve stimulation (PNS) or release.[3,4] As with any injection, the risk of bleeding and hematoma formation, infection, reaction to medication (including elevated blood glucose from steroid), potential motor weakness or sensory loss, and nerve or tissue damage should be discussed with the patient before proceeding.[3] Additional risks unique to each injection are described in their respective section.

Head and neck

Peripheral nerve blocks can serve as adjuncts in the management of headache disorders and cranial neuralgias and can reduce oral medication requirements and polypharmacy. They can provide analgesic benefits for weeks to months after the local anesthetic.

Gasserian Ganglion Injections: The Gasserian ganglion, also known as the trigeminal ganglion, is a common target for facial pains emanating from the trigeminal distribution, especially for trigeminal neuralgia. Although Gasserian ganglion radiofrequency ablation, microvascular decompression, and radiotherapy treatments are more commonly reported, nerve injections with local anesthetic, steroid, and dehydrated alcohol have been described.[5,6]

Technique: Because of the risk of cerebrospinal fluid leak and/or damage to neural structures causing neuritis, dysesthesia, or sensory loss, this procedure should be done with imaging guidance, typically by computerized tomography (CT), although fluoroscopic approaches have been described. A small needle is advanced percutaneously toward the zygoma to the opening of the foramen ovale. Aspiration is performed to confirm lack of cerebrospinal fluid return, and contrast is used to outline Meckel cave, which contains the trigeminal nerve branches. Although this is commonly an outpatient procedure, the patients are often observed for a prolonged period for any neurologic complications.[5]

Patient selection criteria: Patients with disorders of the trigeminal ganglion unresponsive to conventional therapies can be considered.

Risks and contraindications: As above, there is the risk of CSF leak, neuritis, dysesthesia, and sensory loss. More concerning complications include paralysis, facial weakness, infection, paralysis, stroke, and infarction.[5]

Outcome data: A 2017 case series of 465 patients receiving fluoroscopy-guided trigeminal nerve blocks (with needle directed at V2 and V3 portions and combined with infraorbital and supraorbital nerve blocks) with dehydrated alcohol demonstrated that 99% had immediate and complete pain relief, and this pain relief lasted for at least 1 year in 86.2% of patients.[6] An ultrasound-guided technique using local anesthetic and steroids via the pterygopalatine fossa has been described, with the majority of the 15 subjects receiving benefit for at least 15 months.[7]

Maxillary nerve injections: The maxillary nerve is the V2 branch of the trigeminal ganglion, which innervates the skin of the maxilla. Intraoral maxillary injections for dental anesthesia and percutaneous blocks for facial surgery are outside the scope of this article.

Technique: Ultrasound-guided techniques via the pterygopalatine fossa have been reported, with percutaneous needle approaches either at the posteroinferior zygoma, anteroinferior zygoma, or suprazygomatic.[8,9]

Patient selection criteria: Patients with facial pain in the V2 distribution can be considered for this injection.

Risks and contraindications: Risks and contraindications are the same as for Gasserian ganglion injections.

Outcome data: A 2020 literature review described the ultrasound target as easily accessible. There are no long-term outcome data on maxillary nerve injections alone for chronic pain syndromes.[8]

Mandibular nerve injections: The mandibular nerve is a branch of the V3 portion of the trigeminal ganglion, which innervates the skin of the mandible. Case reports of mandibular nerve injections for trigeminal neuralgia in this distribution have been described.

Technique: As the mandibular nerve is the V3 (lowermost) portion of the trigeminal nerve, the technique is similar to that of a Gasserian ganglion injection with the needle directed at the midportion of the lower rim of the foramen ovale. Ultrasound techniques have also been described.[9]

Patient selection criteria: Patients with facial pain in the distribution of V3 could be considered for this injection.

Risks and contraindications: Risks and contraindications are the same as for Gasserian ganglion injections.

Outcome data: A 2010 case series of 120 Gasserian ganglion blocks with dehydrated alcohol showed 99% of patients with complete and immediate pain relief lasting a mean of 46 months, however 20% of patients experienced complications, mainly related to dysesthesias.[10]

Occipital Nerve Injections: The greater occipital nerve (GON) arises from the dorsal ramus of C2 with contribution from C3, supplying sensation to the medial aspect of the posterior scalp. It may be palpated 2 to 2.5 cm below the external occipital protuberance, approximately 1.5 cm lateral to the midline. The lesser occipital nerve (LON) arises from the ventral ramus of C3 and is located in the lateral third of an imaginary line between the occipital protuberance and mastoid process.[11-13]

Technique of injection, non-image guided: A small-caliber needle is advanced subcutaneously along the occipital protruberance, and local anesthetic and/or steroid are injected in a fan-like distribution. Bilateral injections may be done. *Image-guided:* The GON can be identified under ultrasound by scanning from the cranium caudally until the bifid C2 spinous process is identified. The probe is slid laterally and rotated until the C2 lamina and overlying internal obliquus muscle (IOM) is identified. The GON lies superficially to the IOM and deep to the semispinalis capitis and longissimus capitis muscle.[13]

Patient selection criteria: Blocking the GON and LON is used for diagnostic and therapeutic purposes both for primary headache disorders (migraines, cluster headaches) and secondary headache disorders (cervicogenic headaches).

- *Occipital neuralgia:* Patients have pain in the distribution of the GON and/or the LON. Palpation of these nerves elicits the pain and paresthesia may also occur. Relief of pain with local anesthetic block of the occipital nerves is diagnostic.[14]
- *Chronic migraines:* Patients will often have pain on palpation of peripheral nerves because of central sensitization at the level of the trigeminocervical complex. Blocking the GON and LON can reduce the frequency, duration, and intensity of migraine attacks.[14]
- *Cluster headache:* These headaches are characterized by hemicranial pain, cluster headaches can be aborted by ipsilateral GON and LON block.[14]

- *Cervicogenic headaches:* These headaches typically arise in the cervical spine or soft tissues of the neck and are characterized by painful palpation of the region of the GON and LON.[14]

Risks and Contraindications: Risks include hematoma formation, especially for those on anticoagulant or antiplatelet therapy, vasovagal and syncopal episodes, infection, injury to the occipital artery, which is located lateral to the GON, and local anesthetic intravascular injection.[14–16] Corticosteroids can cause alopecia, cutaneous atrophy, and hyperpigmentation. *Contraindications:* Although the literature does not describe absolute contraindications, one needs to be aware of an open skull defect or craniotomy that can lead to an intracranial local anesthetic diffusion.[17]

Outcome data: Ashkenazi and colleagues in a systematic review on peripheral nerve injections for headache management found few randomized controlled studies.[16] The majority of the literature was on GON injections, but most studies were small and noncontrolled. The conditions treated included both primary (eg, migraine, cluster headache) and secondary (eg, cervicogenic) disorders. Overall, the results were positive and the procedures were well tolerated.[14] In 2013, the American Headache Society found that the evidence was strongest for cluster headaches, but there was otherwise a paucity of evidence[14,18] (**Fig. 1**).

Supraorbital/supratrochlear nerve injections: The *supratrochlear nerve (STN)* arises from the frontal nerve, which is the largest branch of the ophthalmic nerve (V1). It enters the orbit via the superior orbital fissure. It innervates the inferomedial section of the forehead, the bridge of the nose, and the medial portion of the upper eyelid. It runs medially to the supraorbital nerve.[19]

Technique: The supraorbital ridge is palpated, and a small caliber needle is inserted lateral to the junction where the bridge of the nose and the supraorbital ridge meet and advanced medially.

Patient selection criteria: Patients with pain in the V1 distribution or specifically the STN distribution.

Risks: There is risk of dissection of the local anesthetic due to the loose tissue that may cause periorbital hematoma. Corticosteroids may cause atrophy or abnormal pigmentation in this region.

Supraorbital nerve injection (SON): The SON is the larger of the two terminal branches of the frontal nerve. It runs through the supraorbital foramen and supplies sensation to the upper eyelid and conjunctiva. It also supplies the forehead and the skin of the scalp up to the lambdoid suture. It also contains postganglionic sympathetic fibers that innervate the sweat glands of the supraorbital area. The supraorbital foramen lies on the superior aspect of an imaginary line course that intersects the pupil, the infraorbital foramen, and the mental foramen.[19]

Technique: The supraorbital notch is palpated at the superior margin of the orbit in the midpupillary line along the eyebrow. The needle is advanced medially at a shallow angle along the supraorbital ridge. The nerve can also be identified by ultrasound with the probe over the supraorbital notch. Color Doppler can be used to identify the supraorbital artery and avoid it.[9]

Patient selection criteria: This injection can be used to relieve pain in the V1 region, for example, due to trigeminal neuralgia, postherpetic neuralgia, or migraine headaches.

Risks: Because of the superficial nature of the injection, facial skin and small muscle atrophy may occur from corticosteroid use.

Outcome data: SON and STN are used for pain in the V1 distribution; however, there is a paucity of data regarding their efficacy.

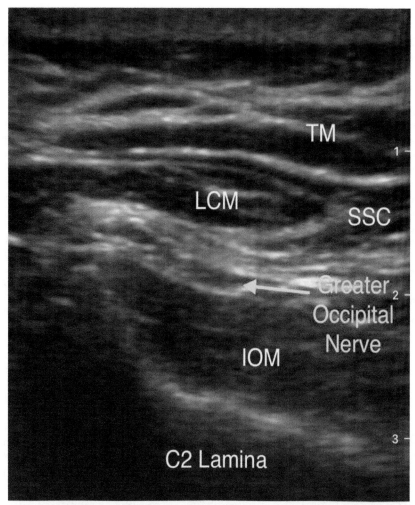

Fig. 1. GON at the level of C2. The lateral edge of the ultrasound is rotated caudally to identify the LCM and SSC muscles in this view. IOM, inferior obliquus capitis; LCM, longissimus capitis; SSC, semispinalis capitis; TM, trapezius muscle. Note the bifid spinous process of C2. (*Image courtesy of* Amy Pearson, MD, Iowa City.)

Greater auricular nerve (GAN) Injections: The GAN arises from the primary ventral ramus of C2 and C3. It is located inferior and lateral to the LON and provides sensory innervation to the ear, external auditory canal, angle of the jaw, and skin overlying the parotid gland.[20]

Technique: The mastoid process is palpated, and the needle is advanced and directed toward the ear lobe and injected in a fan-like distribution. This injection can also be done under ultrasound guidance, where the sternocleidomastoid is identified at roughly the level of C3-4 and the nerve is observed wrapping around the posterior border of the muscle superficially.[15]

Patient selection criteria: Pain in the distribution of the GAN (posttrauma/surgery—cervical lymph node dissection, facelift, carotid endarterectomy) and pain due to herpes zoster.[20]

Risks: Due to the proximity to the brachial plexus (BP) and carotid triangle, there is risk of hematoma formation and injury to neck vessels or BP.

Outcome data: There is a paucity of large-scale data assessing the efficacy of GAN. A case report has described effective use of the GAN injection for Ramsay Hunt syndrome, a form of postherpetic neuralgia affecting the geniculate ganglion and facial nerve, causing otalgia.[21]

Upper brachial plexus injections

Upper extremity BP injections involve injection around the nerves arising from different levels of the BP. The BP is a group of nerves formed by the ventral rami of C5-T1 that innervate the upper extremity. These five nerve roots join to form superior, middle, and inferior trunks. Each trunk divides into anterior and posterior divisions, these divisions rearrange to form three cords posterior, medial, and lateral and finally give rise to terminal branches. Numerous anatomic variations exist, which are beyond the scope of this article.[22] Anatomy, risks, and contraindications are summarized in the table below.

Interscalene brachial plexus injection: The C5-T1 nerve roots emerge between anterior scalene muscles (ASM) and middle scalene muscles (MSM) in the interscalene groove as they exit the foramina. The interscalene injection allows for coverage of the lateral two-thirds of the clavicle, shoulder, and proximal humerus. The inferior trunk (C8-T1) is often inadequately blocked in this approach (**Fig. 2**).

Patient selection criteria:
Before PNS:
- Complex regional pain syndrome (CRPS) of upper extremity
- Scapular and upper chest pain due to cervical radiculopathy
- Phantom limb pain refractory to conservative management
For continuous infusion
- Cancer related pain (neoplastic brachial plexopathy [NBP])
- CRPS of shoulder joint
Outcome data:
- For CPRS: About 59% patients had greater than 50% improvement in pain even after a mean of 27.5 months.[23]

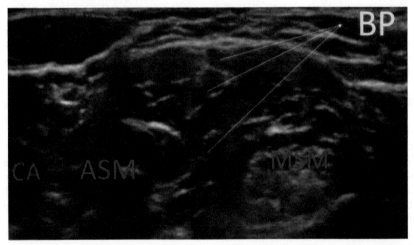

Fig. 2. Interscalene brachial plexus injection. ASM, Anterior scalene muscle; BP, brachial plexus; CA, carotid artery; MSM, middle scalene muscle. (*Image courtesy of* Dr Aparna Jindal, MBBS, Iowa City.).

- For cervical radiculopathy: significant decrease in visual analogue scale (VAS) was noted (with 7 mL of 1% lidocaine and 3.3 mg dexamethasone).[24]
- One week continuous infusion of bupivacaine with rehabilitation showed improvement in pain and range of motion in greater than 80% patients with CRPS of shoulder at 6 months.[25]

Supraclavicular injection: This injection targets the distal trunks/proximal divisions of the BP dorsal to the clavicle and just superficial to the first rib. Typically, these are done under ultrasound guidance with the supraclavicular artery in view[26,27] (**Fig. 3**).

Infraclavicular approach: As the BP passes behind the clavicle in the infraclavicular fossa, the divisions reorganize to form posterior, medial, and lateral cords, named according to their position relative to the axillary artery[22,28] (**Figs. 4** and **5**).

Axillary approach (axillary nerve [AN] injection described separately): The three cords enter the axilla arranged around AA, at the lateral border of pectoralis minor, and divide into terminal branches—musculocutaneous nerve (MCN), median nerve (MN), ulnar nerve (UN), radial nerve (RN), medial cutaneous nerve of arm, and medial cutaneous nerve of forearm.[28,29]

Outcome data for BP injections (**Table 1**):

- Although a number of approaches to the BP can be taken, there is a paucity of data on the advantages of any particular approach. Case reports describe potential benefit primarily in the context of CRPS or brachial plexopathies. For cervical radiculopathy, significant decrease in visual analog scores was noted (with 7 mL of 1% lidocaine and 3.3 mg dexamethasone) with interscalene BP block.[24]
- One week continuous infusion of bupivacaine in the interscalene BP with rehabilitation showed improvement in pain and range of motion in greater than 80% patients with CRPS of shoulder at 6 months.[25]
- NBP: In a case series of eight patients with cancer-related pain originating from the BP underwent either interscalene or supraclavicular BP blocks with a combination of local anesthetic and steroid. Patients reported a sustained decrease in their pain (lasting from 2 weeks to 10 months), a significant decrease in their

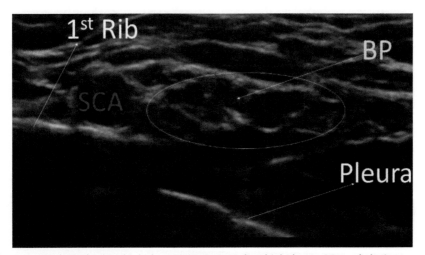

Fig. 3. Supraclavicular brachial plexus injection. BP, brachial plexus; SCA, subclavian artery. (*Image courtesy of* Dr Aparna Jindal, MBBS, Iowa City.)

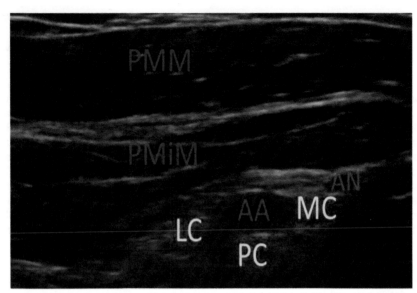

Fig. 4. Infraclavicular brachial plexus block. AA, axillary artery; LC, lateral cord; MC, medial cord; PC, posterior cord; PMiM, pectoralis minor muscle; PMM, pectoralis major muscle. (*Image courtesy of* Dr Aparna Jindal, MBBS, Iowa City.)

opioid and nonopioid (ketamine, gabapentin) consumption, overall satisfaction with the block.[34]

AN injection (axillary approach to the BP addressed separately): The AN is the terminal branch of the posterior cord of the BP branching off at the level of axilla. The nerve exits the axilla posteriorly via the quadrangular space along with the posterior circumflex humeral artery. The borders of this space are superior: teres minor, inferior: teres major, lateral: humerus, and medial: triceps brachii.[35]

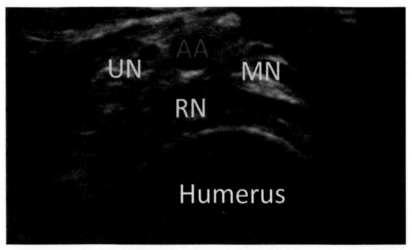

Fig. 5. Axillary brachial plexus block. AA, axillary artery; MN, median nerve; RN, radial nerve; UN, ulnar nerve. (*Image courtesy of* Dr Aparna Jindal, MBBS, Iowa City.)

Table 1
Outcome data for brachial plexus injections

Injection	Level of the Brachial Plexus	Anatomy	Risks/Complications	Contraindications
Interscalene	Roots	Between ASM and MSM [30,31]	Infection, bleeding/hematoma, puncture of a vascular structure, epidural/subarachnoid injection, local anesthetic systemic toxicity, permanent nerve injury, Horner syndrome, hemiparesis of the diaphragm, pneumothorax [32]	Pulmonary disease, heart disease, cellulitis/abscess over the injection site, patient refusal, allergy to the local anesthetic. Morbid obesity may be a relative contraindication as respiratory insufficiency can result in hemidiaphragmatic paralysis Respiratory insufficiency is a contraindication as there is a high likelihood of ipsilateral diaphragmatic hemiparesis (25% decrease in pulmonary function). Existing contralateral vocal cord palsy is also a contraindication as the recurrent laryngeal nerve could be blocked as well leading to complete airway obstruction [32,33]
Supraclavicular	Distal Trunks/Proximal Divisions	Targets the distal trunks/proximal divisions of the BP dorsal to the clavicle and just superficial to the first rib	Pneumothorax and subclavian arterial puncture are the major risks. There is still a risk of causing ipsilateral hemidiaphragmatic paralysis with this injection, although the risk is much lower than ISB. UN sparing may occur if the full	Cellulitis/abscess over the site of injection. Use caution in patients with poor pulmonary reserve, as a resultant pneumothorax may significantly worsen their respiratory status (eg, known pneumonia on the contralateral side) [33]

(continued on next page)

Table 1
(continued)

Injection	Level of the Brachial Plexus	Anatomy	Risks/Complications	Contraindications
			spread of anesthetic is not achieved between the first rib and the plexus	
Infraclavicular	Cords	The infraclavicular fossa boundaries are: pectoralis major muscle (PMM) and minor (PMiM) muscles anteriorly, clavicle superiorly, pleura posteromedially, serratus anterior muscle posteriorly[28]	Because it is a deep injection, arterial compression is difficult if arterial puncture occurs. Anticoagulation is a contraindication for this nerve injection	Cellulitis/abscess over the site of injection
Axillary	Nerves	The boundaries are anterior: pectoralis muscles, posterior: subscapularis, teres major and latissimus dorsi, medial: chest wall and serratus anterior, lateral: humerus and attached muscles. The neurovascular bundle is incompletely surrounded by fascial sheath with the MCN outside the sheath, between biceps and coracobrachialis or within the body of coracobrachialis. In relation to the AA, MN: lateral and superficial, UN: medial and superficial, RN: posterior. Significant variation exists[29]	This is a relatively safer approach for BP blockade as pleura and phrenic nerve are spared	Cellulitis/abscess over the injection site, inability to visualize a clear needle path through the highly vascular region

Patient selection criteria:[4,36,37]

- Before axillary PNS for refractory hemiplegic shoulder pain (HSP) (see outcomes below)
- Chronic shoulder pain: Subacromial impingement syndrome/rotator cuff pathologic condition, glenohumeral joint arthritis, acromioclavicular joint arthritis, adhesive capsulitis, or biceps tendinopathy.

Outcome data: As this injection is typically done as diagnostic before PNS, the following outcomes are for PNS:

- With implantable generators: Greater than 50% improvement in pain at 6 and 12 months, at least 50% improvement at 24 months.[35]
- HSP: PNS of the AN (along with the suprascapular nerve [SSN])—fair-to-moderate evidence to treat HSP with limited evidence for chronic shoulder pain due to other degenerative pathologies.[37]
- Chronic shoulder pain: About 88% responders (decreased pain scores greater than 50% on trial) had average pain reduction by 70%, decreased opioid consumption in 100%.[36]

SSN injection: SSN is a branch of the superior trunk of BP and provides sensory supply to 70% of the shoulder joint.[38]

Technique: Anterior or posterior approach. *Anterior:* Position: similar to supraclavicular injection, the subclavian artery (SCA) and BP are identified with US along with overlying omohyoid muscle (OM). SSN identified deep to OM, lateral and superficial to BP. Needle inserted from lateral to medial side. *Posterior:* Position-sitting, with the probe parallel to scapular spine with slight anterior tilt to see the supraspinous fossa. The needle is inserted lateral to medial in plane.

Patient selection: Chronic shoulder pain etiologies: adhesive capsulitis, arthritis, rheumatologic disorders, trauma, postoperative pain, neoplasm, and HSP. PNS can be considered for chronic refractory neuropathic pain.[23,39,40]

Risks and contraindications: Due to the proximity to the pleura and neurovascular structures, pneumothorax, injury to SSN, or vessels should be considered.

Outcome data:

- A US-guided SSN block using 0.25% bupivacaine and 40 mg triamcinolone decreased pain scores at 72 hours, 1, 3, and 6 months. About 43.7% patients had total pain remission.[39]
- Pulsed radiofrequency (PRF) neuromodulation of SSN combined with short acting steroids resulted in sustained pain relief for up to 24 weeks.[41]
- PRF to the SSN with physical therapy (PT) was superior to SSN nerve block and PT.
- SSN PNS was effective and safe for refractory upper extremity neuropathic pain with greater than 50% improvement in pain after a mean of 27.5 months.[42]
- PNS of the SSN (along with AN): Fair-to-moderate evidence to treat shoulder pain in HSP patients with limited evidence for chronic shoulder pain due to other degenerative pathologies[37] (**Fig. 6**).

Median, Ulnar, and Radial Nerves

Patient selection criteria: neuropathy of the RN

Median nerve: The MN travels inferior to brachial artery (BA) in the arm and lies medial to BA in antecubital fossa. It lies deep to flexor digitorum superficialis muscle as it travels toward the wrist. In the wrist, it is present under the flexor retinaculum in the carpal tunnel.

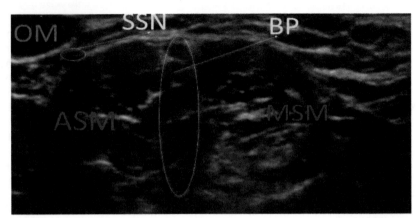

Fig. 6. Anterior approach to SSN block. ASM, anterior scalene muscle; BP, brachial plexus; MSM, middle scalene muscle; OM, omphyoid; SSN, suprascapular nerve. (*Image courtesy of* Dr Aparna Jindal, MBBS, Iowa City.)

Technique: For injections proximal to elbow, the patient is positioned supine with shoulder abducted 90°. The MN is scanned proximal to distal on the medial aspect of the arm with ultrasound as it travels with the AA. For injections distal to elbow, the arm is supinated. MN is scanned proximal to distal from elbow along with BA.[26]

Outcome data: Injection at the distal MN for carpal tunnel syndrome is common, with good results with either the landmark-based or the ultrasound injections.[43] A meta-analysis of corticosteroid injection versus decompression surgery for carpal tunnel syndrome revealed similar efficacy at 3 and 12 months.[44]

Ulnar nerve: The UN courses superficial to the medial head of triceps brachii, through the cubital tunnel, and enters the forearm to lie medial to the ulnar artery.

Technique: The transducer is placed transversely on the wrist, ulnar artery is identified on the medial side of wrist and scanned proximally. The flexor carpi ulnaris tendon is seen superficially.[26]

Radial Nerve: The RN courses in radial (spiral) groove on the lateral surface on midhumerus along with deep branches of BA. At the level of the midforearm, it lies lateral to the radial artery.

Technique: The transducer is placed transversely on wrist, RA identified on lateral side, and scanned proximally.[26]

Outcome data: As these injections can be done as diagnostic before PNS,[4] see PNS article. There are no large-scale outcome data on the efficacy of radial or UN blocks for chronic pain.

Truncal Injections

Intercostal nerve injections

Intercostal nerve injections are a useful tool in the treatment of intercostal neuralgia when conservative management is unsuccessful.[45] Intercostal neuralgia is characterized by sharp, stabbing pain in the dermatomal distribution of the intercostal nerve. The intercostal nerves arise from the ventral rami of thoracic nerves T1 to T11.

Injection: Usually three levels are injected to cover the area of pain due to overlapping innervation. Both ultrasound and fluoroscopic guidance can be used. The nerve is injected posteriorly about 7 to 10 cm from the midline. Using the fluoroscopic technique, the needle is advanced until it contacts the inferior border of the rib. It is then directed caudally so that is inferior to the rib and slightly deep. With US guidance, a probe is placed longitudinally, and the needle is advanced directed to the inferior border of the corresponding rib. Solution can be visualized beneath the fascia of the internal intercostal as the nerve itself cannot be seen.

Patient selection criteria: Postthoracotomy pain syndrome (PTPS; 50% of patients develop chronic pain after thoracotomy)[46]

Postherpetic neuralgia

Risks and contraindications: Due to the proximity of underlying pleura, the risk of pneumothorax should be considered.

Outcome data: Repeated intercostal blocks with local anesthetic have been described to provide a long-lasting benefit for chronic pain conditions.[47] INB have useful diagnostic value and can be used to predict the efficacy of more lasting procedures such as cryoanalgesia that can be used to treat pain from rib fractures.[48] There is a paucity of data on the efficacy of PRF for chronic intercostal neuralgia; however, anecdotal reports have shown radiofrequency lesioning to be a promising treatment of chronic intercostal neuralgia.[49]

Paravertebral nerve injection

Technique: This injection provides analgesia to the thoracic and upper abdominal areas and has been used increasingly in the last decade during breast surgery, thoracic surgery, and the management of rib fractures.[50] The paravertebral space is bounded by the costotransverse ligament and the parietal pleura anteriorly and transverse process and ribs posteriorly. The space is continuous with the intercostal space. Paravertebral block (PVB) involves a needle being inserted just lateral to the vertebral spinal process, injecting local anesthetic into a space where the spinal nerves emerge from the intervertebral foramina.[26] The result is a somatic and sympathetic nerve blockade of four to five dermatomes if using a volume of 15 mL or more. The advantages of PVB over epidural include a lower incidence of side effects like hypotension.

Patient selection criteria: Chest wall pain and intercostal neuralgia (after rib fractures or breast surgery), see later discussion.

Risks and contraindications: There is an additional risk of pneumothorax due to the proximity to the pleura. Patients with lung compromise on the contralateral lung may be at greater risk should a pneumothorax occur.

Outcome data: Thoracic PVBs have been shown to reduce postoperative pain and decrease opioid consumption in patients undergoing breast surgery.[51] In addition, there is evidence that PVBs may prevent chronic pain after breast surgery.[52] Kairaluoma and colleagues followed patients who received PVBs for breast surgery for 1 year, and at 12 months, the PVB group had less motion-related pain and less pain at rest.[53] Karmakar and colleagues also found that PVBs prevent and reduce the severity of chronic pain after breast surgery.[54,55] A total of 180 women undergoing modified radical mastectomy were randomized to either a standardized general anesthesia (GA), GA with a single-injection thoracic paravertebral nerve block (TPVB) or a placebo paravertebral infusion) or GA with a continuous PVB. Although they concluded that there was no significant difference in the incidence or relative risk of chronic pain at 3 and 6 months when PVB was used in conjunction with GA, patients who received TPVBs reported less severe chronic pain, showed fewer symptoms and signs of chronic pain, and also experienced better physical and mental health-related quality of life.[54]

Chronic nonsurgical pain such as postherpetic neuralgia, cancer pain, or chronic pain after rib fractures can benefit from PVBs. Makharita and colleagues compared PVBs with traditional treatment of patients with active herpes zoster and postherpetic neuralgia. A total of 180 patients with acute thoracic herpetic eruption were randomly assigned to receive a PVB using either saline or bupivacaine, and 8 mg dexamethasone in a total volume of 10 mL. Incidence of postherpetic neuralgia was comparable in both groups after 3 months but significantly lower at 6 months.[56]

Transverse abdominus plane (TAP) injections

TAP is useful for the treatment of chronic abdominal wall pain after abdominal surgeries including laparotomy, hernia repair, appendectomy, cesarean section, abdominal hysterectomy, and prostatectomy when other treatment methods have failed. The sensory innervation of the anterior abdominal wall arises from the anterior rami of spinal nerves T7 to L1. Local anesthetic is injected between the transversus abdominis (TA) and internal oblique (IO) muscles.

Technique: With the patient in a supine position, the probe is placed in the transverse plane of the lateral abdominal wall in the midaxillary line between the costal margin and the iliac crest. The needle is advanced between the IO and TA muscles.

Patient selection criteria: Patients with chronic abdominal pain following surgery benefit from these blocks (see later discussion).

Risks: Some complications have been reported in the literature include bowel perforation, hematoma, intrahepatic injection, transient femoral nerve blockage, and intravascular injection.[57]

Outcome data: A retrospective analysis reviewed of 92 patients receiving TAP blocks over 5 years for chronic abdominal pain refractory to conventional treatment. TAP blocks were associated with a statistically significant improvement in abdominal pain scores in 81.9% of procedures. Improvement was 50.3% $\pm$ 39.0% with an average duration of 108 days after procedures with ongoing pain relief at time of follow-up. There was a significant reduction in emergency department visits for abdominal pain before and after the procedure ($P \leq .05$)[58,59] (**Fig. 7**).

Ilioinguinal and iliohypogastric nerve injections: The ilioinguinal and iliohypogastric nerves arise from the first lumbar spinal root and run superomedial to the anterior superior iliac spine (ASIS) and through the TA muscle. They then pierce the external oblique muscle to provide cutaneous sensation. The ilioinguinal nerve provides sensation to the superomedial aspect of the thigh, and the iliohypogastric nerve provides sensation to the skin over the inguinal region. Blockade of the ilioinguinal and iliohypogastric nerves has been shown to be efficacious in providing pain relief for patients with chronic pain following inguinal hernia repair, abdominal hysterectomy, or cesarean section.[60]

Injection technique: Needle insertion is performed 2 cm medially and 2 cm superior to the ASIS to the plane between the IO and TA muscles. Color Doppler imaging can identify a branch of the deep circumflex iliac artery lying in the same anatomic plane and parallel to the ilioinguinal nerve. Injection adjacent to the artery will block both the ilioinguinal and iliohypogastric nerves.[61]

Patient selection criteria: Ilioinguinal neuralgia, iliohypogastric neuralgia, groin pain, pelvic pain, postherpetic neuralgia, and abdominal wall pain postsurgery.[61]

Risks: These include bowel perforation and hematoma formation.

Contraindications: Infection, anticoagulant therapy, and severe scarring over the area to be injected.

Outcome data: Positive diagnostic injections can be followed with an ablation procedure using pulsed mode radiofrequency (RF), cryoanalgesia, or phenol or alcohol. Pulsed RF can provide 6 to 18 months of at least 50% relief.[62,63] In the past, phenol has been shown to provide good relief, although there is possibility of necrosis on and around the nerve.[64] (**Fig. 8**)

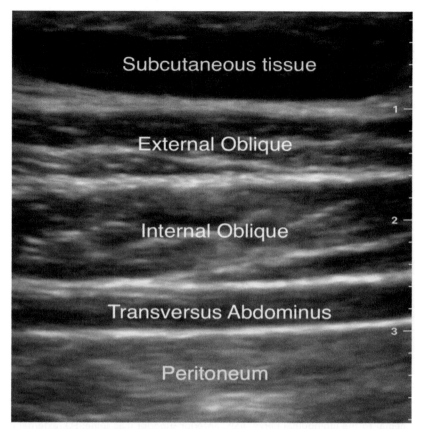

Fig. 7. TAP block at the lateral abdominal wall. The needle is advanced to the plane between the IO and the TA muscles. (*Image courtesy of* Tristan Pearson.)

Lower extremity

Lateral femoral cutaneous: The lateral femoral cutaneous nerve (LFCN) is formed from the posterior divisions of L2-3 nerve roots. It enters the pelvis lateral to the psoas major before crossing the iliacus muscle and exiting superficially at the level of the ASIS. As it descends, it passes under the inguinal ligament below the fascia iliaca before dividing into its terminal branches. The branching pattern and location are highly variable, but most commonly the LFC divides approximately 5 cm below the ASIS on the surface of the sartorius muscle into anterior and posterior branches. The anterior branch provides sensory innervation to the anterolateral thigh and the posterior branch to the lateral thigh.[65] The LFCN is often subject to entrapment due to its superficiality at the level of the inguinal ligament. This neuropathy is commonly referred to as meralgia paresthetica. Although this is mostly a clinical diagnosis, ultrasound examination at the time of nerve injection can aid in confirming the diagnosis (ie, nerve enlargement, nerve hypoechogenicity, and neuroma).[65]

Technique: The LFCN is typically blocked 2 to 5 cm medial and inferior to the ASIS. The LFCN lies atop the sartorius muscle medial to the tensor fascia lata.

Patient selection criteria: Meralgia paresthetica, neuropathic pain along the lateral thigh.

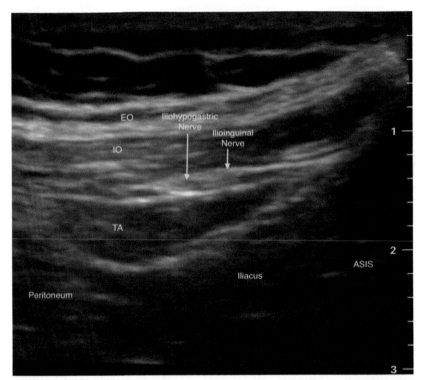

Fig. 8. Ilioinguinal and iliohypogastric nerves. This image is slightly caudad to the top of the ASIS. At this level, the EO starts to thin into its aponeurosis and the Iliacus muscle between the TA and the ASIS comes into view. The deep circumflex iliac artery can occasionally be seen medial to the ilioinguinal nerve. ASIS, anterior superior iliac spine; EO, external oblique; IO, internal oblique; TA, transversus abdominus. (*Image courtesy of* Amy Pearson, MD, Iowa City.)

Outcome data: LFCN injection is a safe alternative to conservative management in patients with neuropathic meralgia paresthetica.[65] In 2016, Klauser and colleagues reported that 15/20 patients with meralgia paresthetica had complete resolution of symptoms after ultrasound-guided injection of the LFCN and 5/20 reported partial resolution (mean VAS score from 92 to 42).[66] A meta-analysis of literature to compare ultrasound-guided injection of LFCN versus surgery found that there was no statistically significant difference between the two techniques.[67]

Sciatic: The sciatic nerve is the largest single nerve in the body. It originates from the ventral rami of nerve roots L4-S3 (ie, lumbosacral plexus) which fuse together on the anterior surface of the lateral sacrum. As the sciatic nerve exits the pelvis, it passes through the greater sciatic foramen just below the piriformis muscle before coursing inferiorly between the greater trochanter and the ischial tuberosity. The tibial nerve and common fibular nerve remain distinct within the sciatic nerve.[55] The sciatic nerve innervates the distal femur, knee, leg, ankle, and foot (except for the medial leg and proximal foot, which are innervated by the saphenous nerve) (**Figs. 9** and **10**).

Technique: The sciatic nerve is typically blocked either proximally in the transgluteal or subgluteal region, or distally in the popliteal region depending on the level of the lesion.

In the ultrasound-guided transgluteal approach, a probe is placed over the buttock. The sciatic nerve is visualized midway between the ischial tuberosity and the greater trochanter of the femur, deep to the gluteus maximus muscle. In the subgluteal approach, the probe is moved distally and, using the same landmarks, the sciatic nerve is visualized directly below the gluteus maximus muscle. Dynamic scanning can help distinguish the sciatic nerve from surrounding tissue and musculature. An in-plane or out-of-plane needle advancement technique can be used. CT-guided techniques have also been described.[68]

Patient selection criteria: Chronic pain of the leg and foot (eg, piriformis syndrome, residual limb pain following amputation, CRPS).

Risks and contraindications: However, use of high doses of local anesthetic in this application is usually avoided due to the nerve's mixed motor and sensory function.[69]

Outcome data: There are no long-term outcome data for sciatic nerve injection for chronic pain, however, it is commonly used as a diagnostic injection before PNS, which may have a role in disabling foot pain in patients with CRPS 1 and also alleviated autonomic symptoms.[70]

Tibial: In the thigh, the sciatic nerve gives off branches to the adductor magnus and hamstring muscles. In most patients, the sciatic nerve splits into two branches, tibial and common fibular, just above the popliteal crease; however, in some patients these branches remain separate along its course.[71] The tibial nerve continues its posterior course to innervate the distal portion of the leg, whereas the common fibular nerve courses laterally to innervate a portion of the knee joint as well as the posterolateral calf.

Technique: The sciatic nerve is visualized superficial to the popliteal vessels when the ultrasound probe is placed above the popliteal crease, lying between the biceps femoris laterally and semimembranosus and semitendinosus muscles medially.[55] Distally, the sciatic branches into the common fibular laterally and the larger tibial nerve medially. The tibial nerve can be injected at this point.

The tibial nerve can also be injected at the ankle dorsal to the medial malleolus; the tibial nerve lies posterior to the tibial artery and vein. The flexor digitorum longus, flexor hallucis longus, and tibialis posterior tendons are identified to avoid tendon injury. The

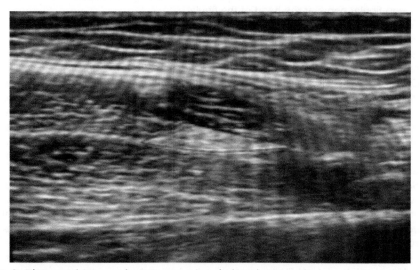

Fig. 9. Ultrasound image of sciatic nerve in subgluteal region. (*Image courtesy of* Nenna Nwazota, MD, Dallas, Texas.)

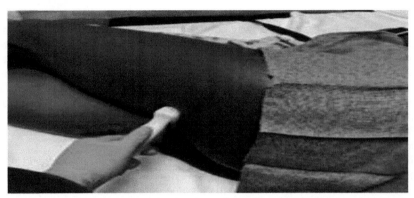

Fig. 10. Subgluteal sciatic nerve injection is performed with a probe placed beneath the gluteal fold. (*Image courtesy of* Nenna Nwazota, MD, Dallas, Texas)

tibial nerve can also be injected proximal to the malleolus, but the results are less reliable.[72]

Patient selection criteria: This injection is more commonly done for surgeries of the foot and ankle, but there is interest in performing this injection for treatment of tibial neuropathy (eg, that caused by nerve entrapment such as tarsal tunnel or soleal sling syndrome) and/or for diagnostic purposes before peripheral nerve stimulator implant.[73]

Risks and contraindications: Similar to other sciatic nerve injections, consideration should be taken of the effect of local anesthetic on motor weakness.

Outcome data: There is limited large-scale outcome data for this injection in the management of chronic pain. One series of nine patients showed a short-term pain relief in six and nerve conduction improvement in two[74] (**Fig. 11**).

Common fibular (also known as common peroneal): Although the tibial nerve courses more medially, the common fibular nerve wraps anteriorly around the lateral tibial plateau before dividing into the superficial fibular (superficial peroneal) nerve and the deep fibular nerve at the head of the fibula.

Technique: Similar to blockade of tibial in the popliteal fossa (above).

Patient selection criteria: Pain in the distribution of the common fibular nerve.

Risks and contraindications: Nerve injury to the common fibular results in foot drop (loss of ankle dorsiflexion), loss of eversion, and loss of toe flexion.[75]

Outcome data: Case report of ultrasound (US) injection of plasma rich in growth factors intraneural for fibular nerve palsy in a patient with foot drop resulted in partial useful recovery. electromyogram (EMG) controls showed complete reinnervation of the tibialis anterior muscle.[76] Local anesthetic injection has also been used diagnostically before surgery.[75] There are limited large-scale outcome data for this procedure in chronic pain although it is commonly used for surgical analgesia along with the tibial nerve (**Fig. 12**).

Superficial fibular (also known as superficial peroneal): The common fibular nerve bifurcates into the superficial and deep fibular nerves at the fibular head. From there, the superficial fibular nerve runs subcutaneously along the anterolateral lower leg until it divides into the intermediate dorsal and medial dorsal cutaneous nerves just caudad to the lateral malleolus.

Technique: The superficial fibular nerve is injected along the lateral border of the fibula. At midcalf, the lateral fibula creates a crisp border between the peroneus brevis posteriorly and the extensor digitorum longus anteriorly. The nerve can be identified

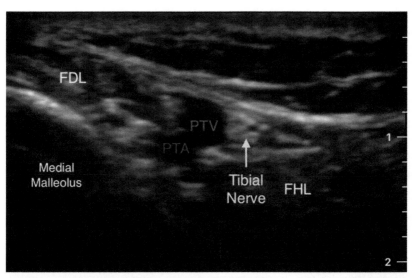

Fig. 11. Tibial nerve at the medial ankle. FDL, flexor digitorum longus; FHL, flexor hallicus longus; PTA, posterior tibial artery; PTV, posterior tibial vein. (*Image courtesy of* Annika Pearson.)

just superficial to the intermuscular septum and deep to the crural fascia.[77] More distally, the nerve sits directly superficial to the crural fascia at its bifurcation.[78]

Patient selection criteria: This injection is typically done for pain in the region of the superficial fibular nerve.

Risks and contraindications: Considering the function of the superficial fibular nerve, the patient should be counseled that motor weakness of the lower extremity causing weakness on eversion of the ankle can occur during the local anesthetic phase and appropriate precautions should be followed.

Outcome data: There are no large-scale studies of outcomes for this intervention. Case reports describe the use of this injection for diagnostic purposes and for the treatment of peripheral mononeuropathy and CRPS[79,80] (**Fig. 13**).

Saphenous nerve: The saphenous is the distal branch of the femoral nerve, innervating the medial lower leg to the ankle. At the knee, the saphenous nerve branches to the infrapatellar nerve and then travels along the medial leg providing sensory innervation to the medial knee, foot, and ankle.

Technique: The saphenous nerve can be approached at the adductor canal, superficially below the knee or at the medial ankle. The adductor canal contains the superficial femoral artery and the saphenous nerve. It is bordered superficially by the sartorius muscle, anteriorly by the vastus medialis, and posteriorly by the adductor magnus muscle and can be found at the mid-to-distal medial thigh.[78,81] The saphenous nerve at the knee is found medially just anterior to the tibia. It can be identified next to the saphenous vein.[82]

Patient selection criteria: It is commonly used to provide analgesia to the medial position of the knee, lower leg, and foot.

Outcome data: There are limited large-scale outcome data on isolated saphenous nerve injection for chronic pain management. A case series has described successful injection of the saphenous nerve in 2 of 16 patients for the treatment of posttotal knee arthroplasty pain[83] (**Fig. 14**).

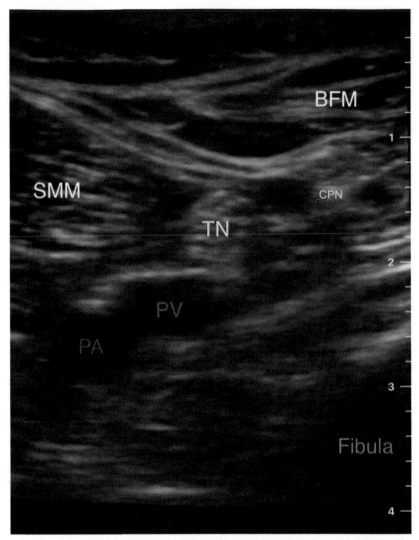

Fig. 12. Bifurcation of the tibial nerve and common fibular nerve superior to the popliteal fossa. BFM, biceps femoris muscle; CPN, common fibular nerve; PA, popliteal artery; PV, popliteal vein; SMM, semimembranosus muscle; TN, tibial nerve. (*Image courtesy of* Annika Pearson.).

Sural nerve: The sural nerve is formed by the fusion of the medial sural cutaneous nerve (terminal branch of tibia) and lateral sural cutaneous nerve (one of the terminal branches of the common fibular). They join in the midcalf and the nerve runs down the posterolateral leg and posterior to the lateral malleolus and anterior to the Achilles and adjacent to the small saphenous vein distally.

Technique: A linear high-frequency ultrasound probe is placed between the Achilles tendon and lateral malleolus, and the small saphenous vein is identified. The sural nerve runs close to the small saphenous vein.[78,81]

Patient selection criteria: Neuropathic pain in the posterolateral calf and fifth digit of the foot.

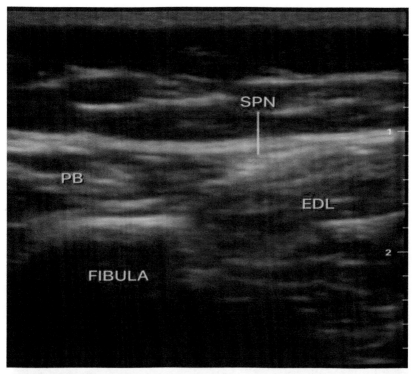

Fig. 13. Superficial fibular (superficial peroneal) nerve (SPN) coursing superficial to the fibula and the intermuscular septum between the peroneus brevis (PB) and extensor digitorum longus (EDL). (*Image courtesy of* Amy Pearson, MD, Iowa City.)

Outcome data: There are limited large-scale outcome data. These blocks are being used diagnostically before percutaneous PNS or surgical nerve release to manage chronic pain in the distribution of the sural nerve[84,85] (**Fig. 15**).

DISCUSSION

Although there are generally few long-term outcome studies for individual peripheral nerve injections, there is small-scale evidence that these interventions may be advantageous for some peripheral mononeuropathies and nerve entrapment syndromes. There is a role for peripheral nerve injections in the management of headache disorders such as migraine, cluster headaches, and painful cranial neuralgias.[60] Occipital nerve injections have been described for the use of primary and secondary headache disorders. The supraorbital nerve injection is effective to anesthetize the forehead. Together with the STN injection, it is used to treat headache disorders and cranial neuralgias in the V1 distribution. It is effective when used in conjunction with occipital nerve injections.

The upper extremity is supplied by nerves that arise from the BP (ventral rami of C5-T1).[26] The interscalene provides analgesia to the shoulder and upper arm. It is associated with Horner syndrome, hemidiaphragmatic paresis and is contraindicated in patients with severe respiratory insufficiency. The supraclavicular BP injection is associated with a risk of injury to the pleura, recurrent laryngeal nerve and dorsal scapular artery. The supraclavicular, infraclavicular, and axillary approaches to the BP injection

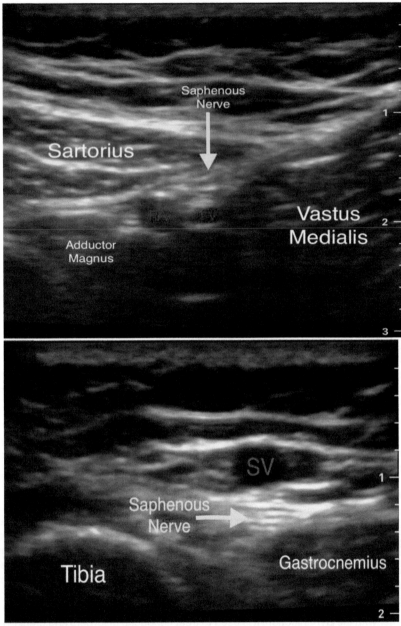

Fig. 14. The saphenous nerve at the adductor canal above the medial knee (top) and below the medial knee. FA, femoral artery; FV, femoral vein; SV, saphenous vein. (*Image courtesy of* Annika Pearson.)

are used in the management of NBP.[26] Suprascapular and axillary nerve injections are used in the management of chronic shoulder pain.

PVBs provide analgesia to the thoracic and upper abdominal areas and have been shown to reduce postoperative pain and decrease opioid consumption in

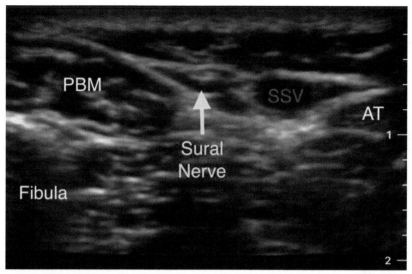

Fig. 15. The sural nerve at the lateral ankle. AT, Achilles tendon; PBM, peroneus brevis muscle; SSV, small saphenous vein. (*Image courtesy of* Annika Pearson.)

patients undergoing breast surgery. In addition, there is evidence to suggest that they may have a role in preventing chronic pain after surgery.[54] Transverse abdominis plane injections are useful in the treatment of chronic abdominal wall pain after abdominal surgeries including laparotomy, hernia repair, appendectomy, cesarean section, abdominal hysterectomy, and prostatectomy when other treatment methods have failed.[58] Ilioinguinal and iliohypogastric nerves arise from the first lumbar spinal root and the Ilioinguinal nerve provides sensation to the superomedial aspect of the thigh, whereas the iliohypogastric nerve supplies the skin over the inguinal region. Blockade of the ilioinguinal and iliohypogastric nerves has been shown to be efficacious in providing pain relief for patients with chronic pain following inguinal hernia repair, abdominal hysterectomy, or cesarean section.

Lower extremity injections include the femoral, sciatic, tibial, common fibular, superficial fibular, and lateral cutaneous nerve of the thigh. The nerves that supply the lower extremity arise from the lumbosacral plexus L2-S2 nerve roots. The area of the patient's pain determines the choice of nerve and level of blockade. Peripheral nerve injections can be therapeutic for lower extremity pain and also diagnostic before PNS for conditions such as limb pain postamputation, CRPS, and entrapment neuropathies.[4,68] These injections may also be beneficial for entrapment neuropathies of the lower extremity such as the common fibular/peroneal (most common), lateral femoral cutaneous (meralgia paresthetica), sural, and tibial nerve (tarsal tunnel).[68,81]

SUMMARY

In summary, the areas of pain should be identified accurately. The knowledge of anatomy and distribution patterns is paramount for optimal use of peripheral nerve injections in the management of chronic pain conditions. They are an important tool in an interventional pain physician's armamentarium and can be integrated into pain practices effectively to offer patients pain relief.

CLINICS CARE POINTS

- Occipital nerve injections have been used in the treatment of migraines, occipital neuralgia, cluster headaches, and cervicogenic headaches. Physical examination should confirm tenderness to palpation of the occipital nerve. The duration of relief can last well beyond the local anesthetic duration and corticosteroids may be added for those who do not respond to local anesthetics alone. There is a paucity of data, but outcomes are positive, and the injections are well tolerated.

- SON and STN are useful injections to be used in conjunction ONB to treat headache disorders and cranial neuralgias, for example, chronic migraines and trigeminal neuralgia. However, there is a paucity of data regarding their efficacy.

- GAN injections can be useful in the treatment of neuralgias in the distribution of the GAN and may be used in conjunction with LON injections.

- Interscalene injections cause phrenic nerve blockade and respiratory insufficiency is a contraindication as there is a high risk of ipsilateral diaphragmatic hemiparesis. Existing vocal cord palsy is also a contraindication as the recurrent laryngeal nerve can be blocked as well, leading to complete airway obstruction.

- Indications for BP injections include NBP as well as CRPS of the upper extremity.

- Axillary nerve block (terminal branch of posterior cord of the BP) and SSN blocks are used to provide analgesia in patients with HSP as well as shoulder pain of other causes—adhesive capsulitis, arthritis, trauma, and rheumatological conditions.

- The intercostal nerves arise from the ventral rami of thoracic nerves T1 to T11 and are a useful tool in the treatment of intercostal neuralgia not responsive to conservative management. The two most common causes of intercostal neuralgia are PTPS and postherpetic neuralgia. The standard of care is using image guidance, and either fluoroscopy or ultrasound-guided techniques may be used. In both techniques, the nerve is blocked posteriorly about 7 to 10 cm from the midline. The risks of INB include pneumothorax, hematoma, local anesthetic toxicity, muscle trauma, nerve damage, and infection. Anticoagulation and patients who are pulmonary compromised are relative contraindications to this injection.

- Paravertebral injections have been used during breast surgery, thoracic surgery, and the management of rib fractures. The target is the paravertebral space adjacent to the vertebral bodies where the spinal roots exit the intervertebral foramina. The paravertebral space is bounded by the costotransverse ligament and the parietal pleura anteriorly and transverse process and ribs posteriorly. The space is continuous with the intercostal space laterally. Thoracic PVBs have been shown to not only reduce postoperative pain and decrease opioid consumption in patients undergoing breast surgery, but there is evidence that they may also prevent chronic pain after breast surgery.

- Ilioinguinal and iliohypogastric nerve injections are relatively simple procedures that usually provide near-complete pain relief for patients with chronic pain after inguinal hernia repair, cesarean section or abdominal hysterectomy. These injections can be diagnostic and therapeutic. The patients with positive diagnostic but not therapeutic response are candidates for an ablation procedure using pulsed mode RF, cryoanalgesia, or phenol or alcohol.

- The femoral nerve arises from the posterior branches of L2-4 nerve roots. It innervates the knee joint, anteromedial thigh and medial leg. It provides motor innervation to the muscles that control hip flexion and knee extension. Femoral nerve injection is associated with quadriceps weakness.

- The sciatic nerve is the largest single nerve in the body and originates from ventral rami of L4-S3. It innervates the distal femur, knee, leg, ankle, and foot. Residual limb pain postamputation, CRPS of the lower extremity, and piriformis syndrome are indications for the sciatic nerve injection.

- The sciatic nerve splits into the tibial and common peroneal, just above the popliteal crease. The tibial nerve is the largest terminal branch of the sciatic. The common peroneal/common fibular nerve is derived from the posterior branches of L4-S2 nerve roots.

- Superficial fibular nerve injections are used to treat pain due to trauma, nerve entrapment, and CRPS of the leg/foot.

- LFCN is formed from the posterior divisions of L2-3 nerve roots. The anterior division provides sensory innervation to the anterolateral thigh and the posterior branch sensory innervation to the lateral thigh. LFCN injection is performed in patients with meralgia paresthetica.

REFERENCES

1. Chang A, Dua A, Singh K, et al. Peripheral nerve blocks. In: . Treasure Island (FL): StatPearls; 2022.
2. Orebaugh SL, McFadden K, Skorupan H, et al. Subepineurial injection in ultrasound-guided interscalene needle tip placement. Reg Anesth Pain Med 2010;35(5):450–4.
3. Wiederhold BD, Garmon EH, Peterson E, et al. Nerve block anesthesia. Treasure Island (FL): StatPearls; 2022.
4. Nayak R, Banik RK. Current innovations in peripheral nerve stimulation. Pain Res Treat 2018;2018:9091216.
5. Candido KD, Germanovich A, Ghaly RF, et al. Case report: computed tomography scan-guided Gasserian ganglion injection of dexamethasone and lidocaine for the treatment of recalcitrant pain associated with herpes simplex type 1 infection of the ophthalmic division of the trigeminal nerve. Anesth Analg 2011;112(1): 224–7.
6. Han KR, Chae YJ, Lee JD, et al. Trigeminal nerve block with alcohol for medically intractable classic trigeminal neuralgia: long-term clinical effectiveness on pain. Int J Med Sci 2017;14(1):29–36.
7. Nader A, Kendall MC, De Oliveria GS, et al. Ultrasound-guided trigeminal nerve block via the pterygopalatine fossa: an effective treatment for trigeminal neuralgia and atypical facial pain. Pain Physician 2013;16(5):E537–45.
8. Anugerah A, Nguyen K, Nader A. Technical considerations for approaches to the ultrasound-guided maxillary nerve block via the pterygopalatine fossa: a literature review. Reg Anesth Pain Med 2020;45(4):301–5.
9. Allam AE, Khalil AAF, Eltawab BA, et al. Ultrasound-guided intervention for treatment of trigeminal neuralgia: an updated review of anatomy and techniques. Pain Res Manag 2018;2018:5480728.
10. Han KR, Kim C. Brief report: the long-term outcome of mandibular nerve block with alcohol for the treatment of trigeminal neuralgia. Anesth Analg 2010; 111(2):550–3.
11. Brown DL. Atlas of regional anesthesia. 4th edition. ed.
12. Fishman S, Ballantyne J, Rathmell JP, Bonica JJ. Bonica's management of pain. 4th edition. ed.
13. Greengrass RA, Narouze S, Bendtsen TF, et al. Cervical plexus and greater occipital nerve blocks: controversies and technique update. Reg Anesth Pain Med 2019;44(6):623–6.
14. Blumenfeld A, Ashkenazi A, Napchan U, et al. Expert consensus recommendations for the performance of peripheral nerve blocks for headaches–a narrative review. Headache 2013;53(3):437–46.

15. Platzgummer H, Moritz T, Gruber GM, et al. The lesser occipital nerve visualized by high-resolution sonography–normal and initial suspect findings. Cephalalgia 2015;35(9):816–24.

16. Ashkenazi A, Blumenfeld A, Napchan U, et al. Peripheral nerve blocks and trigger point injections in headache management - a systematic review and suggestions for future research. Headache 2010;50(6):943–52.

17. Okuda Y, Matsumoto T, Shinohara M, et al. Sudden unconsciousness during a lesser occipital nerve block in a patient with the occipital bone defect. Eur J Anaesthesiol 2001;18(12):829–32.

18. Ambrosini A, Vandenheede M, Rossi P, et al. Suboccipital injection with a mixture of rapid- and long-acting steroids in cluster headache: a double-blind placebo-controlled study. Pain 2005;118(1–2):92–6.

19. Fernandes L, Randall MMF, Idrovo LDF. Peripheral nerve blocks for headache disorders. Pract Neurol 2020;23. https://doi.org/10.1136/practneurol-2020-002612.

20. Katta-Charles SD. Craniofacial neuralgias. NeuroRehabilitation 2020;47(3): 299–314.

21. Kim YS, Son JS, Lee H, et al. A case report of refractory otalgia after Ramsay Hunt syndrome successfully treated by applying pulsed radiofrequency to the great auricular nerve: A CARE-compliant article. Medicine (Baltimore) 2021; 100(39):e27285.

22. Orebaugh SL, Williams BA. Brachial plexus anatomy: normal and variant. ScientificWorldJournal 2009;9:300–12.

23. Bouche B, Manfiotto M, Rigoard P, et al. Peripheral nerve stimulation of brachial plexus nerve roots and supra-scapular nerve for chronic refractory neuropathic pain of the upper limb. Neuromodulation 2017;20(7):684–9.

24. Murata Y, Kanaya K, Wada H, et al. Interscalene brachial plexus block for scapular and upper chest pain due to cervical radiculopathy: a randomized controlled clinical trial. J Orthop Sci 2012;17(5):515–20.

25. Detaille V, Busnel F, Ravary H, et al. Use of continuous interscalene brachial plexus block and rehabilitation to treat complex regional pain syndrome of the shoulder. Ann Phys Rehabil Med 2010;53(6–7):406–16.

26. Hadzic A, Lopez A, Balocco AL, et al, New York School of Regional Anesthesia. . Hadzic's peripheral nerve blocks and anatomy for ultrasound-guided regional anesthesia. 3rd edition. New York: McGraw Hill; 2020.

27. Oliver-Fornies P, Espinosa Morales K, Fajardo-Perez M, et al. Modified supraclavicular approach to brachial plexus block. J Clin Anesth 2022;76:110585.

28. Kumar A, Kumar A, Sinha C, et al. Topographic Sonoanatomy of Infraclavicular Brachial Plexus: Variability and Correlation with Anthropometry. Anesth Essays Res 2018;12(4):814–8.

29. Berthier F, Lepage D, Henry Y, et al. Anatomical basis for ultrasound-guided regional anaesthesia at the junction of the axilla and the upper arm. Surg Radiol Anat 2010;32(3):299–304.

30. Franco CD, Williams JM. Ultrasound-Guided Interscalene Block: Reevaluation of the "Stoplight" Sign and Clinical Implications. Reg Anesth Pain Med 2016;41(4): 452–9.

31. Tsui BC, Lou L. Learning the 'traceback' approach for interscalene block. Anaesthesia 2014;69(1):83–5.

32. Bergmann L, Martini S, Kesselmeier M, et al. Phrenic nerve block caused by interscalene brachial plexus block: breathing effects of different sites of injection. BMC Anesthesiol 2016;16(1):45.

33. Zisquit J, Nedeff N. Interscalene block. Treasure Island (FL): StatPearls; 2021.
34. Zinboonyahgoon N, Vlassakov K, Abrecht CR, et al. Brachial plexus block for cancer-related pain: a case series. Pain Physician 2015;18(5):E917–24.
35. Wilson RD, Bennett ME, Nguyen VQC, et al. Fully implantable peripheral nerve stimulation for hemiplegic shoulder pain: a multi-site case series with two-year follow-up. Neuromodulation 2018;21(3):290–5.
36. Mansfield JT, Desai MJ. Axillary peripheral nerve stimulation for chronic shoulder pain: a retrospective case series. Neuromodulation 2020;23(6):812–8.
37. Mazzola A, Spinner D. Ultrasound-guided peripheral nerve stimulation for shoulder pain: anatomic review and assessment of the current clinical evidence. Pain Physician 2020;23(5):E461–74.
38. Brown DE, James DC, Roy S. Pain relief by suprascapular nerve block in glenohumeral arthritis. Scand J Rheumatol 1988;17(5):411–5.
39. Sa Malheiro N, Afonso NR, Pereira D, et al. [Efficacy of ultrasound guided suprascapular block in patients with chronic shoulder pain: retrospective observational study]. Braz J Anesthesiol 2020;70(1):15–21.
40. Yasar E, Vural D, Safaz I, et al. Which treatment approach is better for hemiplegic shoulder pain in stroke patients: intra-articular steroid or suprascapular nerve block? A randomized controlled trial. Clin Rehabil 2011;25(1):60–8.
41. Sinha P, Sarkar B, Goswami S, et al. Effectiveness of combination of ultrasonography-guided pulsed radiofrequency neuromodulation with steroid at the suprascapular nerve in chronic shoulder pain. Pain Pract 2020;20(1):16–23.
42. Alanbay E, Aras B, Kesikburun S, et al. Effectiveness of suprascapular nerve pulsed radiofrequency treatment for hemiplegic shoulder pain: a randomized-controlled trial. Pain Physician 2020;23(3):245–52.
43. Schwartz RH, Urits I, Viswanath O. Carpal tunnel injection. Treasure Island (FL): StatPearls; 2022.
44. Shi Q, Bobos P, Lalone EA, et al. Comparison of the short-term and long-term effects of surgery and nonsurgical intervention in treating carpal tunnel syndrome: a systematic review and meta-analysis. Hand (N Y) 2020;15(1):13–22.
45. Lee HJ, Park HS, Moon HI, et al. Effect of ultrasound-guided intercostal nerve block versus fluoroscopy-guided epidural nerve block in patients with thoracic herpes zoster: a comparative study. J Ultrasound Med 2019;38(3):725–31.
46. Diwan S, Staats P. Atlas of pain medicine procedures. New York: McGraw-Hill Companies, Inc.; 2015.
47. Perkins FM, Kehlet H. Chronic pain as an outcome of surgery. A review of predictive factors. Anesthesiology 2000;93(4):1123–33.
48. Abram SE. Neural blockade for neuropathic pain. Clin J Pain 2000;16(2 Suppl): S56–61.
49. Abd-Elsayed A, Lee S, Jackson M. Radiofrequency ablation for treating resistant intercostal neuralgia. Ochsner J 2018;18(1):91–3.
50. Ben Aziz M, Mukhdomi J. Thoracic paravertebral block. Treasure Island (FL): StatPearls; 2022.
51. Qian B, Fu S, Yao Y, et al. Preoperative ultrasound-guided multilevel paravertebral blocks reduce the incidence of postmastectomy chronic pain: a double-blind, placebo-controlled randomized trial. J Pain Res 2019;12:597–603.
52. Hussain N, Shastri U, McCartney CJL, et al. Should thoracic paravertebral blocks be used to prevent chronic postsurgical pain after breast cancer surgery? A systematic analysis of evidence in light of IMMPACT recommendations. Pain 2018; 159(10):1955–71.

53. Kairaluoma PM, Bachmann MS, Rosenberg PH, et al. Preincisional paravertebral block reduces the prevalence of chronic pain after breast surgery. Anesth Analg 2006;103(3):703–8.

54. Karmakar MK, Samy W, Li JW, et al. Thoracic paravertebral block and its effects on chronic pain and health-related quality of life after modified radical mastectomy. Reg Anesth Pain Med 2014;39(4):289–98.

55. Karmakar MK, Reina MA, Sivakumar RK, et al. Ultrasound-guided subparaneural popliteal sciatic nerve block: there is more to it than meets the eyes. Reg Anesth Pain Med 2021;46(3):268–75.

56. Makharita MY, Amr YM, El-Bayoumy Y. Single paravertebral injection for acute thoracic herpes zoster: a randomized controlled trial. Pain Pract 2015;15(3): 229–35.

57. Mavarez AC, Ahmed AA. Transabdominal plane block. Treasure Island (FL): Stat-Pearls; 2022.

58. Abd-Elsayed A, Luo S, Falls C. Transversus abdominis plane block as a treatment modality for chronic abdominal pain. Pain Physician 2020;23(4):405–12.

59. Abd-Elsayed A, Malyuk D. Efficacy of transversus abdominis plane steroid injection for treating chronic abdominal pain. Pain Pract 2018;18(1):48–52.

60. Fernandes HDS, Azevedo AS, Ferreira TC, et al. Ultrasound-guided peripheral abdominal wall blocks. Clinics (Sao Paulo) 2021;76:e2170.

61. Gofeld M, Christakis M. Sonographically guided ilioinguinal nerve block. J Ultrasound Med 2006;25(12):1571–5.

62. Karaman H, Tufek A, Kavak GO, et al. Would pulsed radiofrequency applied to different anatomical regions have effective results for chronic pain treatment? J Pak Med Assoc 2011;61(9):879–85.

63. Trescot AM. Cryoanalgesia in interventional pain management. Pain Physician 2003;6(3):345–60.

64. Klippel JH, Dieppe P. Rheumatology. 2nd edition. London (United Kingdom); Philadelphia (PA): Mosby; 1998.

65. Powell GM, Baffour FI, Erie AJ, et al. Sonographic evaluation of the lateral femoral cutaneous nerve in meralgia paresthetica. Skeletal Radiol 2020;49(7):1135–40.

66. Klauser AS, Abd Ellah MM, Halpern EJ, et al. Meralgia paraesthetica: Ultrasound-guided injection at multiple levels with 12-month follow-up. Eur Radiol 2016;26(3): 764–70.

67. Tagliafico AS, Torri L, Signori A. Treatment of meralgia paresthetica (Lateral Femoral Cutaneous Neuropathy): A meta-analysis of ultrasound-guided injection versus surgery. Eur J Radiol 2021;139:109736.

68. Wadhwa V, Scott KM, Rozen S, et al. CT-guided perineural injections for chronic pelvic pain. Radiographics 2016;36(5):1408–25.

69. Rodziewicz TL, Stevens JB, Ajib FA, et al. Sciatic Nerve Block. Treasure Island (FL): StatPearls; 2021.

70. Buwembo J, Munson R, Rizvi SA, et al. Direct sciatic nerve electrical stimulation for complex regional pain syndrome Type 1. Neuromodulation 2021;24(6): 1075–82.

71. Varenika V, Lutz AM, Beaulieu CF, et al. Detection and prevalence of variant sciatic nerve anatomy in relation to the piriformis muscle on MRI. Skeletal Radiol 2017;46(6):751–7.

72. Benimeli-Fenollar M, Montiel-Company JM, Almerich-Silla JM, et al. Tibial Nerve Block: Supramalleolar or Retromalleolar Approach? A Randomized Trial in 110 Participants. Int J Environ Res Public Health 2020;17(11):3860.

73. Hanyu-Deutmeyer A, Pritzlaff SG. Peripheral nerve stimulation for the 21st century: sural, superficial peroneal, and tibial nerves. Pain Med 2020;21(Suppl 1): S64–7.

74. Urits I, Smoots D, Franscioni H, et al. Injection techniques for common chronic pain conditions of the foot: a comprehensive review. Pain Ther 2020;9(1):145–60.

75. Nirenberg MS. A simple test to assist with the diagnosis of common fibular nerve entrapment and predict outcomes of surgical decompression. Acta Neurochir (Wien) 2020;162(6):1439–44.

76. Sanchez M, Yoshioka T, Ortega M, et al. Ultrasound-guided platelet-rich plasma injections for the treatment of common peroneal nerve palsy associated with multiple ligament injuries of the knee. Knee Surg Sports Traumatol Arthrosc 2014; 22(5):1084–9.

77. Chin KJ. Ultrasound visualization of the superficial peroneal nerve in the mid-calf. Anesthesiology 2013;118(4):956–65.

78. Lopez AM, Sala-Blanch X, Magaldi M, et al. Ultrasound-guided ankle block for forefoot surgery: the contribution of the saphenous nerve. Reg Anesth Pain Med 2012;37(5):554–7.

79. Jaffe JD, Henshaw DS, Nagle PC. Ultrasound-Guided Continuous Superficial Peroneal Nerve Block below the Knee for the Treatment of Nerve Injury. Pain Pract 2013;13(7):572–5.

80. Nageeb RS, Mohamed WS, Nageeb GS, et al. Role of superficial peroneal sensory potential and high-resolution ultrasonography in confirmation of common peroneal mononeuropathy at the fibular neck. Egypt J Neurol Psych 2019;55(1).

81. De Maeseneer M, Madani H, Lenchik L, et al. Normal anatomy and compression areas of nerves of the foot and ankle: US and MR imaging with anatomic correlation. Radiographics 2015;35(5):1469–82.

82. Iida H, Ohseto K, Uchino H. Nerve blockade and interventional therapy. 1st edition. Tokyo (Japan): Springer Japan : Imprint: Springer; 2019.

83. Clendenen S, Greengrass R, Whalen J, et al. Infrapatellar saphenous neuralgia after TKA can be improved with ultrasound-guided local treatments. Clin Orthop Relat Res 2015;473(1):119–25.

84. Fabre T, Montero C, Gaujard E, et al. Chronic calf pain in athletes due to sural nerve entrapment. A report of 18 cases. Am J Sports Med 2000;28(5):679–82.

85. Abd-Elsayed A. Wireless Peripheral Nerve Stimulation for Treatment of Peripheral Neuralgias. Neuromodulation 2020;23(6):827–30.

Peripheral Joint Radiofrequency Ablation

Maxim S. Eckmann, MD[a], Brian T. Boies, MD[a], David J. Carroll, MD[a,*],
Lorne D. Muir II, DO[a]

KEYWORDS

- Radiofrequency • Ablation • Hip • Knee • Shoulder • Chronic • Pain

KEY POINTS

- Chronic pain associated with major peripheral joints such as the knee, hip, and shoulder is a major source of morbidity.
- Descriptions of neuroanatomical targets and radiofrequency ablation techniques exist for the treatment of chronic knee, hip, and shoulder pain.
- Peripheral joint radiofrequency ablation is generally well tolerated and shows reliable improvement in commonly assessed pain scales.

INTRODUCTION

Chronic joint pain is common and associated with functional limitations and reduced quality of life.[1] Arthritis alone, the most common cause of chronic joint pain, is projected to have a prevalence of nearly 67 million in the United States by 2030.[2] In addition, many other important causes of chronic joint pain exist, including trauma, osteonecrosis, infectious coxarthrosis, joint instability, impingement syndromes, and persistent pain following joint replacement.

Conservative treatments for chronic joint pain include exercise, weight loss, physical therapy, topical analgesics (nonsteroidal antiinflammatory drugs [NSAIDs], capsaicin cream), oral analgesia (NSAIDs, serotonin and norepinephrine reuptake inhibitors), intraarticular steroid injections, and surgical interventions such as joint arthroplasty.

Radiofrequency ablation (RFA) is a procedure that has been used in the treatment of many medical conditions since d'Arsonval first described the thermal effect generated by radiofrequency energy on soft tissue in 1891.[3] Despite the production of the first continuous radiofrequency lesion generator by Cosman and colleagues in 1950s, its use did not appear in the management of chronic pain until 1974.[4] Initially limited primarily to the treatment of cervical and lumbar facet disease, RFA has since been used

---

[a] Department of Anesthesiology, University of Texas Health Science Center at San Antonio, 5282 Medical Drive, Suite 180, San Antonio, TX 78229, USA
* Corresponding author.
E-mail address: carrolld1@uthscsa.edu

Phys Med Rehabil Clin N Am 33 (2022) 519–531
https://doi.org/10.1016/j.pmr.2022.02.003
1047-9651/22/© 2022 Elsevier Inc. All rights reserved.

pmr.theclinics.com

to treat a multitude of chronic conditions including facial and occipital neuralgia, cervicogenic headaches, radicular pain, intercostal neuralgia, postsurgical pain, and myofascial pain syndromes.[4–6] More recently, its use has gained popularity in the treatment of chronic pain associated with major peripheral joints. Herein the authors review its application in chronic shoulder, hip, and knee pain. Special attention is given to relevant anatomy, patient selection, procedural technique, and relevant outcome data.

The application of radiofrequencies to treat chronic pain comes in 2 principal forms, continuous RF (CRF) and pulsed RF (PRF).

Both techniques use an electrode and grounding pad to deliver an alternating current through the patient. The current in turn generates an electromagnetic field in the vicinity of the electrode that's typically in the 420 to 500 kHz range.[1–3,7] This electromagnetic field causes adjacent molecules to oscillate. Subsequent frictional heat produced by adjacent molecules rubbing into one another causes an increase in temperature of the target tissue that depending on the selected technique may be of clinical significance.

In CRF, continuous alternating current is used to achieve electrode temperatures in the range of 60°C to 90°C[8]; this heats adjacent tissue, including neuronal tissue, past the neurodestructive threshold of 45°C to 50°C, resulting in coagulative necrosis.[1,3,6] Actual lesion size generated by this process has been shown to correlate positively with electrode diameter, length, temperature, and total application time.[1] In addition, the specific electrode shape and type selected (ie, monopolar, bipolar, or cooled electrode) will also influence the size and shape of the lesion generated.

Bipolar electrodes complete the electrical circuit by having one electrode act as the cathode for the circuit and the other the anode, thereby obviating a grounding pad. Relative to monopolar lesions, bipolar lesions can be larger and produce a rounded brick-shaped lesion.[2] Alternatively, cooled RF catheters use chilled water or saline pumped through the chamber shaft of the electrode to create relatively larger lesion sizes when compared with monopolar RF[1,3]; this is because one of the limitations of RF ablation is the electrical and thermal conductivity of human tissue. If power through the electrode increases too fast, the tissue closest to the electrode increases temperature abruptly, resulting in microbubbles and charring that acts as an insulating sleeve around the electrode[3]; this limits the transmission of thermal energy and restricts further expansion of desired tissue destruction. Cooled RF allows for a slower increase in temperature in the tissue adjacent the electrode, enlarging lesion size and creating an oblate ellipsoidal shape.[1,3]

In contrast to CRF, PRF uses radiofrequency current in short (5–50 ms), high-voltage bursts with a frequency of 1 to 10 Hz.[6] The intrinsic oscillation frequency of each pulse, however, is still around 420 kHz, which is similar to that used for CRF.[6] Because the actual burst duration is only a fraction of each second, the tissue is allowed to cool between pulses. As a result, average target tissue temperature never exceeds the neurodestructive threshold of 45°C to 50C.[5,6] The exact mechanism by which PRF modulates pain perception from afferent nerve fibers remains a subject of some debate. Currently, most studies suggest PRF induces an alteration in synaptic transmission via a neuromodulatory-type effect.[5]

PATIENT SELECTION CRITERIA

Currently, there are no published guidelines concerning patient selection criteria for RFA of articular nerve branches of the shoulder, hip, or knee joints. Although diagnostic nerve blocks have been shown to predict who will benefit from RFA in the management of facet joint–related pain of the spine, the prognostic value of these techniques for peripheral joints remains controversial.[8,9] In addition, there is no consensus on the optimal number of blocks, amount of anesthetic to use, or pain reduction achieved to indicate RFA success following the block.[10] Current international consensus guidelines for lumbar facet joint pain advocate for a single prognostic medial branch nerve block with at least 50% or more relief of pain to qualify for RFA.[11] Given the lack of existing guidance, many practitioners have adopted the spinal facet joint RFA selection criteria to the application of their peripheral joint RFA procedures.[12] Further research is needed to evaluate additional variables that could potentially affect treatment success, such as patient demographics, clinical factors, and underlying diagnosis.[13]

RISK AND CONTRAINDICATIONS

Absolute contraindication to peripheral joint RFA includes proximate infection and patient refusal. Relative contraindications include bleeding disorders, drug-induced coagulopathies, uncontrolled diabetes, pregnancy, unstable joints, and predominate psychological cause of pain.[14] In addition, caution should be used in patients with implantable cardiac defibrillators, spinal cord stimulators, pacemakers, or peripheral nerve stimulators. Most modern cardiac and stimulator devices are safe for use during the procedure if they are placed in surgery safe modes beforehand. Peripheral joint RFA is a generally well-tolerated procedure. However, as with any intervention complications can occur. Adverse events reported in the literature include skin burns, hematoma, hemarthrosis, septic arthritis, paresthesia, interference with implanted devices, and muscular weakness secondary to inadvertent ablation of motor containing nerve branches.[9,13]

To minimize the risks inherent to RFA, a variety of strategies are used. Peripheral joint RFA is almost universally done under fluoroscopic guidance. In addition, some investigators to avoid inadvertent puncture of vasculature promote ultrasound guidance. However, actual data to support improved procedural safety with ultrasound have yet to be shown.[13] Finally, most investigators use sensory and motor stimulation before ablation to improve accuracy and avoid inadvertent motor nerve ablation.[15]

ANATOMY AND INNERVATION OF THE KNEE JOINT

The knee joint is a hinge joint that is composed of 2 boney articulations: the tibiofemoral joint and patellofemoral joint. These articulations are continuous with one another through a joint capsule composed of an inner synovial membrane and outer fibrous layer. This outer fibrous layer is primarily a composite of the adjacent long bone periosteum, tendinous extensions of adjacent muscles, and extracapsular ligaments. Similar to the hip, anterior knee joint innervation is typically divided into quadrants. Innervation of the joint capsule is complex with a high degree of anatomic variability.[14] There are 10 nerves innervating the anterior knee joint and 14 in total. Recently, Fonkoue and colleagues identified 5 constant articular branches in their neuroanatomic studies, which could act as potential targets for therapeutic interventions: superomedial genicular nerve (SMGN), inferomedial genicular nerve (IMGN), superolateral genicular nerve (SLGN), inferolateral genicular nerve (ILGN) and the infrapatellar branch of the saphenous nerve (IPBSN).

Although it was previously thought that the SMGN was a branch of the tibial nerve, research has shown that it is a terminal branch of the nerve to vastus medialis.[14] This distal branch joins the descending geniculate artery and descends with it in a bundle on the adductor magnus tendon toward the adductor tubercle. It ultimately makes boney contact with the medial condyle of the femur just anterior the adductor tubercle.

Although historically debated in the literature, contemporary neuroanatomical studies suggest the SLGN and IMGN are branches of the sciatic nerve.[14] The SLGN extends laterally under the biceps femoris muscle toward the posterosuperior angle of the lateral femoral condyle where it contacts the periosteum before giving off several branches. The IMGN arises from the posterior articular nerve (a branch off the sciatic nerve) at the level of the popliteal vessels. This nerve then joins the infero-medial genicular vessels to course around the medial tibial condyle from posterior to anterior following a recurrent trajectory. The nerve then travels proximal along the deep surface of the medial collateral ligament adjacent the tibial metaphysis and then ascends anteriorly toward the anteromedial part of the joint capsule.

The ILGN is generally accepted to be a branch of the common fibular nerve. It orig-inates at the level of the fibular neck and descends forward giving off several muscular branches. The terminal nerve then joins the lateral recurrent genicular vessels at the junction of the lateral condyle and the shaft of the tibia. They ascend together on the periosteum and pass between the tibial tuberosity and Gerdy tubercle to innervate the inferolateral aspect of the knee capsule.[16]

Finally, the IPBSN arises from the saphenous nerve as it leaves the adductor canal at the medial aspect of the distal third of the thigh. From here the nerve curves into the subcutaneous layer from posteromedial to anterior, toward the inferomedial aspect of the knee. The nerve then gives off several branches, some of which extend toward the tibial tuberosity, other cross the patellar ligament or ascend toward the patella.[17] The typical anterior and lateral views with nerve targets are shown in **Figs. 1** and **2**, respectively.

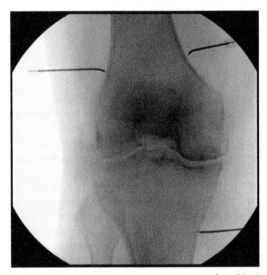

Fig. 1. Anteroposterior (AP) view of RFA cannulae placement for ablation of the SLGN (*top left*), SMGN (*top right*), and IMGN/infrapatellar branch of saphenous nerve (*bottom right*), respectively. Of note, the image does not include the ILGN catheter placement from an AP view.

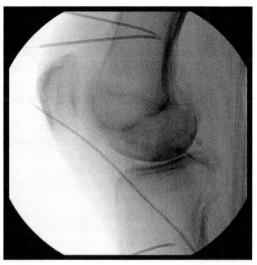

Fig. 2. Lateral view of RFA cannulae placement for the (from superior to inferior) SLGN, SMGN, IMGN/infrapatellar branch of saphenous, and ILGN, respectively. Of note, the initial lesion for the IMGN described by McCormick and colleagues is not depicted here.

KNEE RADIOFREQUENCY ABLATION OUTCOMES

Genicular nerve RFA outcomes have been well studied in many randomized controlled trials (RCTs). Recently, a meta-analysis by Zhang and colleagues looked at the safety and efficacy of genicular RFA in the treatment of osteoarthritis. Their analysis included 9 randomized controlled trials and evaluated pain scores and WOMAC index in patients treated with RFA versus those treated with placebo. The study found a significant difference in pain scores and was associated with improvement in WOMAC index at 4, 12, and 24 weeks between the RFA and placebo group.[18] It is worth noting, however, that the studies considered in their analysis only looked at the classically ablated nerves (SMGN, IMGN, SLGN) and not the additional nerve targets suggested by Fonkoue. Further research is needed to elucidate the effect of targeting additional genicular nerves on pain outcomes.[17]

A retrospective study by Kapural and colleagues showed clinical effectiveness of cooled RFA (CRFA) for treatment of chronic knee pain from osteoarthritis. This study had 183 patients with an average baseline pain score of 8.5/10, which decreased to 4.2/10 following CRFA. Sixty-five percent of patients had greater than 50% pain relief.[19]

In addition, a prospective, multicenter, RCT by Davis and colleagues that compared CRFA and intraarticular steroid (IAS) injection for chronic knee pain secondary to osteoarthritis showed that at 6 months the CRFA had more favorable outcomes with pain reduction of 50% or greater. Pain reduction of 74.1% in CRFA and 16.2% for IAS ($P < .0001$).[20]

ANATOMY AND INNERVATION OF THE HIP JOINT

The hip is a synovial ball and socket joint, which connects the femur to the pelvic girdle and allows for motion in multiple planes. The principal components of the joint consist of the head of the femur articulating with the acetabulum of the pelvis and bound by the manubrium. Several major ligaments then encase this structure to form the joint capsule. More than 20 muscles and their associated neurovascular structures cross this joint.[15,21] Although many potential pain generators exist within and around the joint, most hip pain is thought to originate at the anterior joint capsule.[13,15] Joint capsule innervation is complex but is primarily the result of articular branches from named peripheral nerves. In addition, small accessory articular branches from nerves within the substance of muscles surrounding the joint capsule represent a lesser contribution.

Chronic pain literature typically divides the anterior joint capsule into 4 distinct quadrants: superolateral, inferolateral, superomedial, and inferomedial.[15,22,23] Articular branches of the femoral nerve (FN), obturator nerve (ON), and accessory obturator nerves (AON) primarily innervate the anterior joint capsule. Their anatomic courses and distributions have been described in human cadaver studies. The FN supplies most of the superolateral and inferolateral joint capsule, as well as contributes to the innervation of the superomedial and inferomedial joint capsule; this is accomplished through FN branches designated as high or low depending on whether they originate above or below the inguinal ligament.[15,22,23] FN high branches arise distal to the lateral border of the psoas muscle and travel within iliacus deep to the inguinal ligament before innervating the capsule. FN low branches pierce the iliopsoas to supply the capsule directly or can course inferiorly before recurring to innervate all quadrants of the anterior joint capsule.

The ON supplies the inferomedial and inferolateral section of the anterior joint capsule and similar to the FN has branches designated high or low.[15,22] ON high branches arise proximal to or within the obturator canal and directly supply the inferomedial quadrant. ON low branches arise from the posterior branch of the ON and travel either directly to the capsule or form a fine plexus before supplying both the inferomedial and inferolateral capsule.[15,22] Finally, the AON arises as a single nerve from branches of the lumbar plexus and courses deep to the psoas along its medial margin to pass over the iliopubic eminence before supplying the inferomedial and superomedial quadrants.[15,21] As evident from the discussion, the inferomedial joint capsule is unique from the other 4 quadrants in that it receives innervation from all 3 nerves.

Unlike its anterior counterpart, posterior joint capsule innervation has not been as well characterized by the literature and is considered to be an area of minimal sensory innervation. The posterior joint capsule is frequently divided into posteromedial, lateral, and inferior parts. Articular branches of the sciatic nerve as well as the nerve to the quadratus femoris supply the posteromedial capsule. Small articular branches of the superior gluteal nerve supply the posterolateral capsule.[22] Finally, the posteroinferior joint capsule is innervated by articular branches of the inferior gluteal and obturator nerves. However, there is no clear description in the existing literature regarding the specific anatomic course taken by these nerves to supply the posteroinferior region of the capsule.[22] The ON and FN targets are shown in **Fig. 3**.

OUTCOMES: HIP RADIOFREQUENCY ABLATION

Despite heterogeneity in patient selection, procedural detail, and outcome assessment, hip RFA literature shows reliable improvement in commonly assessed pain scales such as visual analog scale and numerical rating scales.[13] Specific follow-up intervals vary greatly in the literature but range from 3 to 36 months. For example, a recent narrative review of hip RFA literature by Nagpal and colleagues showed a 30% to 80% reduction in pain scores over a variable time period (3 months to 3 years)

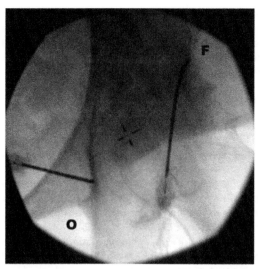

Fig. 3. Left hip RFA cannulae placement for ablation of the obturator (O) and femoral (F) nerve targets.

in the 9 studies they reviewed. Functional outcomes in the literature generally improved as well following RFA.

Kapural and colleagues used RFA for the articular sensory branches of obturator and femoral nerves and published an observational study showing that among the 23 patients involved the change in pain score was from 7.61 ± 1.2 to 2.25 ± 1.4 ($P < .01$). They also cite that the time interval of pain relief was longer with ablation; however, the duration is not stated specifically.[24]

A retrospective analysis performed by Tinnirello and colleagues published on pulsed RFA of the obturator and femoral nerve with a 12-month follow-up showed 57% of patients had a pain reduction greater than 50% at 1-month postprocedure, which lasted until 6 months. However, although scores remained significantly lower at 12 months than baseline, only 21% of the patients continued to have greater than 50% reduction.[25]

ANATOMY AND INNERVATION OF THE SHOULDER JOINT

Similar to the hip, the shoulder joint is a ball and socket joint. It is composed of 3 major bones: the humerus, clavicle, and scapula. These bones and the ribcage create 4 major articulations: the glenohumeral joint (GHJ), acromioclavicular joint, sternoclavicular joint, and the scapulothoracic joint.[26] The stabilization of the joint is primarily created by the rotator cuff muscles, which include the supraspinatus, the infraspinatus, teres minor, and the subscapularis. The supraspinatus, infraspinatus, and teres minor are innervated by the suprascapular nerve from C5 and C6, whereas the subscapularis is innervated by the superior and inferior subscapular nerve from C4 to C7.[26]

There are 4 nerves that have been identified as supplying the most clinically relevant innervation to the GHJ and subdeltoid bursa, although others may also contribute: are the suprascapular nerve, axillary nerve, upper (superior) subscapular nerve, and lateral pectoral nerve.[26] Location of the pain may indicate which nerves should be targeted for therapy, although this concept requires further validation. If the pain is posterolateral in the shoulder, theoretically the suprascapular and axillary nerves should be the target. If the pain is in anterior shoulder, then the lateral pectoral nerve and upper sub-scapular nerve should also be targeted.[26] Full denervation of the entire GHJ may require all 4 nerves to be blocked; whereas the subacromial bursa may primarily require the suprascapular nerve, axillary nerve, and lateral pectoral nerve. To ensure safety, the primary safe zones are noted in **Fig. 4**.

SHOULDER RADIOFREQUENCY ABLATION OUTCOMES

Because of our reliance on shoulder mobility for activities of daily living, it is important for us to find ways to combat chronic shoulder pain. Improved range of motion has been seen in a small case series following palliative ablation of the proximal supra-scapular nerve, with pain duration of up to 18 months.[27,28] Case series of articular shoulder ablation suggests at least 5 to 6 months of greater than 50% pain relief possible in patients with chronic shoulder pain from various causes, predominantly OA.[27,28] Metanalysis of predominantly pulsed RFA of the suprascapular nerve does not show superiority over more conservative medical management at 3 months in terms of pain and function, although significant study heterogeneity is a challenge in interpretation of these outcomes.[29] As of now, there are no RCTs for shoulder abla-tion; this is a relatively new technique, and further research needs to be done to estab-lish if there is long-term benefit.

TECHNICAL ASPECTS AND CONSIDERATIONS

Technical aspects and anatomic landmarks for all 3 joints can be referenced in **Table 1**.

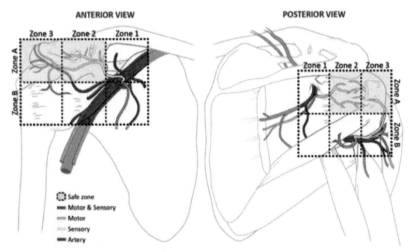

Fig. 4. Safe zones (2,3 A) to avoid motor denervation and reduce chance of vascular injury are lateral to the spinoglenoid notch posteriorly (suprascapular nerve branches, zone 2A), at the inferior-posterior portion of the greater tubercle (axillary nerve branches, zone 3A), and over the midpoint of the coracoid process (lateral pectoral nerve branches, zone 2A). The upper subscapular nerve could also be denervated at the superior anterior neck (zone 2A) of the glenoid, which would avoid the axillary artery, biceps tendon, and brachial plexus. Avoiding the joint line can protect the labrum. (*From* Eckmann MS, Bickelhaupt B, Fehl J, Benfield JA, Curley J, Rahimi O, Nagpal AS. Cadaveric Study of the Articular Branches of the Shoulder Joint. Reg Anesth Pain Med. 2017 Sep/Oct;42(5):564-570. https://doi.org/10. 1097/AAP.0000000000000652. PMID: 28786899.)

Table 1
Summary of current technical methods and landmarks used for articular joint denervation of the knee,[1,9,15–17] hip,[2,13,15] and shoulder[23]

Joint	Articular Nerve Targets	Imaging Landmarks for Articular (Predominantly Sensory) Denervation	Radiofrequency Considerations
Knee[9,15–17]	*Classic:* SMGN, SLGN, IMGN *Emerging:* ILGN	*SMGN:* Confluence of medial femoral shaft and epicondyle *SLGN:* Confluence of lateral femoral shaft and epicondyle *IMGN:* Confluence of medial tibial shaft and flare	*Common approach:* supine with knee flexed 25–30 deg, anterior to posterior trajectory *Recommended cannula:* 18G or greater, 10 cm active tip (standard) or 4–5 mm cooled active tip. Multiple lesions considered. *Stimulation pattern to exclude:* ankle movement w ILGN
Hip[13,15,30]	*Classic:* ON, FN *Theoretic:* N to quadratus femoris, superior gluteal nerve	*ON:* Inferior to the incisura acetabula, confluence of proximal ischium and inferior acetabulum. *FN:* inferomedial to the anterior inferior iliac spine near the anterolateral margin of the acetabulum	*Common approach:* supine, with oblique trajectory (FN) and caudal to cranial trajectory (ON). Consider ultrasound imaging or finder needle to avoid femoral artery and vein. *Recommended cannula:* 18G or greater, 10 cm active tip (standard) or 4–5 mm cooled active tip. Multiple lesions considered. *Stimulation pattern to exclude:* hip adduction or flexion.
Shoulder[26]	*Classic:* suprascapular (SN), axillary (AN), lateral pectoral nerve (LPN). *Emerging:* upper subscapular nerve (USN)	*SN:* upper posterior glenoid neck and anterior neck just posterior to the coracoid process *AN:* posterolateral humerus, near the inferior portion of the greater tubercle and cranial to the surgical neck	*Common approach:* prone (SN, AN), supine (LPN, USN), with oblique trajectory *Recommended cannula:* 18G or greater, 5–10 cm active tip (standard) or 2–5 mm cooled active tip.

(continued on next page)

Table 1 *(continued)*			
Joint	Articular Nerve Targets	Imaging Landmarks for Articular (Predominantly Sensory) Denervation	Radiofrequency Considerations
		LPN: midpoint of the superficial aspect of the coracoid process *USN:* anterior glenoid neck posterior to the coracoid process Safe zones noted in **Fig. 4.**	Multiple lesions considered. *Stimulation pattern to exclude:* supraspinatus/ infraspinatus (SN); deltoid/teres minor (AN); pectoralis major (LPN); subscapularis (USN)

DISCUSSION

Healthy movement of our joints allow for a large range of motion and enables patients to perform their daily activities. However, chronic pain of the hip, knee, and shoulder often limit these activities. Traditional chronic pain treatments include exercise, weight loss, physical therapy, topical analgesics, oral analgesics, intraarticular steroid injections, and surgical interventions.

However, even with all of these options, pain is still often poorly controlled. RFA can provide some relief to those with refractory pain.

RFA of the SMGN, IMGN, SLGN, ILGN, IPBSN, and genicular branches of the knee can provide greater than 50% pain reduction in 65% of patients.[24] Hip ablation of ON and FN showed greater than 50% pain reduction for 6 months in 57% of patients.[25] Because of the novel techniques of shoulder RFA, more research needs to be done to determine long-term efficacy and possible outcomes.

Overall, RFA has been shown to reduce pain significantly in patients who have refractory pain in their hip, knee, and shoulder. It is hope that continued research and adjustment of technique will guide future treatments and improve patient outcomes.

SUMMARY

This article provides a detailed description of peripheral joint RFA and its contemporary use in the treatment of chronic knee, hip, and shoulder pain. Special attention is given to anatomy and innervation, technical approach, selection criteria, contraindications, and patient outcomes. Greater than 50% pain reduction was shown in all 3 joints with variable duration. The shoulder RFA is the least studied joint at this time compared with the knee and hip, and more studies need to be conducted to determine long-term significance of ablation to the articular nerves of the shoulder.

CLINICS CARE POINTS

- Sensory testing to confirm correct cannula placement before ablation is desirable but not absolutely required. Testing is typically done at 50 Hz and cannula considered appropriately placed if the patient's typically experienced knee pain is reproduced.

- Motor testing is conducted following localization via sensory stimulation and accomplished at approximately 2V and 2 Hz. Evidence of motor fiber activity during stimulation should prompt cannula repositioning.
- Cannula placement should be as parallel to target nerve locations as possible during thermal ablation to maximize lesion spread along the length of targets. Not doing so can result in inadequate ablation of target nerves.

DISCLOSURE

Maxim S. Eckmann: funded research from SPR Therapeutics Educational Grants from Medtronic, Abbot, and Boston Scientific. Technical consultant to Abbot, AVANOS. The remaining authors have nothing to disclose.

REFERENCES

1. Cosman ER Jr, Dolensky JR, Hoffman RA. Factors that affect radiofrequency heat lesion size. Pain Med 2014;15(12):2020–36.
2. Neogi T. The epidemiology and impact of pain in osteoarthritis. Osteoarthritis Cartil 2013;21(9):1145–53.
3. Hong K, Georgiades C. Radiofrequency ablation: mechanism of action and devices. J Vasc Interv Radiol 2010;21(8 Suppl):S179–86.
4. Vanneste T, Van Lantschoot A, Van Boxem K, et al. Pulsed radiofrequency in chronic pain. Curr Opin Anaesthesiol 2017;30(5):577–82.
5. Chua NH, Vissers KC, Sluijter ME. Pulsed radiofrequency treatment in interventional pain management: mechanisms and potential indications-a review. Acta Neurochir (Wien) 2011;153(4):763–71.
6. Byrd D, Mackey S. Pulsed radiofrequency for chronic pain. Curr Pain Headache Rep 2008;12(1):37–41.
7. Usmani H, Dureja GP, Andleeb R, et al. Conventional Radiofrequency Thermocoagulation vs Pulsed Radiofrequency Neuromodulation of Ganglion Impar in Chronic Perineal Pain of Nononcological Origin. Pain Med 2018;19(12): 2348–56.
8. Manchikanti L, Kaye AD, Soin A, et al. Comprehensive Evidence-Based Guidelines for Facet Joint Interventions in the Management of Chronic Spinal Pain: American Society of Interventional Pain Physicians (ASIPP) Guidelines Facet Joint Interventions 2020 Guidelines. Pain Physician 2020;23(3S): S1–127.
9. McCormick ZL, Cohen SP, Walega DR, et al. Technical considerations for genicular nerve radiofrequency ablation: optimizing outcomes. Reg Anesth Pain Med 2021;46(6):518–23.
10. Roberts SL, Stout A, Dreyfuss P. Review of Knee Joint Innervation: Implications for Diagnostic Blocks and Radiofrequency Ablation. Pain Med 2020;21(5): 922–38.
11. Cohen SP, Bhaskar A, Bhatia A, et al. Consensus practice guidelines on interventions for lumbar facet joint pain from a multispecialty, international working group. Reg Anesth Pain Med 2020;45(6):424–67.
12. Kidd VD, Strum SR, Strum DS, et al. Genicular Nerve Radiofrequency Ablation for Painful Knee Arthritis: The Why and the How. JBJS Essent Surg Tech 2019; 9(1):e10.

13. Cheney CW, Ahmadian A, Brennick C, et al. Radiofrequency Ablation for Chronic Hip Pain: A Comprehensive, Narrative Review. Pain Med 2021;22(Suppl 1): S14–9.

14. Fonkoué L, Behets C, Kouassi JK, et al. Distribution of sensory nerves supplying the knee joint capsule and implications for genicular blockade and radiofrequency ablation: an anatomical study. Surg Radiol Anat 2019;41(12):1461–71.

15. Kumar P, Hoydonckx Y, Bhatia A. A Review of Current Denervation Techniques for Chronic Hip Pain: Anatomical and Technical Considerations. Curr Pain Headache Rep 2019;23(6):38. Erratum in: Curr Pain Headache Rep. 2019;23(6):45. PMID: 31044316.

16. Fonkoue L, Behets CW, Steyaert A, et al. Accuracy of fluoroscopic-guided genicular nerve blockade: a need for revisiting anatomical landmarks. Reg Anesth Pain Med 2019;100451, rapm-2019.

17. Fonkoue L, Behets CW, Steyaert A, et al. Current versus revised anatomical targets for genicular nerve blockade and radiofrequency ablation: evidence from a cadaveric model. Reg Anesth Pain Med 2020;45(8):603–9.

18. Zhang H, Wang B, He J, et al. Efficacy and safety of radiofrequency ablation for treatment of knee osteoarthritis: a meta-analysis of randomized controlled trials. J Int Med Res 2021;49(4). 3000605211006647.

19. Kapural L, Lee N, Neal K, et al. Long-Term Retrospective Assessment of Clinical Efficacy of Radiofrequency Ablation of the Knee Using a Cooled Radiofrequency System. Pain Physician 2019;22(5):489–94.

20. Davis T, Loudermilk E, DePalma M, et al. Prospective, Multicenter, Randomized, Crossover Clinical Trial Comparing the Safety and Effectiveness of Cooled Radiofrequency Ablation With Corticosteroid Injection in the Management of Knee Pain From Osteoarthritis. Reg Anesth Pain Med 2018;43(1):84–91.

21. Bowman KF Jr, Fox J, Sekiya JK. A clinically relevant review of hip biomechanics. Arthroscopy 2010;26(8):1118–29.

22. Short AJ, Barnett JJG, Gofeld M, et al. Anatomic Study of Innervation of the Anterior Hip Capsule: Implication for Image-Guided Intervention. Reg Anesth Pain Med 2018;43(2):186–92.

23. Bhatia A, Hoydonckx Y, Peng P, et al. Radiofrequency Procedures to Relieve Chronic Hip Pain: An Evidence-Based Narrative Review. Reg Anesth Pain Med 2018;43(1):72–83.

24. Kapural L. Cooled radiofrequency neurotomy of the articular sensory branches of the obturator and femoral nerves – combinded approach using fluoroscopy and ultrasound guidance: Technical report, and observational study on safety and efficacy. Pain Physician 2018;1(21;1):279–84.

25. Tinnirello A, Todeschini M, Pezzola D, et al. Pulsed Radiofrequency Application on Femoral and Obturator Nerves for Hip Joint Pain: Retrospective Analysis with 12-Month Follow-up Results. Pain Physician 2018;21(4):407–14.

26. Eckman Maxim, Joshi Mihir, Bickelhaupt Brittany. How I Do it: Shoulder Articular Nerve Blockade and Radiofrequency Ablations. Am Soc Reg Anesth Pain Med 2020.

27. Eckmann MS, Johal J, Bickelhaupt B, et al. Terminal Sensory Articular Nerve Radiofrequency Ablation for the Treatment of Chronic Intractable Shoulder Pain: A Novel Technique and Case Series. Pain Med 2020;21(4):868–71.

28. Eckmann MS, Lai BK, Uribe MA 3rd, et al. Thermal Radiofrequency Ablation of the Articular Branch of the Lateral Pectoral Nerve: A Case Report and Novel Technique. A Pract 2019;13(11):415–9.

29. Pushparaj H, Hoydonckx Y, Mittal N, et al. A systematic review and meta-analysis of radiofrequency procedures on innervation to the shoulder joint for relieving chronic pain. Eur J Pain 2021;25(5):986–1011.
30. Locher S, Burmeister H, Böhlen T, et al. Radiological anatomy of the obturator nerve and its articular branches: basis to develop a method of radiofrequency denervation for hip joint pain. Pain Med 2008;9(3):291–8.

Novel Technologies in Interventional Pain Management

Yashar Eshraghi, MD[a,b,c], Jay D. Shah, MD[a,*],
Maged Guirguis, MD[a,b,c]

KEYWORDS

- Basivertebral nerve ablation • Percutaneous lumbar decompression
- Ligamentum flavum dissection • Superion • Intracept
- mild (minimally invasive lumbar decompression) • Emerging technologies
- Lumbar spinal stenosis

KEY POINTS

- Novel technologies aimed at reducing the burden of chronic low back pain continue to emerge.
- Direct and indirect lumbar decompression techniques have emerged over the past decade as nonsurgical procedural alternatives to open decompression for lumbar spinal stenosis.
- Long-term follow-up data on direct and indirect lumbar decompression procedures have shown noninferiority to open procedures, with sustained symptomatic and functional relief.
- Identification of basivertebral nerve as a driver of vertebrogenic back pain (a specific subset of chronic low back pain) has led to the emergence and establishment of novel radiofrequency ablation technique. Short and long-term follow-up on this technique has demonstrated excellent safety profiles and sustained functional and symptomatic improvement.
- Emerging technologies in interventional pain management should be carefully evaluated for safety, effectiveness, and sustained impact. Cost of procedure and insurance coverage criteria also need to be considered as gateways to widespread adoption of novel technologies.

INTRODUCTION

As the health care costs and burden of disease for chronic pain continue to rise, so does the amount of research and innovation in pharmacologic and procedural strategies used to treat patients. The National Pain Strategy and Federal Pain Strategy in the mid-2010s served as the first coordinated and comprehensive approach for

[a] Department of Anesthesiology & Interventional Pain Management, Ochsner Health System, 2820 Napoleon Avenue, Ste. 900, New Orleans, LA 70115, USA; [b] University of Queensland - Ochsner Clinical School, Australia; [c] Louisiana State University School of Medicine, School of Medicine, New Orleans, LA 70112, USA
* 215 Postoffice Street, Apartment 1004, Galveston, TX 77550, USA
E-mail address: jay.dipesh.shah@gmail.com

Phys Med Rehabil Clin N Am 33 (2022) 533–552
https://doi.org/10.1016/j.pmr.2022.01.006
1047-9651/22/© 2022 Elsevier Inc. All rights reserved.

addressing the burden of chronic pain and a game-plan for advances in research. Additionally, the National Institutes of Health launched "Helping to End Addiction Long-Term" (HEAL) as a multi-organization effort to advance research into nonopioid solutions and interventions for chronic pain.[1] Before this, the total NIH funding dedicated to innovations in chronic pain was less than 3%.[2]

Recent estimates of annual U.S. health care costs for chronic pain are upwards of $600 million dollars, and the total population affected in some way by chronic pain is more than 50 million.[3] Of these patients, 40% suffer from high impact chronic pain which has deleterious effects on their day-to-day lifestyle.[4] As the treatment of chronic pain continues to evolve and explore novel opioid-sparing methods of management, minimally invasive techniques have risen to the forefront of the conversation. Techniques such as fluoroscopic guided nerve blocks, intrathecal drug delivery systems, and implantable neuromodulation devices have altered the chronic pain experience for many patients and have allowed them to attempt resuming their daily lives.[5]

The true effectiveness of certain approaches (pharmacologic, interventional, and surgical) for managing chronic pain is constantly debated. However, this has not impeded innovation, as advances in minimally invasive techniques and regenerative medicine have gained significant popularity in recent years. The purpose of this article is to synthesize evidence for a few of the emerging technologies in pain medicine and provide a guide for strategizing the best way to incorporate these innovations into everyday patient care. While this list is not comprehensive and management approaches are bound to constantly evolve over time, we chose to focus on a few novel procedures that have the potential to disrupt our current patient care framework. As the management of chronic pain requires an integrative biopsychosocial approach, key aspects to consider for every new procedure or innovation include appropriate patient selection, rigorous preprocedure planning, and comprehensive evaluation of varying surgical techniques. The focus of the article will be in 3 main spaces: (1) minimally invasive lumbar spinal stenosis (LSS) management (including the use of percutaneous interspinous spacers as well as direct percutaneous lumbar decompression), (2) intraosseous basivertebral nerve ablation, and (3) regenerative medicine for lumbosacral degeneration. Considerations for evaluating and incorporating novel technologies into interventional pain management practice will also be discussed.

LUMBAR SPINAL STENOSIS

Symptomatic LSS is a degenerative narrowing of the spinal canal, nerve roots, or foramen that has the potential to lead to debilitating neurogenic claudication. The proposed pathophysiology of LSS is either hypertrophy of the ligamentum flavum or facet, osteophyte formation, or intervertebral disc bulge, any of which can lead to compression, claudication, and functional limitation.[6] LSS is the most common cause of spinal surgery in patients greater than 50 years of age, and due to increased life expectancy, the number of cases continues to rise.[6] The current estimated prevalence of LSS in the United States is 400,000, with 47% in the mild-moderate category and 20% in the severe category.[7,8] Mainstays of initial conservative management are medical therapy with NSAIDs, diet, and exercise/physical therapy. Epidural steroid injections (ESIs) and percutaneous adhesiolysis have also been shown to provide short to medium-term relief, although a 2014 study on 400 patients showed no additional benefit of ESI's when compared with epidural injections of lidocaine alone.[8,9] A retrospective analysis of patients with degenerative LSS who had undergone caudal ESIs showed functional improvement on long-term follow-up in 35% of patients, with only 12.6 patients ultimately needing surgery.[10] Outcomes were especially positive in patients who had concomitant degenerative spondylolisthesis. However, repeated steroid injections may lead to systemic side effects, including poor wound healing, increased risk of osteoporotic fracture, and deleterious changes to blood sugar, blood pressure, and weight.[8] In cases whereby patients no longer respond to ESI for relief, interventional therapy becomes part of the conversation. Although open lumbar decompression had been the mainstay for patients who had failed conservative management in the past, there was a huge gap in the treatment protocol between nonsurgical and surgical options. Minimally invasive, image-guided interventions have addressed this by expanding the list of conservative treatment methods. The only nonelective indication for open surgical decompression is the manifestation of cauda equina syndrome. All other open laminectomies performed are conducted for symptomatic relief and improvement of patient quality of life.[10,11] However, open laminectomies have had complication rates that range from 12% to 29%, based on patient comorbidities.[10] As the main patient population experiencing LSS is over the age of 50, they often have significant comorbidities that negatively affect their candidacy and postsurgical outcome. This further emphasized a need for minimally invasive procedures which could improve quality of life without as high of a risk of severe complications. In 2018, a group of experts in the management of spinal pathology developed a set of practice guidelines for minimally invasive spinal treatment (MIST.) The MIST protocol allows for physicians to appropriately select patients who would be strong candidates for a minimally invasive intervention.[11] Currently, 2 major options are available: direct and indirect decompression. Direct decompression is usually accomplished through a percutaneous approach and indirect decompression is accomplished via the use of percutaneous interspinous spacers.[11]

PERCUTANEOUS INTERSPINOUS SPACERS
Introduction

One of the main goals of interspinous spacers in the treatment of LSS was to avoid some of the known complications of open decompression—including postlaminectomy syndrome, spinal scarring, and intraoperative direct exposure of the spinal cord. Additionally, as the spacer is placed outside of the spine and opens up the spinal canal from the outside in, the procedure is reversible while a laminectomy or fusion is not. From a physiologic perspective, interspinous spacers essentially prevent extension at specific stenotic levels of the spine, leading to a tightening of the ligamentum flavum and reduction of ligament invasion into the spinal canal.[11–13] Although various interspinous spacers have existed in the market over the years, 2 systems have predominated over the last decade: X-Stop Interspinous Spacer by Medtronic) and Superion Indirect Decompression System by Boston Scientific (S-IDS).[11] Another technology on the market, The MinuteMan, an interspinous-interlaminar fusion device has emerged recently as a minimally invasive solution to LSS. This procedure focuses on temporary fixation and ultimately fusion rather than decompression. Multicenter studies regarding the adoption of this technology are underway.[13] Over the last few years, the X-Stop system has been recalled from the market and the Superion system remains as the main standalone system for minimally invasive indirect lumbar decompression.

Patient Selection Criteria

Currently, based on the MIST guidelines, indirect lumbar decompression is indicated in skeletally mature adult patients experiencing up to symptomatic moderate spinal stenosis, as defined as 25% to 50% reduction in canal area when compared with normal or adjacent areas.[12] Key symptoms to evaluate include neurogenic intermittent claudication due to LSS and moderate-severe impaired physical function, both of which are somewhat relieved with flexion. Patients should be managed with conservative therapy for at least 6 months. The guidelines also suggest that spacers may only be placed at two consecutive levels. Specifically, patients with spinal stenosis anywhere from the L1-L2 level to L4-L5, with central or lateral stenosis and ligamentum flavum hypertrophy greater than 2.5 cm are good candidates for indirect lumbar decompression.[11,12]

Key contraindications for indirect decompression include pain that is not relieved on flexion, L5-S1 stenosis, significant scoliosis with Cobb Angle greater than 10, grade 2 or higher spondylolisthesis, pathologic vertebral fracture, significant lumbar spinal instability, and spinous process, pars, or laminal fracture at the level of proposed intervention.[11,12] These contraindications exist specifically to prevent instability of the device once it is implanted in the spine. Radiologic evaluation of spinal instability is conducted with flexion-extension films, evaluation for spondylolisthesis, and facet joint hypertrophy with cyst or fluid accumulation.[12] In cases of instability, minimally invasive direct decompression or open surgical decompression are preferred. Imaging assessment of spinal pathology, including looking for thin, unstable spinous processes is important to reduce the risk of spinous process fracture. Of note, patients with "kissing spine syndrome" (aka Baastrup's disease), whereby the adjacent spinous processes do not have a physiologic gap (or a very small one), are relatively contraindicated for interspinous spacers for the same risk of fracture.[11]

Body habitus is another key consideration. Outcomes tend to be more optimal in patients with a BMI under 35, so physical therapy and exercise should be a mainstay of conservative treatment. If the patient's body habitus does not meet these criteria, assessment of visualization ability via lateral fluoroscopy is key to determining the feasibility of the procedure.[12]

Outcome Data

As interspinous spacers became a mainstay in the LSS treatment market in the early 2000s, a landmark study was released in 2005 evaluating outcomes in patients with moderate LSS using the X-Stop spacer.[14] This study evaluated 2-year follow-up data on 100 patients who had received the X-Stop spacer against 91 patients who were managed with conservative, nonoperative approaches. Symptom severity score at 2 years improved by 45% in the X-Stop spacer cohort and only 7.9% in the nonoperative cohort. Additionally, members of the X-Stop cohort reported statistically significant higher scores in each domain of the Zurich Claudication Questionnaire (ZCQ) than the nonoperative cohort.[14]

This sentinel report was followed up with a 2013 study comparing X-Stop interspinous spacers against surgical open decompression.[15] This was also a 2-year study with 50 patients receiving the X-Stop spacer and 50 patients undergoing open lumbar decompression with laminectomy. This study not only established noninferiority of interspinous spacers as compared with open decompression but also showed significant improvement from baseline in both groups for ZCQ scores and VAS scores.

When the Superion interspinous spacer was coming to market, the FDA approved a pivotal Investigational Device Exemption (IDE) landmark multicenter (29 sites) trial. Results were published at 2 years, 3 years, and 5 years, and compared clinical outcomes using VAS scores and Oswestry Disability Index (ODI) scores for patients undergoing S-IDS versus patients undergoing X-Stop.[16–21] Patients who had received the X-Stop device were not followed up with beyond 2 years, as the device was removed from the market. The original trial included patients with LSS who had failed at least 6 months of conservative, nonsurgical treatment and randomly assigned them to either X-Stop

(201 patients) or Superion (190 patients). At 2 years, the data showed noninferiority of Superion to X-Stop, with a 15% or higher improvement in ODI scores in 63% of Superion patients.[17,18] Additionally, 77% of patients experienced leg pain relief, and 68% of patients experienced back pain relief, based on VAS scores. At 5 years, however, Superion showed consistency, with 65% of patients experiencing greater than 15% improvement in ODI scores, 84% of patients experiencing significant improvement in at least 2 domains of the ZCQ, and 80% of patients experiencing significant improvement of VAS scores.[19–21] 75% of patients did not experience any complications, reoperations, and additional procedural augmentation, and those who did, primarily had any revisions conducted within the first 2 years. Two 2018 observational studies further showed that patients who had been managed with S-IDS had decreasing opioid use and improved quality-of-life (QOL) scores.[22,23]

Risks and Contraindications

In the pivotal IDE trial, the device and procedure-related serious adverse event rate was 8.4% with a neurologic complication of 3.5%.[16–21] Nonhealing spinous process fracture rate at 2 years was 11% in S-IDS and 3.5% in X-Stop, with 80% of these injuries identified at the 6-week follow-up.[20] However, patients who had experienced spinous process fractures were primarily asymptomatic and had not experienced any major functional limitation as a result of it. Other major complications included implant mal-positioning and increased pain as opposed to pain relief at the level of the procedure. Important potential complications which were not commonly seen included risk of implant breakage, uncontrolled scar formation, and damage to nearby structures from implant migration.[11,24] Especially when compared with open surgery, which poses significant long-term neurologic and functional complication risk (up to 29%), this minimally invasive approach has relatively less downside.[11]

Procedural Highlights

The S-IDS system is delivered percutaneously as a single-piece H-shaped titanium alloy spacer via cannula. Dilators within the cannula delivery system allow for layer-by-layer tissue exposure and introduction of the implant to the interlaminar space. The implant has superior and inferior cam lobes which rotate as they are placed into the space to cover the superior and inferior spinous processes, respectively. The implant itself is well designed, with a high contact surface area to size ratio and 5 options for implant size (8, 10, 12, 14, 16 mm).[10] [**Fig. 1**] Important highlights of the procedure include initial measurement of implant size with the interspinous gauge

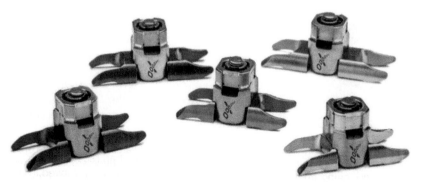

Fig. 1. Percutaneous interspinous spacers. (Image provided courtesy of Boston Scientific. ©2021 Boston Scientific Corporation or its affiliates. All rights reserved.)

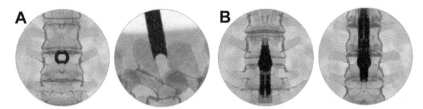

Fig. 2. Fluoroscopic positioning of cannula and interspinous gauge. (*A*): AP and lateral fluoroscopic positioning of cannula: A 12 to 15 mm midline incision is made to expose the superior spinous ligament. Two dilators are provided with the S-IDS system, and the first dilator is advanced to the spino-laminar junction under lateral fluoroscopic guidance. The second, larger dilator is placed over the first dilator and channels are aligned with the superior and inferior spinous processes. The initial dilator should then be removed, and the second dilator advanced with mallet. The cannula is then inserted over the second dilator and advanced to the lateral aspect of the superior spinous ligament with lateral fluoroscopic confirmation. Cannulas should not be passed beyond the interlaminar junction, as this increases the risk of dural injury. (*B*): Superior and Inferior Aspects of Interspinous Gauge Placement. (Images provided courtesy of Boston Scientific. ©2021 Boston Scientific Corporation or its affiliates. All rights reserved.)

followed by deployment via a unique inserter tool and cannula [**Fig. 2**]. Crucial to the process is confirmation via AP and lateral fluoroscopy that the cam lobes are covering the superior and inferior spinous processes and the implant is midline to the spino-laminar junction [**Figs. 3** and **4**].

Cost-Effectiveness

A 2019 review by a team of spine specialists examined the literature on cost-effectiveness of interspinous spacers against that of conservative nonsurgical care and open surgical laminectomy. One of the key takeaways from the review was a reduction of total health care cost when choosing the minimally invasive option because of the indirect peri and postoperative care costs seen in open surgery.[22–28] A 2015 study evaluating procedural considerations for Superion versus open surgery and found shorter procedure times, minimal blood loss, and fewer complications, all of which led to a significantly shorter postoperative rehabilitation time.[26] When

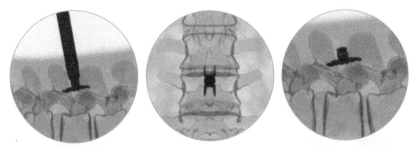

Fig. 3. Fluoroscopic confirmation of implant positioning: (*A*) Lateral fluoroscopic confirmation of implant positioning before the removal of inserter. (*B*) AP fluoroscopic confirmation of implant positioning after removal of inserter. (*C*) Lateral fluoroscopic confirmation of implant positioning after removal of inserter. (Images provided courtesy of Boston Scientific. ©2021 Boston Scientific Corporation or its affiliates. All rights reserved.)

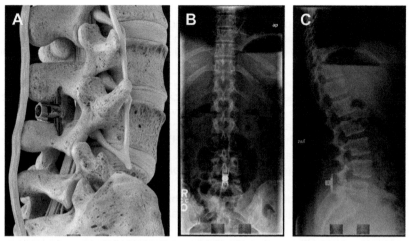

Fig. 4. *Final Interspinous Spacer Implant Views:* The final positioning of the implant should be a deep and anterior position to the lamina, with cam lobes comfortably encompassing the superior and inferior spinous processes. (*A*) Animation of final interspinous spacer viewed from a lateral position. (*B*) Radiographic AP view of final interspinous spacer positioning. (*C*) Radiographic Lateral view of final interspinous spacer positioning. (Image provided courtesy of Boston Scientific. ©2021 Boston Scientific Corporation or its affiliates. All rights reserved.)

comparing direct costs against QALYs, another 2015 analysis showed that conservative care had the lowest cost ($10,540 USD), but also the lowest QALY impact (0.06 improvement). Costs and QALY impact for open surgery and interspinous spacers were similar, with both options costing approximately $14,000 USD and showing QALY bumps of 0.29 and 0.27, respectively.[27,28] However, this study did not take indirect costs such as rehabilitation, peri and postprocedure follow-up, and loss of income due to health care leave. The MIST guidelines support this research and suggest that in the face of similar cost-effectiveness between open surgery and interspinous spacers, physicians should opt to recommend the less invasive, lower complication rate procedure.[11,12] Although the IDE has been the only major clinical trial evaluating outcomes with S-IDS, in the right patient population, the most recent therapeutic guidelines show strong evidence for it to be an effective treatment option.

PERCUTANEOUS LUMBAR DECOMPRESSION
Introduction

Another option for minimally invasive LSS management, which has been heavily evaluated over the last decade, is direct lumbar decompression via a percutaneous approach. The overall goal of percutaneous lumbar decompression is to debulk the ligamentum flavum and lamina using an image-guided dissection and an epidurogram to evaluate the effects of each debulking step.[27]

Patient Selection Criteria

One of the key aspects of the percutaneous lumbar decompression is that the main indication for this procedure is a ligamentum flavum hypertrophy greater than 2.5 cm.[10,11] While LSS may occur due to disk displacement into the canal, facet joint hypertrophy, or other bony, lateral foramen abnormalities, the therapeutic goal of the percutaneous lumbar decompression is the central ligamentum flavum debulking. Thus, the primary patient population who is a good candidate for this procedure is one with central spinal stenosis, with ligamentum flavum hypertrophy, with or without instability, who is not likely to have good surgical outcomes or prefers a less invasive approach.[29,30]

The majority of patients who are candidates for this procedure will have undergone conservative nonsurgical therapy, including physical therapy, medication management, and ESIs.[11] Typically, these approaches would have provided some relief but would not have lasted much longer than 6 months. Imaging confirmation of central spinal stenosis due to ligamentum flavum hypertrophy and reduction in dural sac cross-sectional area are essential to the candidacy for this procedure. Most commonly, patients who have LSS due to central ligamentum flavum hypertrophy will have pathology at the L3-L4 and L4-L5 levels.[31]

Concerns for recommending percutaneous lumbar decompression include significant spinal instability, such as anterior spondylolisthesis greater than 5 mm, prior surgical decompression attempt at the same level, disk protrusion into the spinal canal, and osteophyte formation. Other relative contraindications include patients with lateral foraminal stenosis with minimal ligamentum flavum hypertrophy, as these patients may not experience symptomatic relief from the procedure. However, many patients have lateral foraminal pathology comorbid with ligamentum flavum hypertrophy.[11] The landmark MiDAS Evidence-based Neurogenic Claudication Outcomes Research (ENCORE) study found that while most of patients had comorbid facet hypertrophy, lateral foramen stenosis, or disc bulging, these comorbidities were actually a positive predictor of a better post-procedural outcome.[29] If the patient's body habitus prevents prone positioning, this would be an important perioperative concern for moving forward with this procedure.

Additionally, patients with pain syndromes that coexist with LSS and cause ambiguity as to the origin of pain symptoms are also relatively contraindicated. As mentioned earlier, the only absolute indication for open surgery, as opposed to minimally invasive decompression, is cauda equina syndrome.[11]

Outcome Data

The *MILD* procedure, although having been around for over a decade, has relatively scarce literature regarding its efficacy and outcomes. However, the results available generally show statistically significant improvements in visual analog (VAS) pain scores, functional limitations, and the ODI (Oswestry Disability Index). The initial literature describing the technique and outcomes was published by Deer and Kapural in 2010 as a 90-patient retrospective study that showed no incidents of dural puncture or tear, blood transfusions, nerve injury, or unexpected bleeding or hematoma formation.[30] This was the initial study suggesting that the *MILD* procedure may be a safe and potentially effective alternative to the surgical management of LSS.[30–32] The MiDAS trial was one of the first prospective studies pertaining to the *MILD* procedure, looking at 6-week outcomes for 78 patients. This study was notable for showing improvements in VAS scores from 7.3 to 3.9 at the 6-week follow-up. The disability index (ODI) was significantly improved as well, with baselines at 47.4 and a mean improvement of 17.9 across the entire cohort of patients.[33,34] Longer term (2 years) results reported by this team showed a statistically significant improvement of baseline VAS (7.2) to 4.8 and ODI showed significant Improvement from 48.4 to 39.8.[34] Although pain relief and disability are not as improved as they were in the 6-month follow-up cohort, the ZCQ domains (both pain and neuro-ischemic subdomains) that showed statistically significant improvement at 6 months remained improved at the 2-year follow-up. Patient satisfaction rates hovered around 86% in this cohort, showing the comfort of this patient population with choosing the *MILD* procedure over more invasive lumbar decompression surgery. The MiDAS ENCORE trial mentioned earlier was another major contributor to evidence, as it endeavored to compare outcomes of ESIs against the *MILD* procedure.[29,30] Notably, at 1-year follow-up, *MILD* showed superiority in ZCQ domain improvement, ODI scores, and patient satisfaction scores with no difference in complication rate or safety profile. A study by Mekhail and colleagues evaluated walking distance and standing time in patients at 1-year follow-up and showed a 7x increase in standing time (8 minutes to 56 minutes) and a 16x increase in walking distance (246 feet to 3956 feet). As a lot of our characterization management of patients with LSS is based on functional difficulty, this study was pivotal in showing the anatomic and practical benefits of the *MILD* procedure.[34]

Risks and Contraindications

Importantly, no major complications were reported.[33] The complication profile seems to be advantageous as well, with minimal incidence of direct procedural issues such as dural tear, nerve damage, bleeding, or infection. Intraoperative bleeding was usually controlled with gel foam and postoperative bleeding was not generally difficult to control..[32]

While a three-way outcomes study has not been conducted assessing interspinous spacers and *MILD* against lumbar decompression surgery and fusion surgery, a 2020 review of literature pooled data from multiple trials comparing one procedure against another, which showed that *MILD* had the lowest reoperation rate (5.7%) and lowest rate of device and procedure-related adverse events (1.3%). Additionally, the *MILD* procedure, like the decompression surgery, does not use implants, which reduces the risk of infection and potential "mechanical rejection."[35,36]

To date, there have been 13 peer-reviewed studies that have demonstrated the safety profile, short-and long-term outcomes, and patient comfort with the *MILD* procedure.[28-36] Additional clinical trials are underway to assess the efficacy of the procedure when compared with conservative medical management. One such trial is a multicenter RCT of 150 patients evaluating ODI, ZCQ, and numeric pain scores (VAS). However, the data and outcomes thus far do provide strong support for the *MILD* procedure in patients with LSS and LF thickness greater than 2.5 mm, especially as an alternative to invasive surgery.[28-36]

Procedural Highlights

The primary system used for percutaneous lumbar decompression is the *MILD* system (Vertos Medical, Carlsbad CA). The key components of the *MILD* kit include a 5.1 mm incisional port, a tissue sculpter for ligamentous debulking, and a bone sculpter rongeur to remove pieces of the lamina [**Fig. 5**]. Key components of the procedure include: (1) a baseline epidurogram (for marking of the procedural border and reduction of dural injury risk, (2) identification of the medial-to-lateral trajectory for portal placement, (3) utilization of the bone sculptor rongeur for removal of pieces of superior and inferior lamina, and (4) utilization of the tissue sculptor to debulk the ligamentum flavum. A repeat epidurogram showing improved flow patterns and a less tortuous and dense ligamentum flavum confirms proper debulking and completion of the *MILD* procedure [**Figs. 6** and **7**]. Patients are generally able to resume normal activity within 24 to 48 hours and are assessed for physical therapy 2-weeks postprocedure [**Figs. 8** and **9**].

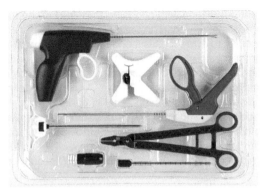

Fig. 5. *mild* Device Kit. (Images provided courtesy of Vertos Medical. ©2021 All rights reserved.)

INTRAOSSEOUS BASIVERTEBRAL NERVE ABLATION
Introduction

Chronic low back pain (CLBP) manifests in patients in a variety of ways, but a common thread is the level of disability that it has the risk of generating. Apart from being the most common cause of activity limitation in individuals younger than age 45, approximately 15% of the patients with CLBP account for greater than 75% of the Medicare

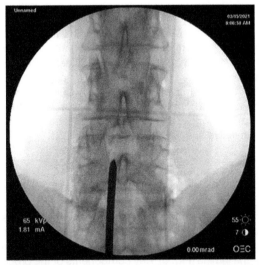

Fig. 6. *AP View of Target Trocar Placement:* A critical procedural step is identifying the medial-to-lateral trajectory for portal placement. This may be mapped topically pre-operatively under fluoroscopic view using a spinal needle or may be conducted intra-operatively. A scalpel (11 blade or 15 blade) is used to make a stab incision and trocar-portal unit (part of the *MILD* kit) is introduced in the same trajectory as the spinal needle. Once the portal is advanced to the superior aspect of the inferior lamina under contralateral oblique fluoroscopy, it is docked, the trocar is removed, and a stabilizing device (also part of the *MILD* kit) is snapped onto the portal to enable tissue removal via cannula. (Images provided courtesy of Vertos Medical. ©2021 All rights reserved.)

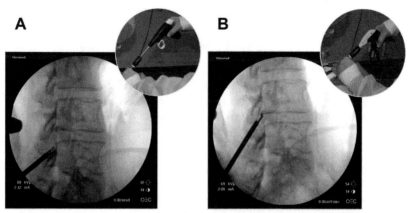

Fig. 7. Oblique fluoroscopic visualization and instrument demonstration of Bone Rongeur and Tissue Sculpter:. (*A*): Bone rongeur: The bone sculptor rongeur is introduced and laminar pieces are removed from both the superior and inferior lamina. Proceduralists may choose to start with the superior aspect of the inferior lamina (access point) and work medially to laterally for both the superior and inferior lamina or remove pieces from the superior lamina first and then work inferiorly. What is important is to clean the rongeur between each bone removal step. (*B*): Tissue Sculpter: After adequate laminar removal, the tissue sculptor is introduced to debulk the ligamentum flavum. The sculptor is introduced inferiorly in the contralateral oblique fluoroscopic view, and a scooping, semi-circular rotation is used for each bite of tissue removal. Again, it is important to clean the tissue sculptor every few bites to ensure adequate removal. (Images provided courtesy of Vertos Medical. ©2021 All rights reserved.)

costs. This is largely due to the fact that CLBP is often diagnosed as nonspecific, and thus treatment is not targeted toward a potential cause (eg, generic options such as exercise, physical therapy, weight loss, core strengthening, chiropractors).[35] In the investigation and study of potential etiologies for CLBP, disk degeneration has been

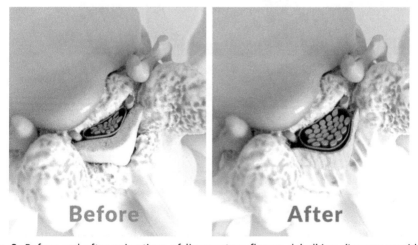

Fig. 8. Before and after animations of ligamentum flavum debulking. (Images provided courtesy of Vertos Medical. ©2021 All rights reserved.)

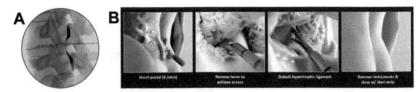

Fig. 9. Animations of Procedural Highlights for *mild*. (*A*): Baseline epidurogram. (*B*): Procedural Steps. (Images provided courtesy of Vertos Medical. ©2021 All rights reserved.)

consistently implicated.[37,38] However, researchers have more recently identified that the vertebral endplates adjacent to each disk also contribute to pathologic disease manifestations. These endplates are rather susceptible to inflammation and injury, as they balance providing vertebral structural support against acting as a primary channel for blood and nutrition supply for the disc.[37]

A 1997 study into etiologies of CLBP evaluated vertebral end plates in disc degeneration patients with and without pain and found that patients experiencing pain also had increased nutrient arterial vascular proliferation at the endplate-disc junction and higher nociceptor density.[38] Further mapping showed that running alongside the nutrient arteries were branches of the sinuvertebral nerve that would course from the vertebral body via the basivertebral foramen (ie, the basivertebral nerves). The basivertebral nerve (BVN) was subsequently found to transmit via high levels of substance P (a pain-associated nociceptor) and found to be PGP 9.5-positive

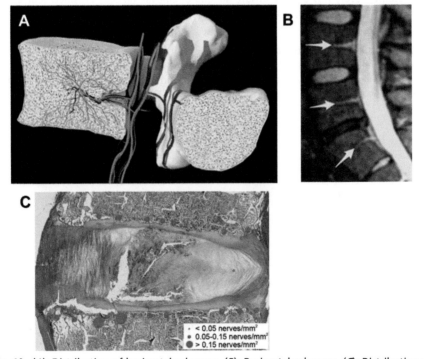

Fig. 10. (*A*): Distribution of basivertebral nerve. (*B*): Basivertebral nerve. (*C*): Distribution of PGP + nerve fibers across endplate. (Images provided courtesy of Relievant Medsystems. ©2021 All rights reserved.)

(immunohistochemical stain for density of pain fibers).[39,40] The pain associated with the BVN was subsequently termed vertebrogenic pain [**Fig. 10**].

One way to characterize the etiology and severity of CLBP and potential vertebrogenic pain was described by Modic and colleagues based on the T1 and T2 weighted signal of the vertebral endplates on MRI. In Modic change 1 (MC1), the endplates seem hypointense in T1 and hyperintense in T2 due to edema and inflammation. Modic change 2 (MC2) shows hyperintensity of signal in both T1 and T2 and is likely due to the conversion of hematopoietic marrow into yellow, fatty marrow. Modic change 3 (MC3) shows hypointensity of signal in both T1 and T2 and is likely due to bony sclerotic changes. Of the 3 types, patients with MC3 are rarely symptomatic, while MC1 is considered to be the most painful and disability inducing.[38,39] Multiple studies have shown the association between Modic I and Modic II changes and the presence and severity of CLBP, especially in the L5-S1 and L4-L5 regions.[41,42] [**Fig. 11**]

Patient Selection Criteria

Interest in potential radiofrequency ablation (RFA) of the basivertebral nerve has grown over the last 7 to 10 years, with the first pilot study and RCT results coming out in the latter half of the 2010s..[39,43,44] Based on these initial studies, inclusion criteria were developed to identify patients who would be good candidates for the RFA procedure. The key criteria include (1) patients with CLBP with greater than 6 months of conservative care attempted and (2) Type 1 or Type 2 Modic changes

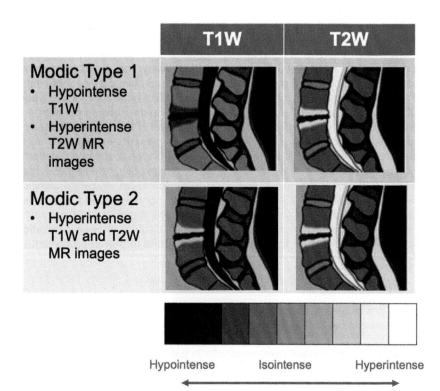

Fig. 11. Modic changes. (Images provided courtesy of Relievant Medsystems. ©2021 All rights reserved.)

at one or more levels from L3-S1. Additionally, some studies suggested a minimum ODI of 30 and VAS of 4 as additional benchmarks for procedure eligibility. Important contraindications to the procedure include cardiopulmonary disability, presence of sensitive structure (eg, spinal canal) < 10 mm from the zone of ablation, active infection, pregnancy, and presence of IPG or pacemakers. Additionally, the effectiveness of the procedure in patient with Modic changes outside of the L3-S1 region has not been reliably proven and reproduced.[43–46] To date, the market leader and primary RFA system for the basivertebral nerve are Intracept, made by Relievent Medsystems.

Outcome Data

Although the procedure is relatively new in the interventional pain management landscape, the studies that have been conducted are very promising. The first human subjects pilot study for BVN ablation was conducted by Becker and colleagues in 2017 on a group of 17 patients with MC1 or MC2 changes and CLBP managed conservatively for 6 months. Baseline ODI of this cohort was 52 and baseline VAS (on a 0–100 scale) was 61. At 3-month postprocedure follow-up, there was a statistically significant improvement in ODI and VAS, with a 29 point decrease in ODI to a mean of 23. This improvement continued into the 12-month follow-up as well.[46,47]

This was followed by the INTRACEPT study, which was a parallel open-label RCT at multiple sites across the United States that monitored 140 patients with CLBP greater than 6 months duration and MC1 or MC2 changes between L3-S1. Patients were randomized between ablation and conservative care and mean ODI changes at 3-months posttreatment was determined as the primary endpoint. The RF ablation at the interim analysis, as well as the 3-month endpoint showed statistically significant superiority in ODI improvement, VAS improvement, and improvement of pain and function in patients with vertebrogenic pain. Specifically, the RF ablation patients experienced an ODI improvement of 25.3, while conservative care patients experienced an ODI improvement of 4.4, giving an adjusted difference of 20.9 points ($P < .001$). VAS scores (0–10 scale) improved by 3.46 in the ablation patients, while conservative care patients experienced an improvement of 1.02, another statistically significant value. Additionally, 74.5% of RF ablation patients experienced an ODI improvement greater than 10, while only 34% experienced a similar improvement with conservative care.[48] The SMART trial, a prospective double-blind sham-controlled RCT, provided short and long-term follow-up showing significant improvement in ODI and VAS. The original patient cohort included 225 patients meeting the eligibility criteria for BVN ablation; this patient population was randomly assigned to the procedure or a sham control. Mean ODI scores showed a statistically significant 48% decrease at the 3-month follow-up and further improvement to a 53.7% decrease at the 24-month follow-up.[38,48]

Risks and Contraindications

No serious procedure-related or device-related adverse events were reported at 12-month follow-up in the SMART trial.[38,48] This trial served as a strong base of evidence for further study into the safety, efficacy, and superior outcomes with BVN ablation as an alternative to conservative care, especially in patients with vertebrogenic pain. A 2021 systematic review of 7 studies evaluating basivertebral nerve ablation showed moderate-quality evidence supporting the reduction of pain and disability in patients with Modic I and II changes and vertebrogenic back pain. Notably, the review found that the effectiveness of the procedure was tied to how accurately the proceduralist was able to locate the basivertebral nerve.[49] This further highlights the importance of proper procedural training before practice adoption.

Procedural Highlights

The key aspect of BVN ablation is accurately and safety identifying and accessing the BVN. This is commonly conducted using a curved cannula-stylet assembly which, when navigated through the vertebral body, will ultimately access the terminus of the BVN at the posterior aspect. The channel this creates is a path for the bipolar probe to access the BVN. Once the probe is in place, it is connected to the RF generator. Ablation should be conducted for 15 minutes at a temperature around 85 C with the end goal of preventing any neuronal transmission from the BVN at that level. Most patients undergo treatment on 2 to 4 vertebral bodies between L3 and S1, which may constitute anywhere from 1 to 3 vertebral motion segments. This procedure is considered especially effective as the likelihood of regeneration after BVN ablation has been shown to be minimal in bovine models.[44,45] [**Fig. 12**]

Evaluating Emerging Technologies

The socioeconomic consequences and quality of life burden caused by chronic pain have, for decades, been a challenge to combat. As we attempt to manage patients' chronic pain issues while being committed to reducing the scale of the opioid epidemic, the paradigm of patient care has shifted from conservative management to more minimally invasive techniques and corrective procedures.

The role of the interventionalist has never been more important as we try to address patients' chronic pain-related needs with opioid-sparing solutions. Certain procedures, such as epidural spinal injections, medial branch blocks, and other fluoroscopic injections have been well described.[12] Recently, newer options like spinal cord and peripheral nerve stimulators, implantable spacers, surgical fusion solutions (eg, Minuteman), and other interventions have emerged onto the market.[12,13,49,50] Adoption of these new technologies varies by center and location. For example, while the annual implantation rate of stimulators is 50,000/year in the United States the procedural volume is much smaller in other countries such as Canada.[51] As the range of evidence increases for each potential intervention, the rate of adoption will increase as well. This article has covered 3 emerging technologies and less commonly performed procedures in interventional pain management, as well as the growing evidence behind them. However, this is not comprehensive nor is this the limit of innovation. The opportunity for disruption in the chronic lower back pain market is massive. A 2018 sizing of the chronic lower back pain market

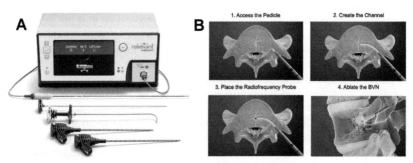

Fig. 12. Intracept procedure. (*A*): Intracept device. (*B*): Intracept Steps. (Images provided courtesy of Relievant Medsystems. ©2021 All rights reserved.)

estimated that it was worth $6.29 billion.[52] With a forecasted 4.97% compounded annual growth rate (CAGR), this number may rise to approximately $9.27 billion in the next 5 years. This is further corroborated by the minimally invasive spine surgery market analysis, which forecasts a similar 4.8% CAGR to a total market size of $550 million. This suggests that currently, 6% of the chronic low back pain market is dominated by minimally invasive procedures.[52] As this number continues to rise, biomedical device companies are well-positioned to enter the market and introduce a variety of innovative solutions. Interventional pain management is a diverse, dynamic, and young specialty and all physicians who practice this continue to add to their arsenal for patient care. We outline some important considerations when evaluating new products.

Our approach to new technology revolves around cautious optimism. We believe that it is important to first judge the body of evidence behind a new technology. Three types of evidence are important to consider: (1) theoretic evidence based on scientific, engineering, and biomechanics principles, (2) concrete, practical evidence from high-level randomized controlled trials (RCTs), and (3) real-world evidence from clinical practice. When evaluating RCTs, things to consider include whereby the RCT was conducted, who led them (ie, investigator-initiated vs sponsored), and whether the premise and volume of patients evaluated was sufficient to extrapolate from. It is important to evaluate both the safety profile (ie, complications, side effects, and so forth) and the effectiveness. Many studies on novel technologies hinge around establishing functional and pain-related noninferiority and superiority of the minimally invasive procedure to the established surgical and medical solutions on the market. This is considered strong evidence in the interventional pain market due to the advantages that minimally invasive procedures provide as far as postoperative disability, pain, and reduced length of inpatient hospital stay. This, in turn, reduces patient and hospital costs, while providing a superior experiential outcome for the patient. The next important thing to consider is the financial factors around new technology. For example, how are insurance companies covering and reimbursing this new procedure or technology? How willing are they to include it in their approved arsenal? Centers for Medicare and Medicaid Services (CMS) usually evaluate new procedures more conservatively before approving them for reimbursement. It is important to note that practices that are early adopters of novel technology have outcomes are vital to the scientific process. Our real-world experiences and real-world evidence are of superior quality and will help guide changes in technique, improvements in patient safety, and reduction of complication rates. Additionally, this evidence will form the body of proof for insurance companies to provide more widespread coverage of a new technology, thus increasing rates of adoption. It is important for interventionalists to be careful when choosing to adopt a technology, however, as they must ensure they are well trained in the techniques of the procedure, and if not, to ensure that the general principles fall within their comfort zone and foundational training. Importantly, they must be confident in their ability to manage complications, should they arise, as this may pose a threat to patient safety.

Two major avenues of innovation moving forward are neuromodulation and corrective solutions for spinal and peripheral joint pathology. Neuromodulation is rapidly expanding its scope of treatment, from neuraxial modulation to peripheral nerves. Continuous innovation in modes of delivery, feedback integration from the patient, and practical implant application will improve the patient experience with modulatory therapies for years to come. Corrective solutions will go beyond modulation and control to techniques such as spacers, guided fusion (minimally invasive fusion plates), annuloplasty (intradiscal electrothermal therapy), kyphoplasty, and so forth. These solutions provide structural improvements that previously were only achievable through invasive surgery and will serve as the foundation for future avenues of innovation.

Our approach to novel technology preaches caution while stewarding well-reasoned innovation. This is a tremendous time to be an interventional pain physician, as the opportunity to expand our procedural arsenal is unparalleled.

CLINICS CARE POINTS

- In the management of LSS, conservative care (exercise, physical therapy, and so forth) is important to try initially, usually for ~6 months. Utilization of ESIs may be effective but are controversial. Recent minimally invasive solutions for definitive LSS management have shown noninferiority, but patient selection is key to clinical decision making.

- Indirect lumbar decompression is indicated in skeletally mature adult patients experiencing up to symptomatic moderate spinal stenosis, as defined as 25% to 50% reduction in canal area when compared with normal or adjacent areas. Additionally, patients with spinal stenosis anywhere from the L1-L2 level to L4-L5, with central or lateral stenosis and ligamentum flavum hypertrophy greater than 2.5 cm are good candidates for indirect lumbar decompression.

- Percutaneous interspinous spacers have shown improvement in VAS and ODI even at the 5-year mark, indicting feasibility and long-term market stability.

- Minimally invasive lumbar decompression, another solution for LSS & LF hypertrophy greater than 2.5 cm, was shown to have the lowest reoperation rate when compared with surgery and implants, and carries a lower infection risk as well.

- Important contraindications to the minimally invasive lumbar decompression include cardiopulmonary disability, presence of sensitive structure (eg, spinal canal) < 10 mm from zone of ablation, active infection, pregnancy, and presence of IPG or pacemakers

- Basivertebral nerve ablation has been shown to promote significantly more pain relief and improvements in VAS, when compared with conservative care, especially in patients with Modic I and Modic II vertebrogenic changes.

- Key selection criteria for basivertebral nerve ablation include: (1) patients with CLBP with greater than 6 months of conservative care attempted and (2) Type 1 or Type 2 Modic changes at one or more levels from L3-S1.

- Emphasis should be placed on patient selection criteria, safety profile, and contraindications when considering the adoption of any novel technology into the interventionalist's practice.

REFERENCES

1. Collins FS, Koroshetz WJ, Volkow ND. Helping to end addiction over the long-term: the research plan for the NIH HEAL initiative. JAMA 2018;320(2):129.
2. Worley SL. New directions in the treatment of chronic pain: National pain strategy will guide prevention, management, and research. P T 2016;41(2):107–14.
3. Gaskin DJ, Richard P. The economic costs of pain in the United States. J Pain 2012;13(8):715–24.
4. Dahlhamer J, Lucas J, Zelaya C, et al. Prevalence of chronic pain and high-impact chronic pain among adults - United States, 2016. MMWR Morb Mortal Wkly Rep 2018;67(36):1001–6.
5. Clarke C. Surgical pain management: A complete guide to implantable and interventional pain therapies: Sanjeet Narang, Alison weisheipl, EL. Ross (editors).

Oxford university press, 2016. ISBN 978-0-199377-37-4. Can J Anaesth. 2017;64(1):114-115.

6. Lurie J, Tomkins-Lane C. Management of lumbar spinal stenosis. BMJ 2016;352: h6234.

7. Helm S 2nd, Racz GB, Gerdesmeyer L, et al. Percutaneous and endoscopic adhesiolysis in managing low back and lower extremity pain: A systematic review and meta-analysis. Pain Physician 2016;19(2):E245–82.

8. Costandi S, Chopko B, Mekhail M, et al. Lumbar spinal stenosis: therapeutic options review. Pain Pract 2015;15(1):68–81.

9. Friedly JL, Comstock BA, Turner JA, et al. A randomized trial of epidural glucocorticoid injections for spinal stenosis. N Engl J Med 2014;371(1):11–21.

10. Barre L, Lutz GE, Southern D, et al. Fluoroscopically guided caudal epidural steroid injections for lumbar spinal stenosis: a restrospective evaluation of long term efficacy. Pain Physician 2004;7(2):187–93.

11. Diwan S, Deer TR, Kapural L, et al. MILD: Percutaneous lumbar decompression for spinal stenosis. In: Diwan Sudhir, editor. Advanced procedures for pain management. Springer International Publishing; 2018. p. 13–25.

12. Deer TR, Grider JS, Pope JE, et al. The MIST guidelines: The Lumbar Spinal Stenosis Consensus Group guidelines for minimally invasive spine treatment. Pain Pract 2019;19(3):250–74.

13. Kaye AD, Edinoff AN, Temple SN, et al. A Comprehensive Review of Novel Interventional Techniques for Chronic Pain: Spinal Stenosis and Degenerative Disc Disease-MILD Percutaneous Image Guided Lumbar Decompression, Vertiflex Interspinous Spacer, MinuteMan G3 Interspinous-Interlaminar Fusion. Adv Ther 2021;38(9):4628–45.

14. Zucherman JF, Hsu KY, Hartjen CA, et al. A multicenter, prospective, randomized trial evaluating the X STOP interspinous process decompression system for the treatment of neurogenic intermittent claudication: two-year follow-up results. Spine (Phila Pa 1976) 2005;30(12):1351–8.

15. Beyer F, Yagdiran A, Neu P, et al. Percutaneous interspinous spacer versus open decompression: a 2-year follow-up of clinical outcome and quality of life. Eur Spine J 2013;22(9):2015–21.

16. Loguidice V, Bini W, Shabat S, et al. Rationale, design and clinical performance of the Superion® Interspinous Spacer: a minimally invasive implant for treatment of lumbar spinal stenosis. Expert Rev Med Devices 2011;8(4):419–26.

17. Patel VV, Whang PG, Haley TR, et al. Superion interspinous process spacer for intermittent neurogenic claudication secondary to moderate lumbar spinal stenosis: Two-year results from a randomized controlled FDA-IDE pivotal trial. Spine (Phila Pa 1976) 2015;40(5):275–82.

18. Patel VV, Nunley PD, Whang PG, et al. Superion(®) InterSpinous Spacer for treatment of moderate degenerative lumbar spinal stenosis: durable three-year results of a randomized controlled trial. J Pain Res 2015;8:657–62.

19. Nunley PD, Patel VV, Orndorff MDD, et al. Five-year durability of stand-alone interspinous process decompression for lumbar spinal stenosis. Clin Interv Aging 2017;12:1409–17.

20. Merkow J, Varhabhatla N, Manchikanti L, et al. Minimally invasive lumbar decompression and interspinous process device for the management of symptomatic lumbar spinal stenosis: A literature review. Curr Pain Headache Rep 2020; 24(4):13.

21. Nunley PD, Patel VV, Orndorff DG, et al. Superion interspinous spacer treatment of moderate spinal stenosis: 4-year results. World Neurosurg 2017;104:279–83.

22. Nunley PD, Deer TR, Benyamin RM, et al. Interspinous process decompression is associated with a reduction in opioid analgesia in patients with lumbar spinal stenosis. J Pain Res 2018;11:2943–8.

23. Nunley PD, Patel VV, Orndorff DG, et al. Interspinous process decompression improves quality of life in patients with lumbar spinal stenosis. Minim Invasive Surg 2018;2018:1035954.

24. Cairns K, Deer T, Sayed D, et al. Cost-effectiveness and safety of interspinous process decompression (Superion). Pain Med 2019;20(Suppl 2):S2–8.

25. Strömqvist BH, Berg S, Gerdhem P, et al. X-stop versus decompressive surgery for lumbar neurogenic intermittent claudication: Randomized controlled trial with 2-year follow-up. Spine (Phila Pa 1976) 2013;38(17):1436–42.

26. Lauryssen C, Jackson RJ, Baron JM, et al. Stand-alone interspinous spacer versus decompressive laminectomy for treatment of lumbar spinal stenosis. Expert Rev Med Devices 2015;12(6):763–9.

27. Zaina F, Tomkins-Lane C, Carragee E, et al. Surgical versus non-surgical treatment for lumbar spinal stenosis. Cochrane Database Syst Rev 2016;1:CD010264.

28. Parker SL, Anderson LH, Nelson T, et al. Cost-effectiveness of three treatment strategies for lumbar spinal stenosis: Conservative care, laminectomy, and the Superion interspinous spacer. Int J Spine Surg 2015;9:28.

29. Benyamin RM, Staats PS, MiDAS Encore I. MILD® is an effective treatment for lumbar spinal stenosis with neurogenic claudication: MiDAS ENCORE randomized controlled trial. Pain Physician 2016;19(4):229–42.

30. Staats PS, Benyamin RM, MiDAS ENCORE Investigators. MiDAS ENCORE: Randomized controlled clinical trial report of 6-month results. Pain Physician 2016; 19(2):25–38.

31. Sakai Y, Ito S, Hida T, et al. Clinical outcome of lumbar spinal stenosis based on new classification according to hypertrophied ligamentum flavum. J Orthop Sci 2017;22(1):27–33.

32. Deer TR, Kapural L. New image-guided ultra-minimally invasive lumbar decompression method: the mild procedure. Pain Physician 2010;13(1):35–41.

33. Chopko B, Caraway DL. MiDAS I (mild Decompression Alternative to Open Surgery): a preliminary report of a prospective, multi-center clinical study. Pain Physician 2010;13(4):369–78.

34. Mekhail N, Costandi S, Abraham B, et al. Functional and patient-reported outcomes in symptomatic lumbar spinal stenosis following percutaneous decompression: Functional outcomes following percutaneous decompression. Pain Pract 2012;12(6):417–25.

35. Jain S, Deer T, Sayed D, et al. Minimally invasive lumbar decompression: a review of indications, techniques, efficacy and safety. Pain Manag 2020;10(5):331–48.

36. Mehra M, Hill K, Nicholl D, et al. The burden of chronic low back pain with and without a neuropathic component: a healthcare resource use and cost analysis. J Med Econ 2012;15(2):245–52.

37. Brown MF, Hukkanen MV, McCarthy ID, et al. Sensory and sympathetic innervation of the vertebral endplate in patients with degenerative disc disease. J Bone Joint Surg Br 1997;79(1):147–53.

38. Lorio M, Clerk-Lamalice O, Beall DP, et al. International Society for the Advancement of Spine Surgery guideline-intraosseous ablation of the basivertebral nerve for the relief of chronic low back pain. Int J Spine Surg 2020;14(1):18–25.

39. Fischgrund JS, Rhyne A, Macadaeg K, et al. Long-term outcomes following intraosseous basivertebral nerve ablation for the treatment of chronic low back pain:

5-year treatment arm results from a prospective randomized double-blind sham-controlled multi-center study. Eur Spine J 2020;29(8):1925–34.

40. Kuisma M, Karppinen J, Niinimäki J, et al. Modic changes in endplates of lumbar vertebral bodies: prevalence and association with low back and sciatic pain among middle-aged male workers: Prevalence and association with low back and sciatic pain among middle-aged male workers. Spine (Phila Pa 1976) 2007;32(10):1116–22.

41. Mok FPS, Samartzis D, Karppinen J, et al. Modic changes of the lumbar spine: prevalence, risk factors, and association with disc degeneration and low back pain in a large-scale population-based cohort. Spine J 2016;16(1):32–41.

42. Modic MT, Steinberg PM, Ross JS, et al. Degenerative disk disease: assessment of changes in vertebral body marrow with MR imaging. Radiology 1988;166(1 Pt 1):193–9.

43. Carragee EJ, Alamin TF, Miller JL, et al. Discographic, MRI and psychosocial determinants of low back pain disability and remission: a prospective study in subjects with benign persistent back pain. Spine J 2005;5(1):24–35.

44. Weishaupt D, Zanetti M, Hodler J, et al. Painful lumbar disk derangement: Relevance of endplate abnormalities at MR imaging. Radiology 2001;218(2):420–7.

45. Truumees E, Macadaeg K, Pena E, et al. A prospective, open-label, single-arm, multi-center study of intraosseous basivertebral nerve ablation for the treatment of chronic low back pain. Eur Spine J 2019;28(7):1594–602.

46. Ae DV, 'agostino GD, 'anna GD, et al. Intra-osseous basivertebral nerve radiofrequency ablation (BVA) for the treatment of vertebrogenic chronic low back pain. Neuroradiology 2021;63(5):809–15.

47. Becker S, Hadjipavlou A, Heggeness MH. Ablation of the basivertebral nerve for treatment of back pain: a clinical study. Spine J 2017;17(2):218–23.

48. Kim HS, Wu PH, Jang I-T. Lumbar degenerative disease part 1: Anatomy and pathophysiology of intervertebral discogenic pain and radiofrequency ablation of basivertebral and Sinuvertebral Nerve treatment for chronic discogenic back pain: A prospective case series and review of literature. Int J Mol Sci 2020; 21(4):1483.

49. Conger A, Schuster NM, Cheng DS, et al. The Effectiveness of Intraosseous Basivertebral Nerve Radiofrequency Neurotomy for the Treatment of Chronic Low Back Pain in Patients with Modic Changes: A Systematic Review. Pain Med 2021;22(5):1039–54.

50. Fischgrund JS, Rhyne A, Franke J, et al. Intraosseous basivertebral nerve ablation for the treatment of chronic low back pain: 2-year results from a prospective randomized double-blind sham-controlled multicenter study. Int J Spine Surg 2019;13(2):110–9.

51. Hong A, Varshney V, Hare GMT, et al. Spinal cord stimulation: a nonopioid alternative for chronic pain management. CMAJ 2020;192(42):E1264–7.

52. DelveInsight Business Research, LLP. Chronic Lower Back Pain market size is expected to increase with a CAGR of 3.55% for the study period, 2017-2030 in the 7MM. PR Newswire. 2020. Available at: https://www.prnewswire.com/news-releases/chronic-lower-back-pain-market-size-is-expected-to-increase-with-a-cagr-of-3-55-for-the-study-period-20172030-in-the-7mm-301057379.html. Accessed September 28, 2021.

Moving?

Make sure your subscription moves with you!

To notify us of your new address, find your **Clinics Account Number** (located on your mailing label above your name), and contact customer service at:

Email: journalscustomerservice-usa@elsevier.com

800-654-2452 (subscribers in the U.S. & Canada)
314-447-8871 (subscribers outside of the U.S. & Canada)

Fax number: 314-447-8029

Elsevier Health Sciences Division
Subscription Customer Service
3251 Riverport Lane
Maryland Heights, MO 63043

*To ensure uninterrupted delivery of your subscription, please notify us at least 4 weeks in advance of move.

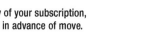

Printed and bound by CPI Group (UK) Ltd, Croydon, CR0 4YY

14/10/2024

01773716-0001